Paradise Found

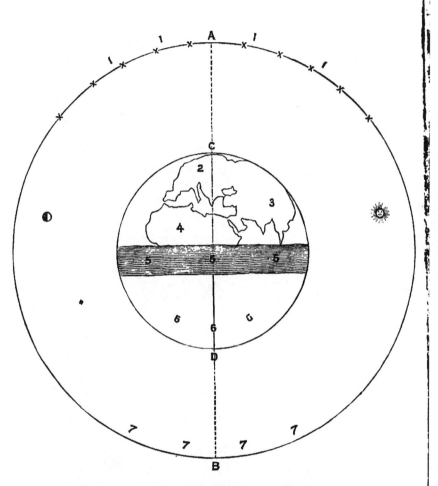

DIAGRAM ILLUSTRATING THE TRUE KEY TO ANCIENT COSMOLOGY AND
MYTHICAL GEOGRAPHY.

Compare p. 479.

A. The Northern celestial Pole in the zenith.
A B. The axis of the heavens in perpendicular position.
C D. The axis of the Earth in perpendicular position.
I I I I. The abode of the supreme God, or gods.
2, 3, 4. Europe, Asia, and the known portion of Africa.
5 5 5. The Earth-surrounding equatorial Ocean-river.
6 6 6 The abode of disembodied human souls.
7 7 7 7. The abode of demons.
C. Location of submerged Eden.
C A. "The Strength of the Hill of Sion."

PARADISE FOUND

THE CRADLE OF THE HUMAN RACE AT
THE NORTH POLE

A Study of the Prehistoric World

BY

WILLIAM F. WARREN, S.T.D., LL.D.

PRESIDENT OF BOSTON UNIVERSITY, CORPORATE MEMBER OF THE AMERICAN ORIEN-
TAL SOCIETY, AUTHOR OF "ANFANGSGRÜNDE DER LOGIK," "EINLEITUNG IN
DIE SYSTEMATISCHE THEOLOGIE," "THE TRUE KEY TO ANCIENT
COSMOLOGY AND MYTHICAL GEOGRAPHY," ETC., ETC.

WITH ORIGINAL ILLUSTRATIONS

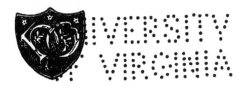

BOSTON
HOUGHTON, MIFFLIN AND COMPANY
New York: 11 East Seventeenth Street
The Riverside Press, Cambridge
1885

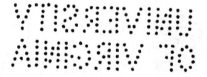

The Riverside Press, Cambridge:
Electrotyped and Printed by H. O. Houghton and Company.

RESPECTFULLY DEDICATED,

WITH FRIENDLY PERMISSION,
TO
PROFESSOR F. MAX MÜLLER,
OF
THE UNIVERSITY OF OXFORD.

PREFACE.

THIS book is not the work of a dreamer. Neither has it proceeded from a love of learned paradox. Nor yet is it a cunningly devised fable aimed at particular tendencies in current science, philosophy, or religion. It is a thoroughly serious and sincere attempt to present what is to the author's mind the true and final solution of one of the greatest and most fascinating of all problems connected with the history of mankind.

That this true solution has not been furnished before is not strange. The suggestion that primitive Eden was at the Arctic Pole seems at first sight the most incredible of all wild and willful paradoxes. And it is only within the lifetime of our own generation that the progress of geological discovery has relieved the hypothesis of fatal antecedent improbability. Moreover, when one considers the enormous variety and breadth of the fields from which its evidences of truth must be derived; when one remembers how recent are those comparative sciences on whose results the argument must chiefly depend; when one observes that many of the most striking of our alleged proofs, both in the physical and in the anthropological domain, are precisely the latest of the conclusions of these most modern of all sciences, — it is easy to see that a generation ago the demonstration here attempted could not have been given. Even five years ago some of the most interesting and cogent of our arguments would as yet have been lacking.

The interest which has so long invested our problem, and which has prompted so many attempts to solve it, was never greater than to-day. The lapse of centuries has rendered many another question antiquated, but not this. On the contrary, the more the modern world has advanced in new knowledge, the more exigent has grown the necessity of finding a valid solution. Men are feeling as never before that until the starting-point of human history can be determined, the historian, the archæologist, and the paleontological anthropologist are all working in the dark. It is seen that without this desideratum the ethnologist, the philologist, the mythographer, the theologian, the sociologist can none of them construct anything not liable to profound modification, if not to utter overthrow, the moment any new light shall be thrown upon the mother-region and the prehistoric movements of the human race. Every anthropological science, therefore, and every science related to anthropology, seems at the present moment to be standing in a state of dubitant expectancy, willing to work a little tentatively, but conscious of its destitution of the needful primal datum, and conscious of its consequent lack of a valid structural law.

To the believer in Revelation, or even in the most ancient and venerable Ethnic Traditions, the volume here presented will be found to possess uncommon interest. For many years the public mind has been schooled in a narrow naturalism, which has in its world-view as little room for the extraordinary as it has for the supernatural. Decade after decade the representatives of this teaching have been measuring the natural phenomena of every age and of every place by the petty measuring rod of their own local and temporary experience. So long and so successfully have they dogmatized on the constancy of Nature's laws and the uniformity of Nature's forces that of late it has required no small degree of courage to enable an intelligent man to stand up in the face of his generation and avow his personal faith in the early existence of men of gigantic stature and of almost millenarian longevity. Especially have clergymen and Christian teachers and writers upon Biblical history been embarrassed by the popular incredulity on these subjects, and not infrequently by a consciousness that this incredulity was in some measure shared by themselves. To all such, and indeed to all the broader minded among the naturalists themselves, a new philosophy of primeval history — a philosophy which for all the alleged extraordinary effects provides the adequate extraordinary causes — cannot fail to prove most welcome.

The execution of the plan of the book is by no means all that the author could desire. To the elaboration of so vast an argument, the materials for which must be gleaned from every possible field of knowledge, the broadest and profoundest scholar might well devote the undistracted labor of a lifetime. To the writer, loaded with the cares of a laborious executive office, there were lacking both the leisure and the equipment otherwise attainable for so high a task. The best he could do was to turn one or two summer vacations into work-time and give the result to the world. Of the correctness of his position he has no doubt, and of the preparedness of the scientific world to accept it he is also confident.

To the foregoing remarks it may be proper to add that apart from its immediate purpose the book has interest, and, it is hoped, value as a contribution to the infant science of Comparative Mythology. By the application of the author's "True Key to Ancient Cosmology and Mythical Geography," it has been possible to adjust and interpret a great variety of ancient cosmological and geographical notions never before understood by modern scholars. For example, the origin and significance of the Chinvat Bridge are here for the first time explained. The indication of the polocentric character common to the mythical systems of sacred geography among all ancient peoples will probably be new to every reader. The new light thrown upon such questions as those relating to the direction of the Sacred Quarter, the location of the Abode of the Dead, the character and position of the Cosmical Tree, the course of the backward-flowing Ocean-river, the correlation of the "Navels" of Earth and Heaven, — not to enumerate other points, — can hardly fail to attract the lively attention of all students and teachers of ancient mythology and mythical geography.

To teachers of Homer the fresh contributions toward a right understanding of Homeric cosmology are sure to prove of value. And if, in the end, the work may only lead to a systematic and intelligent teaching of the long neglected, but most important science of ancient cosmology and mythical geography in all reputable universities and classical schools, it will surely not have been written in vain.

That the author has escaped all errors and oversights while ranging through so numerous and such diverse fields of investigation, many of which are but just opened to the pioneering specialist, is too much to expect. He only asks that any such blemishes which a more competent scholarship may detect, or which the progress of new learning may yet bring to light, may not be allowed to prejudice the force of true arguments, but may be pointed out in the spirit of a candid and helpful criticism.

In conclusion, the author respectfully commits

his work to all truth-seeking spirits, — not less to
the patient investigators of nature than to the students of history, of literature, and of religion. Particularly would he commend it to all those yearning
and waiting *Königssöhnen* whose experience has
been described by Hans Andersen in the words,
" Es war einmal ein Königssohn ; Niemand hatte so
viele und schöne Bücher wie er ; Alles, was in dieser
Welt geschehen, konnte er darin lesen, und die Ab-
bildungen in prächtigen Kupferstichen erblicken.
Von jedem Volke und jedem Lande konnte er
Auskunft erhalten ; aber wo der Garten des Paradieses zu finden sei, davon stand kein Wort darin ;
*und der, gerade der war es, an dem er am meisten
dachte.*" [1]

W. F. W.

Boston.

[1] The same, being interpreted, read as follows : " Once upon a
time there was a king's son ; nobody had so many and such beautiful books as he. In these all that had ever happened in the world
he could read and see depicted in splendid engravings. Of every
people and of every land could he get information, but as to where
the Garden of Eden was, — not a word was to be found therein ;
and this, just this it was, on which he meditated most of all."

TABLE OF CONTENTS.

———◆———

PART FIRST.

THE LOCATION OF EDEN : STATE OF THE QUESTION.

CHAPTER I.

THE RESULTS OF EXPLORERS, HISTORIC AND LEGENDARY.

CHAPTER II.

THE RESULTS OF THEOLOGIANS.

CHAPTER III.

THE RESULTS OF NON-THEOLOGICAL SCHOLARS: NATURALISTS, ETH-
NOLOGISTS, ETC.

PART SECOND.

A FRESH HYPOTHESIS : PRIMITIVE EDEN AT THE NORTH
POLE.

CHAPTER I.

THE HYPOTHESIS, AND THE CONDITIONS OF ITS ADMISSIBILITY.

CHAPTER II.

IMPORTANT NEW FEATURES AT ONCE INTRODUCED INTO THE PROB-
LEM OF THE SITE OF EDEN AND THE SIGNIFICANCE OF THESE FOR
A VALID SOLUTION.

PART THIRD.

THE HYPOTHESIS SCIENTIFICALLY TESTED AND CONFIRMED.

CHAPTER I.

THE TESTIMONY OF SCIENTIFIC GEOGONY.

CHAPTER V.

THE TESTIMONY OF PALEONTOLOGICAL BOTANY.

CHAPTER VI.

THE TESTIMONY OF PALEONTOLOGICAL ZOÖLOGY.

CHAPTER VII.

THE TESTIMONY OF PALEONTOLOGICAL ANTHROPOLOGY AND GENERAL ETHNOLOGY.

CHAPTER VIII.

CONCLUSION OF PART THIRD.

PART FOURTH.

THE HYPOTHESIS CONFIRMED BY ETHNIC TRADITION.

CHAPTER I.

ANCIENT COSMOLOGY AND MYTHICAL GEOGRAPHY.

CHAPTER II.

THE CRADLE OF THE RACE IN ANCIENT JAPANESE THOUGHT.

CHAPTER III.

THE CRADLE OF THE RACE IN CHINESE THOUGHT.

CHAPTER VII.

THE CRADLE OF THE RACE IN ANCIENT EGYPTIAN THOUGHT.

CHAPTER VIII.

THE CRADLE OF THE RACE IN ANCIENT GREEK THOUGHT.

PART FIFTH.

FURTHER VERIFICATIONS OF THE HYPOTHESIS BASED UPON A STUDY OF THE PECULIARITIES OF A POLAR PARADISE.

CHAPTER I.

THE EDEN STARS.

CHAPTER II.

THE EDEN DAY.

CHAPTER III.

THE EDEN ZENITH.

CHAPTER IV.

THE NAVEL OF THE EARTH.

CHAPTER V.

THE QUADRIFURCATE RIVER.

CHAPTER VI.

THE CENTRAL TREE.

CHAPTER VII.

THE EXUBERANCE OF LIFE.

CHAPTER VIII.

REVIEW OF THE ARGUMENT.

PART SIXTH.

THE SIGNIFICANCE OF OUR RESULTS.

CHAPTER I.

THEIR BEARING UPON THE STUDY OF BIOLOGY AND TERRESTRIAL PHYSICS.

CHAPTER II.

THE BEARING OF OUR RESULTS ON THE STUDY OF ANCIENT LITERATURE.

CHAPTER III.

THE BEARING OF OUR RESULTS ON THE PROBLEM OF THE ORIGIN AND EARLIEST FORM OF RELIGION.

CHAPTER IV.

THE BEARING OF OUR RESULTS ON THE PHILOSOPHY OF HISTORY AND ON THE THEORY OF THE DEVELOPMENT OF CIVILIZATION.

APPENDIX.

ILLUSTRATIONS.

——◆——

PART FIRST.

LOCATION OF EDEN: STATE OF THE QUESTION.

You shall understand that no mortal may approach to that Paradise; for by land no man may go, for wild beasts that are in the deserts, and for the high mountains and great huge rocks that no man may pass by for the dark places that are there; and by the rivers may no man go, for the water runs so roughly and so sharply, because it comes down so outrageously from the high places above, that it runs in so great waves that no ship may row or sail against it; and the water roars so, and makes so huge a noise, and so great a tempest, that no man may hear another in the ship though he cried with all the might he could. Many great lords have assayed with great will many times to pass by those rivers towards Paradise, with full great companies; but they might not speed in their voyage; and many died for weariness of rowing against the strong waves; and many of them became blind, and many deaf, from the noise of the water; and some perished and were lost in the waves; so that no mortal man may approach to that place without the special grace of God. — SIR JOHN DE MAUNDEVILLE.

CHAPTER I.

THE RESULTS OF EXPLORERS, HISTORIC AND
LEGENDARY.

Man lernt die Welt am besten durch Reisen kennen.

K. H. W. VÖLCKER.

ONE of the most interesting and pathetic passages to be found in all literature is that in which
Christopher Columbus announces to his royal pa-
trons his supposed discovery of the ascent to the
gate of the long-lost Garden of Eden. With what
emotions must his heart have thrilled as, steering
up this ascent, he felt his " ships smoothly rising
toward the sky," the weather becoming " milder " as
he rose! To be so near the Paradise of God's own
planting, to be the first discoverer of the way in
which the believing world could at length, after so
many ages, once more approach its sacred precincts
even if forbidden to enter, — what an exquisite experience it must have been to the lonely spirit of
that great explorer!

It is his third voyage. He is in the Gulf of Paria
to the north or north-west of the mouth of the Ori-
noco. In his loyal epistle to Ferdinand and Isabella
thus he writes : —

The Holy Scriptures record that our Lord made the
earthly Paradise and planted in it the tree of life ; and
thence springs a fountain from which the four principal rivers of the world take their source ; namely, the

Ganges in India, the Tigris and Euphrates, and the Nile.

I do not find, nor ever have found, any account by the Romans or Greeks which fixes in a positive manner the site of the terrestrial Paradise, neither have I seen it given in any *mappe-monde*, laid down from authentic sources. Some placed it in Ethiopia at the sources of the Nile, but others, traversing all these countries, found neither the temperature nor the altitude of the sun correspond with their ideas respecting it ; nor did it appear that the over-whelming waters of the deluge had been there. Some pagans pretended to adduce arguments to establish that it was in the Fortunate Islands, now called the Canaries.

St. Isidore, Bede, and Strabo[1] and the Master of scho-lastic history,[2] with St. Ambrose and Scotus, and all the learned theologians agree that the earthly Paradise is in the East.

I have already described my ideas concerning this hemisphere and its form,[3] and I have no doubt that if I could pass below the equinoctial line after reaching the highest point of which I have spoken, I should find a much milder temperature and a variation in the stars and in the water: not that I suppose that elevated point to be navigable, nor even that there is water there ; indeed, I believe it is impossible to ascend thither, because I am convinced that it is the spot of the earthly Paradise, whither no one can go but by God's permission ; but this land which your Highnesses have now sent me to explore is very extensive, and I think there are many other countries in the south, of which the world has never had any knowledge.

I do not suppose that the earthly Paradise is in the form of a rugged mountain, as the descriptions of it have made it appear, but that it is on the summit of the spot

[1] Walafried Strabus of Reichenau, Baden.
[2] Petrus Comestor, who wrote the *Historia Scholastica*.
[3] See APPENDIX, Sect. I.

which I have described as being in the form of the stalk [or stem end] of a pear; the approach to it from a distance must be by a constant and gradual ascent; but I believe that, as I have already said, no one could ever reach the top; I think also that the water I have described may proceed from it, though it be far off, and that stopping at the place I have just left, it forms this lake.

There are great indications of this being the terrestrial Paradise, for its situation coincides with the opinions of the holy and wise theologians whom I have mentioned; and, moreover, the other evidences agree with the supposition, for I have never either read or heard of fresh water coming in so large a quantity, in close conjunction with the water of the sea; the idea is also corroborated by the blandness of the temperature; and if the water of which I speak does not proceed from the earthly Paradise, it seems to be a still greater wonder, for I do not believe that there is any river in the world so large and deep.

When I left the Dragon's Mouth, which is the northernmost of the two straits which I have described, and which I so named on the day of our lady of August,[1] I found that the sea ran so strongly to the westward that between the hour of mass,[2] when I weighed anchor, and the hour of complines [3] I made sixty-five leagues of four miles each; and not only was the wind not violent, but on the contrary very gentle, which confirmed me in the conclusion that in sailing southward there is a continuous ascent, while there is a corresponding descent towards the north.

I hold it for certain that the waters of the sea move from east to west with the sky, and that in passing this track they hold a more rapid course, and have thus eaten away large tracts of land, and hence has resulted this great number of islands; indeed, these islands them-

---

[1] The feast of the Assumption.
[2] Probably six A. M.   [3] Nine P. M.

selves afford an additional proof of it, for on the one hand, all those which lie west and east, or a little more obliquely north-west and south-east, are broad; while those which lie north and south or north-east and south-west, that is in a directly contrary direction to the said winds, are narrow; furthermore, that these islands should possess the most costly productions is to be accounted for by the mild temperature, which comes to them from heaven, since these are the most elevated parts of the world. It is true that in some parts the waters do not appear to take this course, but this only occurs in certain spots where they are obstructed by land, and hence they appear to take different directions. . . .

I now return to my subject of the land of Gracia, and of the river and lake found there, which latter might more properly be called a sea; for a lake is but a small expanse of water, which, when it becomes great, deserves the name of a sea, just as we speak of the Sea of Galilee and the Dead Sea; and I think that if the river mentioned does not proceed from the terrestrial Paradise, it comes from an immense tract of land situated in the south, of which hitherto no knowledge has been obtained. But the more I reason on the subject the more satisfied I become that the terrestrial Paradise is situated in the spot I have described; and I ground my opinion upon the arguments and authorities already quoted. May it please the Lord to grant your Highnesses a long life, and health and peace, to follow out so noble an investigation; in which I think our Lord will receive great service, Spain considerable increase of its greatness, and all Christians much consolation and pleasure, because by this means the name of our Lord will be published abroad.[1]

Alas for the hope of settling the problem of Eden's site by actual exploration! Columbus never

---

[1] *Select Letters of Christopher Columbus.* Translated by R. H. Major, F. S. A. 2d ed., London, 1860 : pp. 140–147.

lived to find his Paradise; and geographers have
long ago ascertained that the golden summit of the
world is not in Venezuela, nor in any of its neighbor
states.

Of course Columbus supposed himself to be off
the eastern coast, not of a new continent, but of
Asia. His idea of the location of the terrestrial
Paradise as in, or to the eastward of, Farther India
was the prevailing idea of his age. The Hereford
map of the world, dating from the thirteenth century,
represents the favored spot as a circular island to the
East of India, and as separated from the mainland,
not only by the sea, but also by a battlemented wall,
with its one gate to the West, through which our
first parents were supposed to have been expelled.
Hugo de St. Victor wrote: "Paradise is a spot in
the Orient productive of all kinds of woods and
pomiferous trees. It contains the Tree of Life;
there is neither cold nor heat there, but perpetually
an equable temperature. It contains a fountain
which flows forth in four rivers." So Gautier de
Metz, in a poem written in the thirteenth century,
describes the terrestrial Paradise as situated in
an unapproachable region in Asia, surrounded by
flames, and guarded at its only gate by an armed
angel.

In the year 1322 Sir John de Maundeville made
his memorable pilgrimage to the East. In his account of these travels, after describing the marvelous kingdom of Prester John in India, he says:
"And beyond the land and isles and deserts of
Prester John's lordship, in going straight towards
the East men find nothing but mountains and great
rocks; and there is the dark region where no man

may see, neither by day nor by night, as they of the
country say.   And that desert and that place of
darkness lasts from this coast unto terrestrial Paradise, where Adam, our first father, and Eve were
put, who dwelt there but a little while ; and that is
towards the East, at the beginning of the earth. . . .
Of Paradise I cannot speak properly, for I was not
there.   It is far beyond; and I repent not going
there, but I was not worthy.   But as I have heard
say of wise men beyond I shall tell you with good
will.   Terrestrial Paradise, as wise men say, is the
highest place of the earth ; and it is so high that it
nearly touches the circle of the moon there, as the
moon makes her turn.   For it is so high that the
flood of Noah might not come to it, that would have
covered all the earth of the world all about and
above and beneath except Paradise.   And this Paradise is inclosed all about with a wall, and men know
not whereof it is; for the wall is covered all over
with moss as it seems: and it seems not that the
wall is natural stone.   And that wall stretches from
the South to the North ; and it has but one entry,
which is closed with burning fire, so that no man
that is mortal dare enter.   And in the highest place
of Paradise, exactly in the middle, is a well that
casts out four streams, which run by divers lands,
of which the first is called Pison, or Ganges, that
runs throughout India or Emlak, in which river are
many precious stones, and much lignum, aloes, and
much sand of gold.   And the other river is called
Nile, or Gyson, which goes through Ethiopia, and
after through Egypt.   And the other is called Tigris
which runs by Assyria and by Armenia the Great.
And the other is called Euphrates, which runs

through Media, Armenia, and Persia. And men there beyond say that all the sweet waters of the world, above and beneath, take their beginning from the well of Paradise ; and out of that well all waters come and go." [1]

Various writers and map-makers of the same age seem very evidently to have identified the Paradise of Genesis with the island of Ceylon. Even to this day a mount near the centre of the island bears the name of "Adam's Peak." According to Mohammedan tradition, this was only so called because it was the place where Adam alighted when cast out of the true celestial Paradise in heaven. Nevertheless, Christian tradition or legend long lingered about Ceylon as the genuine site of primitive Eden. [2]

In entire accord with this view is the remarkable story of Prince Eirek, as told in an Icelandic Saga of the fourteenth century. Mr. Baring-Gould, in a style not very reverent, has summarized the tale as follows : —

[1] *Early Travels in Palestine.* Edited by Thos. Wright, London, 1848, p. 276.

[2] Even Maundeville, whose Paradise, as we have seen, was still farther to the East, found here a Fountain of Youth whose head-spring was in Paradise : "Toward the head of that forest is the cytee of Polombe [Columbo], and above the cytee is a great mountayne, also clept Polombe. And of that mount the Cytee hathe his name. And at the foot of that Mount is a fayr welle and a gret, that hathe odour and savour of all spices ; and at every hour of the day he chaungethe his odour and his savour dyversely. And whoso drynkethe 3 times fasting of that watre of that welle, he is hool of alle maner sykenesse that he hathe. And thei that duellen there and drynken often of that welle, thei nevere have sykenesse and thei semen alle weys yonge. I have dronken there of 3 or 4 sithes ; and zit, methinkethe, I fare the better. Some men clepen it the Welle of Youthe ; for thei that often drynken thereat semen alle weys youngly and lyven withouten sykenesse. And men seyn, that that welle comethe out of Paradys ; and therefore it is so vertuous."

Eirek was a son of Thrand, king of Drontheim, and having taken upon him a vow to explore the Deathless Land he went to Denmark, where he picked up a friend of the same name as himself. They then went to Constantinople, and called upon the Emperor, who held a long conversation with them, which is duly reported, relative to the truths of Christianity and the site of the Deathless Land, which, he assures them, is nothing more nor less than Paradise.

"The world," said the monarch, who had not forgotten his geography since he left school, " is precisely 180,000 stages round (about 1,000,000 English miles), and it is not propped up on posts, — not a bit! — it is supported by the power of God ; and the distance between earth and heaven is 100,045 miles (another MS. reads 9382 miles ; the difference is immaterial) ; and round about the earth is a big sea called Ocean." " And what's to the south of the earth ? " asked Eirek. " Oh! there is the end of the world, and that is India." " And pray where am I to find the Deathless Land ? " " That lies — Paradise, I suppose you mean — well, it lies slightly east of India."

Having obtained this information, the two Eireks started, furnished with letters from the Greek Emperor.

They traversed Syria, and took ship, — probably at Balsora ; then, reaching India, they proceeded on their journey on horseback, till they came to a dense forest, the gloom of which was so great, through the interlacing of the boughs, that even by day the stars could be observed twinkling, as though they were seen from the bottom of a well.

On emerging from the forest, the two Eireks came upon a strait, separating them from a beautiful land, which was unmistakably Paradise; and the Danish Eirek, intent on displaying his Scriptural knowledge, pronounced the strait to be the river Pison. This was crossed by a stone bridge, guarded by a dragon.

The Danish Eirek, deterred by the prospect of an en-counter with this monster, refused to advance, and even endeavored to persuade his friend to give up the attempt to enter Paradise as hopeless, after that they had come within sight of the favored land. But the Norseman de-liberately walked, sword in hand, into the maw of the dragon, and the next moment, to his infinite surprise and delight, found himself liberated from the gloom of the monster's interior, and safely placed in Paradise.

The land was most beautiful, and the grass as gor-geous as purple ; it was studded with flowers, and was traversed by honey rills. The land was extensive and level, so that there was not to be seen mountain or hill, and the sun shone cloudless, without night and darkness ; the calm of the air was great, and there was but a feeble murmur of wind, and that which there was breathed red-olent with the odor of blossoms. After a short walk, Eirek observed what certainly must have been a remark-able object, namely, a tower or steeple self-suspended in the air, without any support whatever, though access might be had to it by means of a slender ladder. By this Eirek ascended into a loft of the tower, and found there an excellent cold collation prepared for him. After hav-ing partaken of this he went to sleep, and in vision beheld and conversed with his guardian angel, who promised to conduct him back to his fatherland, but to come for him again and fetch him away from it forever at the ex-piration of the tenth year after his return to Drontheim.

Eirek then retraced his steps to India, unmolested by the dragon, which did not affect any surprise at having to disgorge him, and, indeed, which seems to have been, notwithstanding his looks, but a harmless and passive dragon.

After a tedious journey of seven years, Eirek reached his native land, where he related his adventures, to the confusion of the heathen, and to the delight and edifi-cation of the faithful. And in the tenth year, and at break of day, as Eirek went to prayer, God's Spirit caught him away, and he was never seen again in this world : so here ends all we have to say of him.

Here we get farther than with Columbus, but however beautiful and credible this story of Eden-exploration may have been five hundred years ago, we now know that the only Paradise in Ceylon is a symbolical Buddhist one,[1] as far removed from the primitive garden of Genesis as Roman Catholic "*Calvarios*" in South America are from the primitive Calvary of the crucifixion. Moreover, even the scribes of five hundred years ago, however credulous in other things, seem well to have understood the true character of this story of travel, for "according to the majority of the MSS. the story purports to be nothing more than a religious novel." [2]

As the Keltic terrestrial Paradise, Avalon, was a sea-girt island in the waters of the North, it could of course be reached only by ship. The first to accomplish this feat, so far as Christian legend informs us, was St. Brandan, son of Finlogho, a celebrated saint of the Irish Church, who died A. D. 576 or 577. According to the story an angel brought to this good abbot a book from heaven, in which such marvelous things were narrated concerning the then unknown portions of the world that the honest father charged both angel and book with falsehood,

---

[1] "The Buddhists of Ceylon have endeavored to transform their central mountain, Dêva-kuta (Peak of the Gods), into Meru, and to find four streams descending from its sides to correspond with the rivers of their Paradise." — Obry, *Le Berceau de l'Espèce Humaine.* Amiens, 1858 : p. 118 n. Lassen, *Indische Alterthumskunde.* Bonn, 1862 : Bd. i., 196.

[2] Baring-Gould, *Curious Myths of the Middle Ages.* London, 1866 : p. 236.

and in his righteous indignation burned the latter. As a punishment for his unbelief God sentenced him to recover the book. He must search through hell and earth and sea until he finds the heavenly gift. The token given him by the angel is that when he sees two twin fires flame up he shall know that they are the two eyes of a certain ox, and on the tongue of that ox he shall find the book. For seven long years he sails the Western and the Northern Ocean.[1] He here encounters more marvels than were recorded in the original incredible book, and is even permitted to visit the earthly Paradise. The beauty of the soil, of the fountain with four streams, of the magnificent castle and castle halls lighted with self-luminous stones and adorned with all manner of precious jewels, surpassed description. The stay of the party seems, however, to have been short, and unfortunately just where the island was located — the commander forgets to mention.

A more elaborate and fanciful picture of the same mediæval Paradise is furnished us in the story of Oger, or Holger, a Danish knight of the age of Charlemagne. In a plain prose rendering, this is the style in which a famous court minstrel of six hundred years ago was accustomed to chant the adventure to admiring audiences.

Caraheu and Gloriande were in a boat with a fair company, and Oger had with him a thousand men-at-arms. When they were a certain way on, there arose so mighty a tempest that they knew not what to do, only to commit their souls to God. So great was the storm that the mast of Oger's ship brake, and he was constrained to

---

[1] Carl Schroeder, *Sanct Brandan. Ein lateinischer und drei deutsche Texte.* Erlangen, 1871 : pp. xii., xiii. and *passim.*

embark in a little vessel with a few of his comrades, and the wind struck them with such fury that they lost sight of Caraheu. Caraheu was so sore troubled that he was like to die, and he began to mourn the noble Oger ; for he wist not what was become of the boat. And Oger in like manner lamented Caraheu. Thus grieved Caraheu and the Christians in his company, saying, " Alas ! Oger, what is become of thee ? This is, I ween, the most sudden departure that I heard of ever." " Nay, but cease, my beloved," said Gloriande ; " he will not fail to come again when God wills, for he cannot be far away." " Ah, lady," said Caraheu, " you know not the dangers of the sea ; and I pray God to take him into his keeping." . . .

Now I will leave speaking of Caraheu, and return to Oger, who was in peril, yet was ever grieving for his friend, and saying, " Ah, Caraheu, hope of the remaining days of my life, thou whom I loved next to God ! How has God allowed me to lose so soon you and your lady ? " At that moment the great ship, in which Oger had left his men-at-arms, struck against a rock, and he saw them all perish, at which sight he was like to die of grief. And presently a loadstone rock began to draw towards it the boat in which Oger was. Oger, seeing himself thus taken, recommended his soul to God, saying, " My God, my Father and Creator, who hast made me in Thine image and semblance, have pity on me now, and leave me not here to die ; for that I have used my power as was best to the increase of the Catholic faith. But if it must be that Thou take me, I commit to Thy care my brother Guyou, and all my relatives and friends, especially my nephew Gautier, who is minded to serve Thee, and bring the paynim into Thy Holy Church. . . . Ah, my God ! had I known the peril of this adventure, I should never have abandoned the beauty, sense, and honor of Clarice, Queen of England. Had I but gone back to her, I should have seen, too, my redoubted sovereign, Charlemagne, with all the princes who surround him."

Meanwhile the boat continued to float upon the water till it reached the loadstone castle, which they call the Château d'Avalon, which is but a little way from the earthly Paradise, whither were snatched in a beam of fire Elias and Enoch, and where was Morgue la Fée, who at his birth had given him such great gifts. Then the mariners saw well that they were drawing near to the loadstone rock, and they said to Oger, " My lord, commend thyself to God, for it is certain that at this moment we are come to our voyage's end ;" and as they spake the bark with a swing attached itself to the rock, as though it were cemented there.

That night Oger thought over the case in which he was, but he scarce could tell of what sort it might be. And the sailors came and said to Oger, " My lord, we are held here without remedy ; wherefore let us look to our stores, for we are here for the remainder of our lives." To which Oger made answer, " If this be so, then will I make consideration of our case, for I would assign to each one his share, to the least as to the greatest." For himself Oger kept a double portion, for it is the law of the sea that the master of the ship has as much as two others. But if that rule had not been, he would still have needed a double quantity, for he ate as much as two common men.

When Oger had apportioned his share to each, he said, "Masters, be sparing, I pray you, of your food as much as you may, for so soon as ye have no more be sure that I myself will throw you into the sea." The skipper answered him, "My lord, thou wilt escape no better than we." Their food failed them all, one after another, and Oger cast them into the sea, and he remained alone. Then he was so troubled that he knew not what to do. " Alas ! my God, my Creator," said he, " hast Thou at this hour forsaken me ? I have now no one to comfort me in my misfortune." Thereupon, whether it were his fantasy or no, it seemed to him that a voice replied, " God orders

that so soon as it be night thou go to a castle after thou
hast come to an island which thou wilt presently find.
And when thou art on the island thou wilt find a small
path leading to the castle. And whatsoever thing thou
seest there, let not that affray thee." And Oger looked,
but wist not who had spoken.

Oger waited the return of night, to learn the truth of
that which the voice foretold, and he was so amazed that
he wist not what to do, but set himself to the trial. And
when night came he committed himself to God, praying
Him for mercy ; and straightway he looked and beheld the
Castle of Avalon, which shone wondrously. Many nights
before he had seen it, but by day it was not visible.
Howbeit, so soon as Oger saw the castle he set about to
get there. He saw before him the ships that were fastened
to the loadstone rock, and now he walked from ship to
ship, and so gained the island ; and when there he at once
set himself to scale the hill by a path which he found.
When he reached the gate of the castle, and sought to
enter, there came before him two great lions, who stopped
him and cast him to the ground. But Oger sprang up
and drew his sword, Curtain, and straightway cleft one of
them in twain ; then the other sprang and seized Oger
by the neck, and Oger turned round and struck off his
head.

When Oger had performed this deed, he gave thanks
to our Lord, and then he entered the hall of the castle,
where he found many viands, and a table set as if one
should dine there ; but no prince nor lord could he see.
Now he was amazed to find no one, save only a horse,
which sat at the table as if it had been a human being.
This horse, which was called Papillon (Psyche ?), waited
upon Oger, gave him to drink from a golden goblet, and
at length conducted him to his chamber, and to a bed
whose fairy-made coverlet of cloth of gold and ermine
was *la plus mignonne chose qui fut jamais vue.*

When Oger awoke he thought to see Papillon again,

but could see neither him, nor man, nor woman, to show him the way from the room. He saw a door, and, having made the sign of the cross, sought to pass out that way; but as he tried to do this he encountered a serpent, so hideous that the like has scarce been seen. It would have thrown itself upon Oger, but that the knight drew his sword and made the creature recoil more than ten feet; but it returned with a bound, for it was very mighty, and the twain fell to fight. And now, as Oger saw that the serpent pressed hard upon him, he struck at it so doughtily with his sword that he severed it in twain. After that Oger went along a path which led him to a garden, so beauteous that it was in truth a little paradise; and within were fair trees, bearing fruit of every kind, of tastes divers, and of such sweet odors that he never smelt trees like them before.

Oger, seeing these fruits so fine, desired to eat some, and presently he lighted upon a fine apple-tree, whose fruit was like gold, and of these apples he took one and ate. But no sooner had he thus eaten than he became so sick and weak that he had no power nor manhood left. And now again he commended his soul to God and prepared to die. . . . But at this moment turning round, he was aware of a fair dame, clothed in white, and so richly adorned that she was a glory to behold. Now as Oger looked upon the lady without moving from his place, he deemed that she was Mary the Virgin, and said, "Ave Maria," and saluted her. But she said, "Oger, think not that I am she whom you fancy; I am she who was at your birth, and my name is Morgue la Fée, and I allotted you a gift which was destined to increase your fame eternally through all lands. But now you have left your deeds of war to take with ladies your solace; for as soon as I have taken you from here I will bring you to Avalon, where you will see the fairest noblesse in the world."

And anon she gave him a ring, which had such virtue

that Oger, who was near a hundred years old, returned
to the age of thirty.   Then said Oger, " Lady, I am more
beholden to thee than to any other in the world.   Blessed
be the hour of thy birth, for, without having done aught
to deserve at your hands, you have given me countless
gifts, and this gift of new life above them all.   Ah, lady,
that I were before Charlemagne, that he might see the
condition in which I now stand ; for I feel in me greater
strength than I have ever known.   Dearest, how can I
make return for the honor and great good you have done
me ?   But I swear that I am at your service all the days
of my life."   Then Morgue took him by the hand, and
said, " My loyal friend, the goal of all my happiness, I
will now lead you to my palace in Avalon, where you will
see of noblesse the greatest and of damosels the fairest."
And she took Oger by the hand and led him to the Castle of Avalon, where was King Artus, and Auberon, and
Malambron, who was a sea fairy.

As Oger approached the castle the fairies came to
meet him, dancing and singing marvellous sweetly.   And
he saw many fairy dames, richly crowned and apparelled.
And presently came Arthur, and Morgue called to him,
and said, " Come hither, my lord and brother, and salute
the fair flower of chivalry, the honor of the French noblesse, him in whom all generosity and honor and every
virtue are lodged, Oger le Danois, my loyal love, my
only pleasure, in whom lies for me all hope of happiness."
Then Morgue gave Oger a crown to wear, which was so
rich that none here could count its value ; and it had beside a wondrous virtue, for every man who bore it on
his brow forgot all sorrow and sadness and melancholy,
and he thought no more of his country nor of his kin that
he had left behind him in the world.

We leave Oger thus " *bien assis et entretenu des dames
que c'était merveilles*," and return to the earth, where
things were not going so well ; for while Oger was in
Fairie the paynim assembled all their forces and took

Jerusalem and proceeded to lay siege to Babylon (that is, Cairo). Then the most valiant knights who were left on earth — Moysant, and Florian, and Caraheu, and Gautier (Oger's nephew) — assembled all their powers to defend this place. But they lamented greatly because Oger was no more. And a great battle took place without the walls of Babylon, in which the Saracens, assisted by a renegade, the Admiral Gandice, gained the victory.

Oger had been long in the Castle of Avalon, and had begotten a son by Morgue, when she, having heard of these doings and of the danger to Christendom, deemed it needful to awake Oger from his blissful forgetfulness of all earthly things, and tell him that his presence was needed in this world once more. Thereupon follows an account of Oger's returning to earth, where no one knew him, and all were astonished at his strange garb and bearing. He inquired for Charlemagne, who had been long since dead ; the generation below Oger had grown to be old men, yet he still had the habit of a man of thirty. We need not wonder that his talk excited suspicion. But at length he made himself known to the King of France, joined his army, and put the paynim to flight. He had now forgotten his life in Fairie ; he was beloved by the Queen of France (the King having been killed), and was about to marry her, when Morgue again appeared and carried him off to Avalon.[1]

Looking back over this long story to see just where it locates its Paradise, and how one could get there, we find the data extremely few and discouraging. And the older story in Plutarch respecting

[1] From Keary's *Outlines of Primitive Beliefs*, pp. 452–458. He remarks, " The account which I here translate is only a sixteenth-century version of the tale, but it is copied directly from the poetic version of the well-known troubadour Adenez, chief minstrel at the court of Henry III. of Bavaria (1248–1261), and for his excellence in his art called Le Roy, or king of all. There can be no doubt that in its chief particulars the story is far older than the days of Adenez."

the same isle of blessedness is not less destitute of indications as to exact locality.[1]

Going some centuries farther back we find another traveler who claims to have been in the terrestrial Paradise. He says, —

As I looked towards the North, over the mountains, I saw seven mountains full of precious balsam and odorous trees and cinnamon and pepper. And from thence I went over the summits of these mountains far towards the East, and passed on still farther over the sea and came far beyond it. And I came into the Garden of Righteousness, and saw a many-colored crowd of trees of every kind; for many and great trees flourish there, very noble and lovely, and the Tree of Wisdom, which gives wisdom to any one who eats of it. It is like the Johannis bread tree; its fruit is like a cluster of grapes, very good; and the fragrance of the tree spreads far around. And I said, "Fair is this tree, and how beautiful and ravishing its look!" And the holy Angel Raphael, who was with me, answered and said to me, "This is the Tree of Wisdom of which thy forefathers, thy hoary first parent and thy aged first mother, ate, and found the knowledge of wisdom, and their eyes were opened, and they knew that they were naked, and were driven out of the garden."

This favored explorer, who had the special advantage of being guided by a holy angel, was the unknown author of the Book of Enoch, which writing is believed by some to be as old as the second century before Christ. No one can read many chapters of his production, however, without arriving at the firm conclusion that sacred geography has very little to hope from such a source, however ancient.[2]

---

[1] "On the Face appearing in the Orb of the Moon," Sect. 26, *Plutarch's Morals.* Goodwin's ed., vol. v., p. 201.

[2] *Das Buch Henoch.* Uebersetzt von Dr. A. Dillmann. Leipsic,

Coming down to the travelers of our own time, we fare no better, even though they do not tax our credulity with stories of angelic guides or of guardian dragons. One, writing only ten years ago, professedly from the very Garden itself, momentarily raises our expectations when he says, "Discoveries made within the last decade tend to confirm the supposition that the primeval abode of man was near the confluence of the Euphrates and the Tigris; and it is not too much to anticipate the exhuming of inscribed tablets which will fully establish this belief." But as suddenly as our hopes are excited, so suddenly do they die away in disappointment. Incredulous critics greet the suggestion of "exhuming inscribed tablets" on the subject with a chorus of derisive laughter. The author himself does not venture to give any of the "discoveries made within the last decade" which tend to confirm the notion that Eden was located at the point described. On the contrary, in the immediately following sentence, he takes leave of the subject, and in so doing gives us over to his own admitted uncertainty in the following terms: "And although, after the lapse of so many centuries, exact correspondence of topography is not to be expected, yet guided by the general features of the scene rather than by the minuter ones, the present traditional Garden of Eden may be accepted until another has been discovered and its identity more clearly proved."[1] In such darkness dies out the kindled hope. Meantime, in a letter to Sir Roderick Murchison, published in "The Athe-

1853. There is an earlier English translation by R. Lawrence (Oxford, 1821, '33, '38).

[1] J. P. Newman, D. D., *A Thousand Miles on Horseback.* New York, 1875 : p. 69.

næum " not far from the same date, the indefatiga-
ble Livingstone disclosed the secret of his tireless
perambulations through Central Africa, — he believed that at the sources of the Nile, could he once
discover them, he would stand upon the site of the
primeval Paradise ! Evidently exploration, wonderful as have been its achievements, has not yet solved
the problem of the site of Eden. To this day the
word of Pindar, uttered half a thousand years before
Christ, has remained true : —

> " Neither by taking ship,
> Neither by any travel on foot,
> To the Hyperborean Field
> Shalt thou find the wondrous way."

CHAPTER II.

THE RESULTS OF THEOLOGIANS.

Some have placed it in the third heaven, some in the fourth, in the heaven of the moon, in the moon itself, on a mountain near the lunar heaven, in the middle region of the air, out of the earth, upon the earth, beneath the earth, in a place that is hidden and separated from man. It has been placed under the northern pole, in Tartary, or in the place now occupied by the Caspian Sea. Others placed it in the extreme south, in the land of fire; others in the Levant, or on the shores of the Ganges, or in the island of Ceylon. It has been placed in China, or in an inaccessible region beyond the Black Sea; by others in America, in Africa, etc. — BISHOP HUET.

An ein Resultat, das auch nur einigermassen befriedigte, ist nicht zu denken. — WETZER UND WELTE, Kirchen-Lexicon.

THEOLOGIANS, Christian and Jewish, have in all ages differed, and irreconcilably differed, as to the location of the cradle of the human race. The evidences of this are so well known, or so easily accessible to every intelligent reader, that they need not be adduced in this place.[1]

The fathers and theologians of the Early Church and of the Middle Ages held many curious and conflicting opinions upon the subject. Some, following the allegorizing method of Philo, interpreted the whole narrative in Genesis as a parable setting forth spiritual things. Eden was not a place, but a state of spiritual blessedness. The four rivers were not rivers, but the four cardinal virtues, etc. The majority, however, held to the historic character of the narrative, and to the strictly geographical reality

[1] See McClintock and Strong, *Cyclopædia of Biblical, Theological, and Ecclesiastical Literature,* Arts. " Eden " and " Paradise."

of Eden. To the question of its location, numberless were the answers. Often it was in the far East,
beyond all lands inhabited by men. Sometimes it
was thought of as perhaps within, or under, the
earth, in the regions of the dead. Sometimes it was
neither on nor below the earth, but high above it, in
the third heaven, or some way associated with the
lunar orbit. Again, it would be stated that there
are two paradises, a celestial and a terrestrial one, —
the one in heaven, the other on the earth. Ter-
tullian, conceiving of the torrid zone as the flaming
sword, which turned every way to keep the way of
the tree of life (Gen. iii. 24), placed Eden beyond
it, in the southern hemisphere. Now it was at the
bottom of the sea ; [1] or again it held a position midway between earth and heaven. Anon, it was on
the summit of a miraculous mountain, which rose to
the height of the moon. Of this mountain only the
base was washed, when by the waters of the Deluge
all other mountains were covered. It was conceived
of as rising in three gigantic stages to its stupendous height. All kinds of marvelous plants and
precious metals and gems adorned it, but its supreme adornment was a divine river, which, starting
from the throne of God in the highest heaven,
descended to the holy garden on the mountain's
head, and thence parting into four, after watering
and beautifying the whole mountain in its descent,
gradually lost more and more of its celestial taste
and vivifying virtues, and became the water system
of the habitable globe. Sometimes the location of

---

[1] "In some legends Eden was submerged by the earliest deluge
that covered the Mount. The happy garden was believed to be lying
at the bottom of Lake Van, in Armenia." — Gerald Massey, *The Natural Genesis*, vol. ii., p. 231.

this mountain was described as in some distant portion of the earth, "where the sea, or earth, and the sky meet."

Impatient of such contradictions, Luther, in his own brusque way, rejected all attempts to locate the primeval garden, declaring that the Deluge had so changed the face of the earth and the course of its original rivers that all search was fruitless.

Calvin, on the contrary, confidently affirmed that the writer of the Genesis narrative must be understood as locating the Garden of Eden near the mouths of the Euphrates. Soon this original diversity of Protestant teaching upon the subject became aggravated by new theories, some of them suggested by orthodox ingenuity, some introduced by rationalistic conceptions of the semi-mythical character of the Bible, until at the present time the state of theological teaching respecting Eden is, if possible, a worse Babel than in any preceding age.

For a partial illustration of the confusion one has only to turn to the most recent and authoritative biblical, theological, and religious encyclopædias. In McClintock and Strong's, the writer on Eden inclines to locate it in Armenia. In Smith's "Bible Dictionary" the problem is abandoned as probably insoluble. In the great German encyclopædia of Herzog it is declared necessary to deny to the story of Eden a strictly historical character; it is "a bit of mythical geography." In the supplement, however, Pressel makes an elaborate argument of many pages in favor of the location at the junction of the Tigris and Euphrates. Dillmann, in Schenkel's "Bibel-Lexicon," places it in the Himalayas, north of India. In the chief Roman Catholic cyclopædia, Wetzel

and Welte's " Kirchen - Lexicon," the writer vacil-
lates between Eastern Asia, taken in a vague and
undefined sense, and an equally undefined North.
In Lichtenberg's just completed " Encyclopédie des
Sciences Religieuses " the whole story in Genesis ii.
is declared a " philosophic myth." Professor Brown,
of New York, in the new work edited by Dr. Schaff,
on the basis of Herzog, enumerates a variety of
opinions advocated by others, but refrains from expressing any opinion of his own. Such is all the
light which contemporary theology seems able to
throw upon our problem.

But here some plain reader of the Bible opens at
the second chapter of Genesis, and reads, " And
the Lord God planted a garden eastward in Eden ;
and there he put the man whom he had formed."
And the plain reader asks how a believer in the
Bible can doubt that this passage fixes the location
of the garden somewhere to the East of Palestine.
But, looking a little more critically, our inquirer
himself quickly sees that the verse does not necessarily affirm anything as to the direction of the garden from the writer. It may naturally mean that the
garden was planted in the eastern part of the land
of Eden, wherever that was ; and turning to the
most careful and orthodox commentators, he finds
that not a few take this view of it. Moreover, *Miqqedem*, here translated " eastward," may be otherwise translated, as it is in King James's Version, in
the passages Ps. lxxiv. 12, lxxvii. 6, and elsewhere.
In fact, in the Vulgate it is here translated, *a prin-
cipio*, " in or from the beginning." Among the
early Greek translators, Symmachus, Theodotion,
and Aquila understand the term in the same way.

Hence, nearly two hundred years ago, the learned Thomas Burnet wrote as follows : " Some have thought that the word *Miqqedem*, Gen. ii. 8, was to be rendered *in the East*, or *Eastward*, as we read it, and therefore determined the site of Paradise ; but 't is only the Septuagint translate it so ; all the other Greek versions, and St. Jerome, the Vulgate, the Chaldee Paraphrase, and the Syriak, render it *from the beginning*, or *in the beginning*, or to that effect. And we that do not believe the Septuagint to have been infallible or inspired have no reason to prefer their single authority above all the rest." [1]

The same writer says again, " We may safely say that none of the Christian Fathers, Latin or Greek, ever placed Paradise in Mesopotamia ; that is a conceit and innovation of some modern authors, which hath been much encouraged of late, because it gave more ease and rest as to further inquiries in an argument they could not well manage." [2]

As to the new source of evidence opened up by the decipherment of the Cuneiform inscriptions, Lenormant says, that in none of these, so far as yet deciphered, has anything been found indicating that the Chaldæo-Babylonians believed that their country was the cradle of the human race. [3]

" But the four rivers," says our inquirer, and he reads verses 10–14 : " And a river went out of Eden to water the garden ; and from thence it was parted and became into four heads. The name of the first is Pison. . . . And the name of the second river is Gihon. . . . And the name of the third river

---

[1] *Sacred Theory of the Earth.* London, 2d ed., 1691 : p. 252.
[2] Ibid., p. 253.
[3] *Les Origines de l'Histoire.* Paris, 1882 : tom. ii. 1, p. 120.

is Hiddekel, . . . and the fourth river is Euphrates."
" Surely here in the fourth river we have *one* undeniable landmark.   However impossible it may be
satisfactorily to identify all four of the primitive rivers of Eden, the mention of the Euphrates at least
restricts the location of the garden to some part of
the region drained by that river."

Consulting the theologians, however, our investigator finds a great variety of serious objections
urged against this short and easy method of settling
the controversy.

First, he is told that some Biblical critics have
expressed doubt as to the genuineness of the verses,
and that as earnest a defender of the Bible as Mr.
Granville Penn considered the whole passage an in-
terpolation.

Secondly, he learns that Perath or Phrath, the
Hebrew name of the river, is from the older form
Buratti or Purattu, a word believed to signify " the
broad," or " the deep." [1]   Of course such a descriptive term may well have been the name of more
than one ancient river, just as " Broad Brook" is the
name of many an American stream.   Indeed, in his
learned work, " Le Berceau de l'Espèce Humaine,"
Obry shows that in ancient times Phrat, or Euphrates, was the name of one, or possibly two, of the
rivers of Persia.[2]   One of these in Pliny's time still
bore the name in the hardly changed form Ophradus.
Lenormant says he does not hesitate to consider the
Phrath of the Khorda-Avesta identical with the Per-

---

[1] Delitzsch, *Wo lag das Paradies?* p. 169. Grill, *Die Erzväter der Menschheit*, Bd. i., p. 230. In Old Persian it is *Ufratu,* " the fair flowing."   F. Finzi, *Antichità Assira*, Turin, 1872: p. 112.

[2] See pp. 95, 136, 140.

sian river Helmend.[1] Africa also had its sacred Euphrates.[2] If therefore the passage in Genesis is genuine, and Moses wrote of the Phrath, it is not absolutely certain what "broad" or "abounding" river he had in mind. Moreover, in any case, the Euphrates of Mesopotamia is not one of four equal offshoots into which the one "river" proceeding "out of Eden" divided itself according to the statement of the text. Its source is not from another river at all, but from ordinary mountain springs.

Thirdly, it must not be forgotten, our friend is told, that all peoples coming into a new country love to name their new rivers and towns after the loved and sacred ones they have left in the elder home. The Thames of New England perpetuates the memory of the Thames of Old England. "It is very seldom indeed," says a late writer, "that a river has no namesakes."[3] Very possibly, therefore, the Phrath of Mesopotamia may have been named for some elder river of the antediluvian world, wherever that may have been. That it was so is the firm belief of various learned writers.[4]

Fourthly, continue the theologians, the language of Ezekiel xxviii. 13–19, and of Proverbs iii. 18 ; xi. 30, etc., shows that poetic and symbolical applications of the name and images of Eden were common.

---

[1] *Origines de l'Histoire*, tom. ii. 1, p. 99.

[2] " Also there is a very sacred river in Hwida called the Euphrates or Eufrates." — Gerald Massey, *The Natural Genesis*. London, 1883: vol. ii., p. 165.

[3] " There is no improbability in supposing that there may have been in Britain two rivers named Trisanton. On the contrary, it is very seldom indeed that a river has no namesakes." — Henry Bradley, in *The Academy*, April 28, 1883, p. 296.

[4] See Grill, *Die Erzväter der Menschheit*, Bd. i., pp. 239, 242.

And if the Hebrews named one of the water-courses
at Jerusalem Gihon, in commemoration of one of the
four Paradise rivers,[1] it is not irrational to suppose
that the inhabitants of Mesopotamia may have called
their chief stream in honor of another of the four.
Lenormant, Grill, Obry, and others support this view.
They might have rendered the probability still
stronger by calling attention to the fact that the
oldest name of Babylon, Tin-tir-ki, was of the same
commemorative or symbolical character, and signified " the place of the Tree of Life." [2]

Finally, pursuing these curious investigations further, our plain reader finds mention in Pausanias, ii.
5, of a strange belief of the ancients, according to
which the Euphrates, after disappearing in a marsh
and flowing a long distance underground, rises again
beyond Ethiopia, and flows through Egypt as the
Nile. This reminds him of the language of Josephus,
according to which the Ganges, the Tigris, the Euphrates, and the Nile are all but parts of "one river
which ran round about the whole earth," — the Oke-
anos-river of the Greeks.[3] And he wonders whether
the old Shemitic term from which the modern Euphrates is derived was not originally a name of the
general water system of the world, — a name of that
Ocean-river which Aristotle describes as rising in
the upper heavens, descending in rain upon the
earth, feeding, as Homer tells us, all fountains and
rivers and every sea, flowing through all these water-

[1] Ewald, *Geschichte des Volkes Israel,* 2d ed., Bd. iii., pp. 321–328.

[2] Lenormant, *Origines de l'Histoire,* vol. i., p. 76. English version,
p. 85. See also Rev. O. D. Miller, " The Symbolical Geography of
the Ancients," in the *American Antiquarian and Oriental Journal,*
Chicago, July, 1881.

[3] Compare Rev. ix. 14.

courses down into the great and "broad" equatorial ocean-current which girdles the world in its embrace, thence branching out from the further shore into the rivers of the Underworld, to be at last fire-purged and sublimated, and returned in purity to the upper heavens to recommence its round.[1] And just as he is wondering over the question, he finds that some of the Assyriologists, in their investigation of pre-Babylonian Akkadian mythology, have found reason to believe this surmise correct, and to say that in that mythology the term Euphrates was applied to "the rope of the world," "the encircling river of the snake god of the tree of life," "the heavenly river which surrounds the earth."[2] Furthermore, as he turns back to the pages of Hyginus, and Manilius, and Lucius Ampelius, and reads of the fall of the "world-egg" at the beginning "into the river Euphrates," he perceives that he is in a mythologic, and not a historic region.[3] And when he lights upon a mutilated fragment of an ancient Assyrian inscription, in which descriptions of the visible and invisible world are mixed up together, and in which the river "of the life of the world" is designated by the name "Euphrates,"[4] he quickly concludes that it will not do to take the term Phrath, or Eu-frata, as always and everywhere referring to the historic river of Mesopotamia.

[1] See below Part V., chapter 5 : "The Quadrifurcate River."

[2] The Rev. A. H. Sayce in *The Academy*. London, Oct. 7, 1882 : p. 263. " Professor Sayce, after recently observing that 'in early Akkadian mythology the mouth of the Euphrates was identified with the River of Death,' adds, ' The Okeanos of Homer had, I believe, its origin in this Akkadian river which coiled itself around the world.'"—Robert Brown, Jun., F. R. S., *The Myth of Kirkê*. London, 1883 : p. 33.

[3] Bryant, *Analysis of Ancient Myths*, vol. iii., pp. 160–162.

[4] *Records of the Past*, x., p. 149.

Hitherto, then, the "results" of the theologians as to the location of Eden are purely negative and mutually destructive. "It would be difficult," says one of their number, "to find any subject in the whole history of opinion which has so invited and at the same time so completely baffled conjecture as this. Theory after theory has been advanced, but none has been found which satisfies the required conditions. The site of Eden will ever rank, with the quadrature of the circle and the interpretation of unfulfilled prophecy, among those unsolved and perhaps insoluble problems which possess so strange a fascination." [1]

[1] William A. Wright, of Trinity College, Cambridge, in Smith's *Dictionary of the Bible*, Art. "Eden."

CHAPTER III.

THE RESULTS OF NON-THEOLOGICAL SCHOLARS : NATURALISTS, ETHNOLOGISTS, ETC.

It is useless to speculate on this subject. — CHARLES DARWIN.

THE location of the cradle of the human race is as much a problem for the ethnologist and anthropologist as it is for the theologian. The archæologist, the zoölogist, and even the biologist, if at all broad and philosophical in their inquiries, cannot ignore the high interest of the questions, Was there for the human race one primitive centre of distribution? and, if so, Where was it located?

Thirty years ago the pretentious American work by Nott and Gliddon, entitled "The Types of Mankind," [1] — a work written in opposition to the doctrine of the unity of the human race, — attracted unusual attention to the former of these questions. The teaching therein put forth was that there are very many types or varieties of men without genealogical connection with each other, and that therefore a great number of primitive centres of distribution must be assumed. The avowed prejudices of the projectors of the work against certain races, particularly the African, would have rendered the influence of the work upon the scientific world extremely slight, had not contributions of some value from Dr. S. G. Morton, and Professor Louis Agassiz

[1] Philadelphia and London, 1854.

3

been incorporated with it. As it was, it gave European ethnologists occasion to form and express very uncomplimentary conceptions of American representatives of ethnological research.[1] Fortunately these crude beginners of the science have had no influential successors of their own sort in this country, and but obscure or half-hearted disciples in any other.[2] The polygeny of the race has at present no respectable support. Even the author of the latest and perhaps ablest of the works on the Preadamite Hypothesis remarks, "The plural origin of mankind is a doctrine now almost entirely superseded. All schools admit the probable descent of all races from a common stock." [3] To the second question, therefore, the attention of the scientific and archæological world is steadily gravitating. Given one primeval point of departure for the race, where shall that point of departure be sought?

The answers which recent biologists, naturalists, and ethnologists have given to this problem are hardly less numerous or less conflicting than are the solutions proposed by theologians. Of these

---

[1] Such references as the following are not uncommon : "Unerlässlich bleibt die Behauptung eines einzigen Ausgangsortes sämmtlicher Menschenrassen, *im Gegensatze zur Anthropologenschule unter den Amerikanern, die vielleicht um ihr Gewissen über die vormalige Negersklaverei und den Rassenmord der Indianer zu beruhigen, in neuster Zeit über hundert Menschenarten, nicht Menschenrassen, überhaupt so viele geschaffen hat als Völkertypen sich aufstellen lassen,*" etc. — O. Peschel, in *Ausland*, 1869, p. 1110. Cited in Caspari, *Die Urgeschichte der Menschheit.* 2d ed., Leipsic, 1877, vol. i., p. 241.

[2] See Simonin, *L'Homme Américain.* Paris, 1870: p. 12. A. Réville, *Les Religions des Peuples non-civilisés.* Paris, 1883: vol. i., p. 196.

[3] Alexander Winchell, *Preadamites ; or a Demonstration of the Existence of Men before Adam.* Chicago, 1880 : p. 297. One of the latest and most authoritative criticisms and refutations of Agassiz's polygenism is found in Quatrefages, *The Human Race.* N.Y., 1879: chap. xiv.

answers Professor Zoeckler, in a late work, enumerates *ten*, each having the support of eminent scientific names.[1] In latitude they range from Greenland to Central Africa, and in longitude from America to Central Asia. Of the whole number, the two which seem to command the widest and weightiest support are, first, the hypothesis that " Lemuria " — a wholly imaginary, now submerged prehistoric continent under the northern portion of the Indian Ocean — was the " mother-region " of the race ; and, secondly, that it was in the heart of Central Asia.

The former of these sites is the one supported by Haeckel, Caspari, Peschel, and many others.[2] Though less positive, Darwin and Lyell seem favorable to the same location or to one in the adjoining portion of Africa. Most of the recent maps of the progressive dispersion of the race over the globe have been constructed in accordance with this theory.[3] Perhaps the best popular summary of the arguments in its favor is that found in Oscar Peschel's " Races of Men." [4]

But while biological speculation, especially in the hands of Darwinists, has strongly inclined toward the chief habitat of the ape tribes in its attempts to find man's primitive point of departure, comparative philologists, mythologists, and archæological

---

[1] *The Cross of Christ.* Translated by Evans. London, 1877. Appendix iii., p. 389.

[2] Ernst Haeckel, *The Pedigree of Man, and other Essays.* London, 1883 : pp. 73–80. Otto Kuntze, *Phytogeogenesis.* Leipsic, 1884 : p. 52, note.

[8] See Caspari's in *Die Urgeschichte der Menschheit*, at the close of vol. i.; Kracher's *Ethnographische Weltkarte* in Novara Expedition, Vienna, 1875 ; Winchell's in his *Preadamites*, p. 1.

[4] New York, Appletons, pp. 26–34.

ethnographers have of late very strongly tended
to place the cradle of mankind on the lofty plateau
of Pamir in Central Asia. For these the eminent
French anthropologist, Quatrefages, is well entitled
to speak.

We know [says this savant] that in Asia there is a
vast region bounded on the south and south-west by the
Himalayas, on the west by the Bolor mountains, on the
north-west by the Alla-Tau, on the north by the Altai
range and its off-shoots, on the east by the Kingkhan, on
the south and south-east by the Felina and Kwen-lun.
Judging of it by what exists at the present day, this great
central region might be regarded as having included the
cradle of the human race.

In fact, the three fundamental types of all the races
of mankind are represented in the populations grouped
around this region. The negro races are the furthest removed from it, but have nevertheless marine stations,
in which they are found pure or mixed, from the Kiussiu
to the Andaman Islands. On the continent they have
mingled their blood with nearly all the inferior castes and
classes of the two Gangetic peninsulas; they are still
found pure in each of them; they ascend as far as Nepâl,
and, according to Elphinstone, spread to the west as far
as the Persian Gulf and Lake Zareh. The yellow race,
pure, or mixed here and there with white elements, seems
alone to occupy the area in question. The circumference
of this region is peopled by it to the north, the east, the
south-east, and the west. In the south it is more mixed,
but it none the less forms an important element of the
population. The white race, by its allophylian representatives, seems to have disputed the possession of even
the central area itself with the yellow race. In early
times we find the Yu-Tchi, the U-Suns, to the north of
Hoang-Ho; and at the present day in Little Thibet, in
Eastern Thibet, small islands of white populations have

been pointed out. The Miao-Tsé occupy the mountainous regions of China; the Siaputhes are proof against
all attacks in the gorges of Bolor. On the confines of
this area we find to the east the Aïnos and the Japanese
of high caste, the Tinguians of the Philippine Islands;
to the south the Hindus. To the south-west and west,
the white element, pure or mixed, is completely predominant. No other region on the face of the globe presents
similar reunion of the extreme types of the human race
distributed around a common centre. This fact of itself
might suggest to the naturalist the conjecture which I
have expressed above; but we may appeal to other considerations.

One of the weightiest of these is drawn from philology. The three fundamental forms of human language
are found in the same regions and in analogous connections. In the centre and the south-east of our area the
monosyllabic languages are represented by the Chinese,
the Annamite, the Siamese, and the Thibetan. As agglu-
tinative languages, we find, from the north-east to the
north-west, the group of the Ugro-Japanese; in the south
that of the Dravidians and the Malays; and in the west
the Turkish languages. Lastly, Sanscrit with its deriva-
tives, and the Iranian languages, represent, in the south
and south-west, the inflectional languages. With the linguistic types accumulated around this central region of
Asia all human languages are connected, either by their
vocabulary or their grammar. Some of these Asiatic languages resemble very closely languages spoken in regions
far removed, or separated from the area in question by
very different languages.

Lastly, it is from Asia, again, that our earliest-tamed
domestic animals have come. Isidore Geoffroy-Saint-
Hilaire is entirely agreed on this point with Dureau de
la Malle.

Thus, taking into account only the present epoch,

everything leads us back to this central plateau, or rather this vast inclosure. Here, we are inclined to say to ourselves, the first human beings appeared, and multiplied down to the moment when the populations overflowed like a bowl which is too full, and poured themselves out in human waves in all directions.[1]

This view of the location of the first centre of the race is very widely accepted. It has the support of ʻmany great names. To its establishment contributions have been made by scholars in a great variety of fields. Among them may be mentioned Lassen, Burnouf, Ewald, Renan, Obry, D'Eckstein, Höfer, Senart, Maspéro, Lenormant, etc. Perhaps the most important single treatise representing the view is Obry's "Cradle of the Human Species," — a work of singular interest to every scholar.[2]

But the latest writers on the question are by no means confined to the two locations just mentioned. The difficulty of accounting for the first advent of human beings in America, without supposing in early times a closer land-connection between the eastern and western hemispheres in the intertropical regions than now exists, has led not a few ethnologists to postulate a lost Atlantis, including perhaps the Canary and Madeira Islands, or the Azores,

---

[1] *The Human Species*, pp. 175-177. — Quatrefages' noteworthy suggestion as to the possibility of a modification of the above conclusion in consequence of the revelations of recent paleontological researches will be noticed in Part III., chapter 7.

[2] *Le Berceau de l'Espèce Humaine selon les Indiens, les Perses et les Hébreux.* Amiens, 1858. See also Lenormant, *Origines de l'Histoire.* Paris, 1882 : tom. ii. 1, pp. 41, 144, 145. (Translated in part in *The Contemporary Review*, Sept. 1881.) *Fragments cosmogoniques de Berose*, pp. 300-333. Renan, *Histoire générale des Langues Semitiques*, pp. 475-484. Wilford, *Asiatic Researches*, vol. vi., pp. 455-536, and the following volumes.

or located to the North or South of them, and to place in it the fountain head of the streams of population which colonized both the Old and the New World.[1]

Another location lately advanced with great confidence and supported with remarkable acuteness and learning is that advocated by Dr. Friedrich Delitzsch in his valuable work entitled " Wo lag das Paradies ? "[2] This site is on the Euphrates between Bagdad and Babylon.[3] In the author's construction the "four rivers" are the great canal west of the Euphrates, called by the Greeks the Pallaco-

---

[1] Unger, *Die versunkene Insel Atlantis.* Vienna, 1860. An American work in advocacy of this theory is Ignatius Donnelly's *Atlantis: The Antediluvian World.* New York, 1882. In Europe the hypothesis has been represented as largely abandoned. See Engler, *Die Entwickelungsgeschichte der Pflanzenwelt.* Leipsic, 1879 : vol. i., p. 82. But a new modification has since appeared in the work of M. Berlioux of Lyons : *Les Atlantes. Histoire de l'Atlantis et de l'Atlas primitif, ou Introduction a l'histoire de l'Europe.* Paris, 1883.

[2] *Wo lag das Paradies ? Eine biblisch-assyriologische Studie. Mit zahlreichen assyriologischen Beiträgen zur biblischen Länder- und Völkerkunde und einer Karte Babyloniens.* Von Dr. Friedrich Delitzsch, Professor der Assyriologie an der Universität Leipzig. Leipsic, 1881. The author is a son of the well-known Biblical scholar Professor Franz Delitzsch, and is himself eminent as an Assyriologist.

[3] Compare the language of his fellow-student in Assyriology, Professor Felice Finzi : " Mentre a cercare la culla degli Ariani dobbiamo volgerci ad Oriente, agli Uttara-Kuru degli Indiani, al mitico paradiso degli nomini del monte Meru, all' Airyanem Vaêdjô degli Irani, al regno di Udyana presso al Caschmir ; mentre in qualche gruppo del sistema uralo-altaico dee forse indicarsi il centro di formazione della famiglia turanica, e la orografia del Caucaso potrà forse sola determinare il sito più opportuno per lo sviluppo delle tribù che se ne attestano autottone ; i Semiti ci si mostrano figli di quella terra ove si sono svolte le pagine più belle della loro storia. È là forse in un angolo di questo paese ricco un tempo dello splendore di una natura lussureggiante che la tribù semita si formò." — *Ricerche per lo Studio dell' Antichità Assira.* Torino, 1872 : p. 433.

pas, the Shat-en-Nil, and the lower Tigris and Euphrates. But despite the conceded ability of the
plea, there seems at present little prospect that it
will secure acceptance among scholars. The distinguished Theodor Noeldeke, in a recent review, while
cordially praising the learning and ingenuity of the
work, professes himself unmoved by its arguments.[1]
Similarly a critic in this country writes : "Unfortunately for the theory so powerfully advanced, almost
all the linguistic evidences by which it is supported
are still of doubtful value, the etymology of the
Babylonian names in most cases, and the reading in
some, being disputed by high authorities in this obscure field of inquiry. Were the linguistic points
proved, it would be hard to resist the power of the
argument, in spite of various difficulties arising from
the scanty text of Genesis itself. As it is, although
all other solutions of the knotty Biblical problem
may be subject to still graver objections, the following questions militate too strongly against Professor
Delitzsch's solution : Why, if the stream of Eden be
the middle Euphrates, is it left unnamed in the narrative, though it is certain that the Hebrews were
perfectly familiar both with the middle and the upper course of that river? Why, if the Pison and
Gihon designate the canals Pallacopas and Shat-en-
Nil, are they said to *compass* lands which the canals
only traverse ? If the *lower* Tigris be meant by the
Hiddekel, why is this river described as flowing in
front of Assyria, which lay *above* the central Meso-

---

[1] "Seine Ansicht zu begründen wendet er sehr viel Gelehrsamkeit
und noch mehr Scharfsinn auf, aber ich fürchte umsonst. Nach sorg-
fältiger Prüfung muss ich festhalten an einer Lage des Paradieses in
'Utopien,' wie er etwas spöttisch sagt." — *Zeitschrift der Deutschen
Morgenländischen Gesellschaft,* 1882, p. 174.

potamian lowland asserted to be Eden? How should
a writer familiar with the whole course of the Tigris
deem its lower part a branch of the Euphrates?
Why should Cush, a name which commonly designated Ethiopia, have been used by the narrator in a
sense in which it nowhere else occurs in the Scriptures, without the least further definition? Why,
on the other hand, is Havilah, if the Arabian border-
land so well known to the Hebrews be meant, so
fully described by its products? Who tells us that
the gold, the bdellium, and the shoham of Babylonia
were also characteristic of the adjoining Havilah?
But whether these objections, in the present stage
of Assyriological studies, be fatal to the theory of
Professor Delitzsch or not, we have no hesitation in
saying that his dissertation, amplified as it is by
supplementary treatises on the ancient geography
and ethnology of the Mesopotamian and neighbor-
ing countries, of Canaan, Egypt, and Elam, is a perfect treasury of knowledge, — made most accessible
by excellent indexes, — and probably the most brilliant production in all Biblico-Assyriological literature." [1]

At the present writing, the latest monograph
upon the subject is the one just published in the
"Revue de l'Histoire des Religions," from the pen of
M. Beauvois.[2] This locates the Eden of ethnic traditions in America, and ascribes to the Keltic race

---

[1] *The Nation.* New York, Mar. 15, 1883. See Lenormant's criticisms in *Les Origines de l'Histoire*, tom. ii. ; and Halévy's in the *Revue
Critique*, Paris, 1881, pp. 457-463, 477-485.

[2] "L'Elysée Transatlantique et l'Eden Occidental," par E. Beauvois. *Revue*, Paris, 1883, pp. 273 ss. See also " L'Elysée des Mexi-
cains comparé a celui des Celtes," by the same author, in same Review, 1884.

no small influence upon the Greco-Roman mythology in the development of such ideas as those pertaining to the Gardens of the Hesperides, the Isles of the Blessed, etc. The site advocated is not new, though the line of argument is fresh and scholarly. The hypothesis that the cradle of the race is to be sought in America has before found advocacy at the hands of J. Klaproth, Gobineau, and others.

That this, however, is not to be the last and only word on the subject is evident from the fact that, in a huge work just from the press, an English writer says: " If there be an earthly original for the heavenly Eden, it will be found in equatorial Africa, the land of seething, swarming, multitudinous, and colossal life, where the mother nature grew great with her latest race ; the lair in which the lusty breeder brought forth her black, barbarian brood, and put forth for them such a warm, welling bosom as cannot be paralleled elsewhere on earth. This was the world of wet and heaven of heat ; the land of equal day and dark ; that supplied the Two Truths of *Uarti* (Egyptian) ; the top of the world ; the very nipple (*Kepa*) of the breast of earth, which is there one vast streaming fount of moisture quick with life. So surely as a topographical Meru is found in Habesh, so surely is the Earthly Paradise, the original of the mythical which was carried forth over the world by the migrations from Kam, to be found there, if at all." [1]

---

[1] *The Natural Genesis, containing an attempt to recover and reconstitute the lost Origins of the Myths and Mysteries, Types and Symbols, Religion and Language, with Egypt for the mouthpiece, and Africa as the birthplace.* By Gerald Massey. London, 1883 : vol. ii., p. 162. It is impossible to understand how Mr. Massey reconciles the foregoing language with that used on p. 28 of the same volume, where

In fine, so resultless seem all discussions and investigations in this field that in his work on "The Patriarchs of Humanity" Dr. Julius Grill, like Noeldeke, prefers to locate lost Paradise "in Utopia," and to deny to it all historic reality.[1] Evidently the naturalists and the ethnologists, the comparative mythologists, and *Kulturgeschichtschreiber*, have not yet solved the problem. Their "mother-region" of the human race is as elusive and Protean as are any of the terrestrial Edens of theology, or of legend, or of poetry.

Thus far, then, all search has been fruitless. Paradise is indeed lost. The explorer cannot find it; the theologian, the naturalist, and the archæologist have all sought it in vain. Representative voices out of every camp are heard confessing utter ignorance as to the region where human history began. "The problem," says Professor Ebers, "remains unanswered."

he speaks of the crooked sword *Khepsh*, "that turned every way, and by its revolution formed the circle of Eden, or, as it was represented, kept the way of the Tree of Life, the POLE, where the happy garden was planted as the primary creation, which was the home of the primeval pair." But in the language of *The Nation* (June 26, 1884) the work is "an enormous conglomeration of facts set down with entire indifference to scientific principles of comparison, . . . and, as far as the author's aim is concerned, absolutely worthless."

[1] "Der Ort, wohin die althebräische Ueberlieferung die Wiege des Menschengeschlechtes verlegt . . . ist also nicht auf der Erde gelegen, und gehört dem Bereich der Wirklichkeit nicht an." — Grill, *Die Erzväter der Menschheit.* Leipzig, 1875 : Abth. I., p. 242.

PART SECOND.

A NEW HYPOTHESIS.

When Newton said "*Hypotheses non fingo*" he did not mean that he deprived himself of the facilities of investigation afforded by assuming in the first instance what he hoped ultimately to be able to prove. Without such assumptions science could never have attained its present state. — JOHN STUART MILL.

In scientific investigations it is permitted to invent any hypothesis, and if it explains various large and independent classes of facts it rises to the rank of a well-grounded theory. — CHARLES DARWIN.

CHAPTER I.

THE HYPOTHESIS.

The golden guess
Is morning star to the full round of truth.
TENNYSON.

FROM the foregoing chapters it would seem as if nearly every imaginable site for the Gan-Eden of Genesis had been proposed, examined, and found unavailable. One, however, remains, — a region of rarest interest in astronomical, physical, and historical geography, — the natural centre of the only historic hemisphere. Considering the fascination of the subject and the inexhaustible ingenuity that has been expended upon it, it seems remarkable that it should be left to the closing years of the nineteenth century to bring forward and seriously to test the proposition THAT THE CRADLE OF THE HUMAN RACE, THE EDEN OF PRIMITIVE TRADITION, WAS SITUATED AT THE NORTH POLE, IN A COUNTRY SUBMERGED AT THE TIME OF THE DELUGE.[1]

[1] As to the alleged "newness" of the above hypothesis, it is proper to say that something like a year elapsed after its full acceptance and public announcement by the writer before he could find any evidence that it had ever been entertained or advocated by any other person. He then met with the allusion in the passage quoted from Bishop Huet as a motto to chapter second of the preceding part, and with a similar allusion in an anonymous article in Dickens' *All the Year Round*. Whether these were more than rhetorical flourishes he was long in doubt. Not until after the manuscript of the present work had been completed, packed, and addressed to the publishers,

This is the hypothesis which it is proposed in the following pages to examine and according to the evidences to adjudge. We propose to make the test both strict and comprehensive. Hypotheses, however promising, must be brought face to face with reality. Ours, like its numberless predecessors, must be rejected if the solid facts of any of the following sciences show that it is inadmissible : —

1. *General Geogony*, or the science of the origin of the earth ;

2. *Mathematical* or *Astronomical Geography*, particularly its teachings as to the inhabitableness or uninhabitableness of the circumpolar region with respect to light ;

3. *Physiographical Geology*, particularly its teachings as to the probability or improbability of the former existence and subsequent submersion of a circumpolar country ;

4. *Prehistoric Climatology*, particularly with reference to the temperature at the Pole at the time of the beginning of human history ;

5. *Paleontological Botany ;*

6. *Paleontological Zoölogy ;*

7. *Paleontological Anthropology* and *Ethnology ;* and

8. *Comparative Mythology*, viewed as the science

was the doubt resolved by finding in an anonymous English magazine article of more than thirty years ago this brief statement : " Pastellus will have it that Paradise was under the North Pole." Who Pastellus was and what he wrote upon the subject remain to be investigated. Suffice to say that up to the date of this writing the author has found no book or tractate in which the above hypothesis has ever been advocated. This fact renders some of the mottoes prefixed to the chapters farther on remarkably significant and impressive. In many cases their authors express truths which they themselves did not perceive.

of the oldest traditionary beliefs and memories of
mankind. On the contrary, if the hypothesis is capable of meeting this eightfold test, and especially
if we can show, not only that it is admissible, but
also that in greater or less degree it is supported by
the positive evidence of the facts in nearly all of
these fields of knowledge, we shall afford a much
more complete and convincing verification than is
at all usual in matters of prehistoric research.

4

CHAPTER II.

IMPORTANT NEW FEATURES AT ONCE INTRODUCED
INTO THE PROBLEM OF THE SITE OF EDEN.   SIG-
NIFICANCE OF THESE FOR A VALID SOLUTION.

It appears, then, to be a condition of a genuinely scientific hypothesis that it be not destined always to remain an hypothesis, but be certain to be either proved or disproved by that comparison with observed facts which is termed verification. . . . Verification is proof; if the supposition accords with the phenomena there needs no other evidence of it. — JOHN STUART MILL.

IT is evident, on a moment's thought, that our hypothesis immediately and materially modifies the whole problem of the location of Paradise.

Given a prehistoric circumpolar continent at the North Pole as the cradle of the race, what must have been marked and memorable features of that primitive abode ?

1. To the first men there would have been but one day and one night in a year.

2. The stars, instead of seeming to rise and set, would have had an apparently horizontal motion round and round the observer from left to right.

3. The Pole, the unmoving centre-point of the heavens directly overhead, would naturally have seemed to be the top of the world, the true heaven, the changeless seat of the supreme, all-ruling God. And if, accordingly, through all the long lifetime of the ante-diluvian world, the *circumpolar* sky was to human thought the true abode of God, the oldest post - diluvian peoples, though scattered down the

sides of the globe half or two thirds the distance to the equator, could not easily have forgotten that at the centre and true top of the rotating sky was the throne of its great Creator, and that there, in the far North, was "the sacred quarter" of the world.

4. Standing at the Pole of the earth, an observer would be not only directly under the centre of the celestial hemisphere, but also directly on the centre of the surface of the terrestrial hemisphere. There, and there alone, the heavenly bodies would move, in horizontal planes, round and round him everywhere at an apparently equal distance, and he would seem to himself to stand on the one precise centre-point of the entire earth. Every departure of a few miles in any direction from this polar position would at once confirm this first impression. If, therefore, primeval Eden was at the Pole, the descendants of the first man, going away from such an original country, could hardly have failed to remember it as the centre of all lands, the *omphalos* of the whole earth.

5. Supposing the first man to have been located in the central and most elevated portion of the hypothetical Eden-land, the streams there originating and flowing seaward would have flowed, not in one but in various opposite directions toward all the cardinal points of the horizon. Moreover, all of these streams being obviously fed, not by each other, but by the rain from heaven, it would not have required a very powerful imagination to conceive of them as parts of a finer and more celestial stream whose head-springs were in the sky.[1] If, finally, the streams

---

[1] Compare the poetic representation of "the river of God," in Ps. lxv. 9, 10. Also the following : " Aristotle, I remember, in his *Me-*

flowing in the opposite directions grew at length into four opposite-flowing rivers, — *flumina principalia*, as many old theologians have called them, — dividing the circumpolar land into four nearly equal quarters, it would have constituted a never-to-be-forgotten feature of that first home of men.

6. In another chapter we shall expose the baselessness of the popular impression that at the Pole six months of every twelve are spent in darkness, and shall show that, on the contrary, less than one fifth of the year is so spent, while more than four fifths are spent in light. This being true, a primitive abode in that part of the world would have been remembered by the descendants of the first man as preëminently a land of beauty, — preëminently the home of the sun. Moreover, Arctic explorers find it impossible to describe the nocturnal splendors of the Aurora Borealis in those regions, — the whole top of the globe ofttimes seeming veiled in and over-canopied with quivering curtains and banners and streamers of living, leaping flame ; — it is therefore easy to believe that, once exiled from such a home, mankind would ever have looked back to it as to an abode of unearthly and preternatural effulgence, — a home fit for the occupancy of gods and holy immortals.

7. Finally, assuming the prevalence of an equable tropical temperature, we find the biological conditions of the region — such as the extraordinary prevalence of daylight, the intenser terrestrial magnetism,

teors, speaking of the course of the Vapours, saith, there is a River in the Air, constantly flowing betwixt the Heavens and the Earth, made by the ascending and descending Vapours." — Burnet, *Sacred Theory of the Earth*, p. 226.

and the unparalleled electric forces which feed the Northern Lights — all combining to raise a high probability that if ever such a land as we have supposed existed, it must have presented forms of life surpassing those with which we are familiar ; a flora and fauna of almost unimagined vigor and luxuriance of development. Under such conditions men themselves may well have had a stature and strength and longevity never attained since the Deluge, which destroyed "the world that then was," and immediately or ultimately occasioned the translocation of the seed of our new post-diluvian humanity into the cold and barren and desolate regions of the Northern Temperate zone. And if the first men were of the stature and strength and longevity supposed, how certainly would traditions of the fact linger in the memory of mankind long after its exile from its earlier and happier home !

Glancing back now over these various points, one instantly sees that they present conditions of human existence totally unlike the conditions of life as we know it, or as it has ever been known in what are called historic ages. They necessarily modify in the profoundest manner the whole problem of the site of Eden. No solution ever heretofore presented exposed itself to refutation at so many points. None ever before postulated so extraordinary an adjustment of both heavens and earth. None ever before required, in order to its establishment, so incredibly wide a concurrency of testimony. Against no other has it ever been possible for the very stars in their courses to fight. If false, it demands of human tradition shadowy recollections of world - conditions which have never existed in human experience. An hypothesis so peculiarly difficult must surely break down, if it be not true. Promising the reader, therefore, not a new *ignis-fatuus* chase, but at least the satisfaction of a definite result as respects one hypothesis, we cordially invite his critical and patient attention to the facts to be presented in the following chapters.

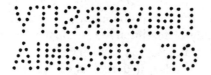

PART THIRD.

THE HYPOTHESIS SCIENTIFICALLY TESTED AND CONFIRMED.

It follows . . . that man, issuing from a "mother-region" still undetermined, but which a number of considerations indicate to have been in the North, has radiated in several directions; that his migrations have been constantly from North to South. — M. LE MARQUIS G. DE SAPORTA, in *Popular Science Monthly*, October, 1883, p. 753.

Eine jede Reise, welche nach der eisumgürteten Inselwelt im Norden Amerikas unternommen wurde, weiss von Anzeichen der ehemaligen Anwesenheit eines Volkes zu erzählen, welches Länder bewohnte, die heute kein menschlicher Fuss mehr zu betreten scheint. — DR. F. BOAS, in *Zeitschrift der Gesellschaft für Erdkunde in Berlin*, Bd. xviii. (1883), p. 118.

CHAPTER I.

THE TESTIMONY OF GEOGONY, OR THE SCIENCE OF THE ORIGIN OF THE EARTH.

Les lois générales de la géogénie favorisent d'une façon remarquable l'hypothèse dont nous venons d'ebaucher les traits. — COUNT SAPORTA.

COULD it once be proven that the Arctic terminus of the earth has always been the ice-bound region which it now is, and which for thousands of years it has been, it would of course be useless to entertain for a moment the hypothesis that the cradle of the human race was there located. Probably the popular impression that from the beginning of the world the far North has been the region of unendurable cold has been one of the chief reasons why our hypothesis is so late in claiming attention. At the present time, however, so far as this difficulty is concerned, scientific studies have abundantly prepared the way for the new theory.

That the earth is a slowly cooling body is a doctrine now all but universally accepted. In saying this we say nothing for or against the so-called nebular hypothesis of the origin of the world, for both friends and foes of this unproven hypothesis believe in what is termed the secular cooling or refrigeration of the earth. All authorities in this field hold and teach that the time was when the slowly solidifying planet was too hot to support any form of life, and that only at some particular time in the cooling process was there a temperature reached which was adapted to the necessities of living things.

On what portion of the earth's surface, now, would this temperature first be reached? Or would it everywhere be reached at the same time?

These are most interesting questions, and the writer has often marveled that in scientific treatises on the cooling globe he could nowhere find them formally discussed. Granting, however, a uniform interior heat and a uniform loss of it in the mode of superficial radiation in all directions into space, it is certain that if these were the only factors in the problem the cooling process would affect every part of the surface in a uniform manner, and we might confidently infer that the temperature compatible with organic life was reached at the same time at all points of the earth's surface. But the factors named are not the only ones of the problem. In those far-off geologic ages the heat received from the great central furnace of our system, the sun, cannot have been less than at the present time. Some astronomers and geologists claim that it was greater.[1] In any case, therefore, as early as the time when the earth's atmosphere became penetrable by the rays of the sun, local differences of temperature must have been produced at the base of the atmosphere, whether the body of the globe was as yet crusted over or not. Then as now, viewed apart from air and water currents, every particular spot on the surface of the globe must have had a temperature determined, first by the fixed and uniform inherent heat of the earth-mass, and secondly by the varying quantity of heat received from the sun. But

[1] See Winchell, *World-Life*, pp. 484–490.

the difference between the solar heat received at a point under the equator and that received at a point at the pole cannot have been less in those ages than at the present time ; and this incessant increment of the equatorial heat of the earth by the direct rays of the sun suggests at once the portions of the globe to which we must look if we would find the regions which first became cool enough to sustain organic life. Then as now the polar regions must have been cooler than the equatorial, and hence, as far as the teachings of theoretical geogony can be trusted, the conclusion is inevitable that there, to wit, in the polar regions, life first became possible.[1]

The bearing of this result upon our central thesis is at once obvious. We asked the geologist this question : " Is the hypothesis of a primeval polar Eden admissible ? " Looking at the slowly cooling earth alone, he replies, " Eden conditions have probably at one time or another been found everywhere upon the surface of the earth. Paradise may have been anywhere." Looking at the cosmic environment, however, he adds, " But while Paradise may have been anywhere, the *first* portions of the earth's surface sufficiently cool to present the conditions of Eden life were assuredly at the Poles."

[1] The similar or identical reasonings of Professor Philip Spiller were unknown to me when the foregoing was written. See the following : *Die Weltschöpfung vom Standpunkte der heutigen Wissenschaft. Mit neuen Untersuchungen*, 1868, 2d ed., 1873. *Die Entstehung der Welt und die Einheit der Naturkräfte. Populäre Kosmogonie*, 1872. *Die Urkraft des Weltalls nach ihrem Wesen und Wirken auf allen Naturgebieten.* Berlin, 1879. In Professor Otto Kuntze's latest work, *Phytogeogenesis : Die vorweltliche Entwickelung der Erdkruste und der Pflanzen*, Leipsic, 1884, I also find traces of a recognition of the truth above set forth. See pp. 51, 52, 53, 60, of the work.

CHAPTER II.

THE TESTIMONY OF ASTRONOMICAL GEOGRAPHY.

The nights are never so dark at the Pole as in other regions, for the moon and stars seem to possess twice as much light and effulgence. In addition, there is a continuous light in the North, the varied shades and play of which are amongst the strangest phenomena of nature. — RAMBOSSON's Astronomy.

The fact which gives the phenomenon of the polar aurora its greatest importance is that the earth becomes self-luminous ; that, besides the light which as a planet it receives from the central body, it shows a capability of sustaining a luminous process proper to itself. — HUMBOLDT.

WE are apt to think of an unbroken night of six months at the Pole. Eminent scientific authorities speak as if this conception were correct. Thus Professor Geikie, in his admirable new manual of Geology, writing of the Arctic flora of the Miocene age, says, "When we remember that this vegetation grew luxuriantly within 8° 15′ of the North Pole, *in a region which is in darkness for half of the year,* . . . we can realize the difficulty of the problem in the distribution of climate which these facts present to the geologist." [1]

In like manner Sir Charles Lyell, discussing the question of the possibility of whales reaching the supposed open sea at the Pole, says, "They could pass under considerable barriers of ice, provided there were openings here and there ; and so they may, perhaps, reach a more open sea near the Pole,

[1] *Text-book of Geology.* By Archibald Geikie, LL. D., F. R. S. London, 1882 : p. 869.

and find sustenance there during a day of more than *five months'* duration." [1]

From such representations as these the reader naturally carries away the impression that daylight lasts at the Pole somewhat over five months, while all the rest of the year the region is shrouded in darkness. Were this true, it would certainly be an unpromising region in which to search for the terrestrial Paradise.

Fortunately for our hypothesis, this conception of the duration of the polar night is very far from true. The half yearly reign of darkness exists only in the uninstructed imagination. Astronomical geography teaches that, as respects daylight, the polar regions are and always have been the most favored portions of the globe. As early a popularizer of natural science as the Rev. Thomas Dick set forth the real facts as follows : " Under the Poles, where the darkness of night would continue six months without intermission if there were no refraction, total darkness does not prevail one half of this period. When the sun sets at the North Pole, about the 23d of September, the inhabitants (if any) enjoy a perpetual aurora till he has descended eighteen degrees below the horizon. In his course through the ecliptic, the sun is two months before he can reach this point, during which time there is a perpetual twilight. In two months more he arrives again at the same point, namely, eighteen degrees below the horizon, when a new twilight commences, which is continually increasing in brilliancy for other two months, at the end of which the body of this luminary is seen rising in all its glory. So that in this

---

[1] *Principles of Geology*, New York ed., vol. i., p. 246.

region the light of day is enjoyed in a greater or
less degree for ten months, without interruption by
the effects of atmospheric refraction ; and during
the two months when the influence of the solar light
is entirely withdrawn, the moon is shining above the
horizon for two half months without intermission ;
and thus it happens that no more than two separate
fortnights are passed in total darkness, and this
darkness is alleviated by the light of the stars and
the frequent coruscations of the Aurora Borealis.
Hence it appears that there are no portions of our
globe which enjoy throughout the year so large a
portion of the solar light as these northern regions." [1]

Striking as is this account of the polar day, it is
noteworthy that experience has repeatedly shown
that the actual duration of light in high latitudes
exceeds even the calculations of the astronomers.
Thus, in the spring of 1873, the officers of the Aus-
trian expedition, under Lieutenants Weyprecht and
Payer, were surprised to behold the sun three days
before the date on which he was expected to rise.
A late writer thus states the case : " In the latitude
(79° 15' N.) in which the Tegethoff was lying, the
sun ought to reappear above the horizon on the 19th
of February ; but, owing to an effect of refraction,
due to the low temperature prevailing, —30° R., the
explorers were able to salute its rays three days earlier." [2]

Lieutenant Payer's own account is as follows :
"Though the sun did not return to our latitude (78°

---

[1] *Works of Thomas Dick, LL. D., The Practical Astronomer*, ch.
ii. Hartford, vol. ii., second half, p. 30.

[2] *Recent Expeditions in Eastern Polar Seas.* London, 1882: p. 83.

15' N., 71° 38' E. long.) till the 19th of February, we were able to greet his beams three days previous to that date, owing to the strong refraction of 1° 40' which accompanied a temperature of — 30° R." [1]

Still more remarkable was the experience of Barentz's Arctic expedition, almost three hundred years ago. Dr. Dick alludes to it as follows: "The refractive power of the atmosphere has been found to be much greater, in certain cases, than what has now been stated. In the year 1595 [1596–97] a company of Dutch sailors having been wrecked on the shores of Novaia Zemlia, and having been obliged to remain in that desolate region during a night of more than three months [it was a little less than three months], beheld the sun make his appearance in the horizon *about sixteen days before the time in which he should have risen according to calculation,* and when his body was actually more than four degrees below the horizon." The only explanation of this astonishing phenomenon which the same writer offers is found in this appended clause, — "which circumstance has been attributed to the great refractive power of the atmosphere in those intensely cold regions." This is so unsatisfactory that not a few prefer to believe, what seems entirely incredible, namely, that Barentz and his men in the short space of less than three months made a blunder of sixteen days in their time record.

Professor Nordenskjöld has recently referred to the case as follows: "On the $\frac{4\text{th}}{}$ November the sun disappeared and was again visible on the $\frac{3d\ Feb.}{24th\ Jan.}$. These dates have caused scientific men much perplexity, because, in latitude 76° North, the upper

---

[1] *New Lands within the Arctic Circle.* Lond. 1876: vol. i., p. 237.

edge of the sun ought to have ceased to be visible when the sun's south declination in autumn became greater than 13°,[1] and to have become visible again when the declination again became less than that figure ; that is to say, the sun ought to have been seen for the last time at Barentz's Ice Haven on the $\frac{27th}{17th}$ October, and it ought to have appeared again there on the $\frac{14th}{4th}$ Feb. It has been supposed that the deviation arose from a considerable error in counting the days, but this was unanimously denied by the crew who wintered."[2] In a foot-note he gives proofs which seem convincing that no such error can have been committed.

But while these experiences of Barentz and the Austrians point to a duration of darkness at the Pole of less than sixty days out of the three hundred and sixty-five, some apparently good authorities extend the period to seventy-six or seventy-seven days. Thus Captain Bedford Pim, of the Royal Navy of Great Britain, makes the following statement: "On the 16th of March the sun rises, preceded by a long dawn of forty-seven days, namely, from the 29th of January, when the first glimmer of light appears. On the 25th of September the sun sets, and after a twilight of forty-eight days, namely, on the 13th of November, darkness reigns supreme, so far as the sun is concerned, for seventy-six days, followed by one long period of light, the sun remaining above the horizon one hundred and ninety-four days. The year, therefore, is thus divided at the Pole : 194 days sun ; 76 darkness ; 47 days dawn ; 48 twilight."[3]

[1] On the assumption of a horizontal refraction of about 45'.

[2] *The Voyage of the Vega.* London, 1882 : p. 192.

[3] Pim's *Marine Pocket Case :* quoted in Kinn's *Harmony of the Bible with Science.* London, 1882 : 2d ed., p. 474.

Even according to this account we should have at the Pole only 76 days of darkness to 289 days of light in the year. In other words, instead of being in darkness little short of half of the time, as at the equator, one would be in darkness but about one fourth of the time. As far as light is concerned, therefore, even on this calculation the polar region is twice as favorable to life as any equatorial region that can be named.

But whence this discrepancy among the astronomers? Why should some of them make the polar night sixteen days longer than others?

The simple answer is that they proceed upon different assumptions as to atmospheric refraction in the region of the Pole. In our latitude twilight is usually reckoned to begin when the centre of the rising sun is yet 18° below the horizon. Starting with this as the limit, and counting sunrise and sunset to be the moments when the sun's upper limb is on the horizon, we arrive at the division of the polar year given by Captain Pim. But astronomers say that in England twilight has been observed when the sun was 21° below the horizon. To be entirely safe some have therefore taken 20° as the limit of solar depression, and reckoning with this datum, instead of the 18° before mentioned, have found that at the Pole the morning twilight would begin January 20th, and the evening twilight would cease November 21st. This would make the period of darkness but 60 days, and the period of light 305. Thus a difference of only two degrees in the assumed limit of solar depression at the beginning and end of the twilights makes the difference of sixteen days in the supposed duration of darkness. " Which of

5

the two calculations," writes an eminent American mathematician, "is the more correct is known, I imagine, by no one." [1]

To us in the present discussion the discrepancy is of very little moment. It is only a question as to whether at the Pole there is daylight three fourths or five sixths of the year. Both suppositions may be and probably are wrong. For if "in tropical climates 16° or 17° is said to be a sufficient allowance for the extreme solar depression, while, on the other hand, it is said in England to vary from 17° to 21°," it certainly looks as though in yet higher latitudes the light of the sun might be discernible when its body is as much as 23° or 24° below the horizon; and this would reduce the annual polar darkness to less than fifty days. This supposition is rendered the more probable by the fact that, while the expeditions already alluded to found much more of daylight than their astronomical calculations had led them to expect, we have no offsetting accounts where the sun was awaited in vain. The final and authoritative settlement of the question can be reached only by actual observation. Among the fascinating problems whose solution awaits the progress of Arctic exploration, we must therefore place the scientific determination of the unknown duration of the polar day.

In view of the foregoing we are certainly safe in conceiving of the polar night as lasting not over four fortnights. During two of these, as Dick reminds us, the moon would be walking in beauty

[1] Professor J. M. Van Vleck, LL. D., of Wesleyan University, in a letter to the author under date of October 11, 1883. Professor Van Vleck was for many years a *collaborateur* upon the *American Ephemeris and Nautical Almanac.* He is the authority for the next quoted statement.

through the heavens, and exhibiting all her changing phases of loveliness in unbroken successions. The other two would be passed beneath the starry arch of heaven, all of whose sparkling constellations would be moving round and round the observer in exactly horizontal orbits.

In such a perfect and regular stellar system kept in view so long and so continuously, the irregular movements of the " planets," or wandering stars, could not possibly escape observation. All their curious accelerations, retardations, conjunctions, declinations, would be perfectly marked and measured on the revolving but changeless dial-plate of the remoter sky. Dwelling in such a natural observatory, any people would of necessity become astronomers.[1] And how magnificent and orderly would the on-goings of the universe appear when viewed from underneath a firmament whose centre of revolution was fixed in the observer's zenith! After long months of unbroken daylight; how would one's soul yearn for a new vision of those stellar glories of the night! Nor would the moon and silent stars be the only attractions of the brief period during which the light of the sun was withdrawn. The mystic play of the Northern Light would transform the familiar daylight world into a veritable fairy-land.

---

[1] Even an equatorial position would probably have been less favorable. "The Peruvians had also their recurrent religious festivals ; . . . but the geographic position of Peru, with Quito, its holy city, lying immediately under the equator, greatly simplified the process by which they regulated their religious festivals by the solstices and equinoxes ; and the facilities which their equatorial position afforded for determining the few indispensable periods in their calendar *removed all stimulus to further progress.*" — Dr. Daniel Wilson on " Pre-Aryan American Man," in *Proceedings and Transactions of the Royal Society of Canada.* Montreal, 1883: vol. i., sect. ii., p. 60.

In our latitude the Aurora Borealis is a comparatively rare and tame phenomenon. In the highest Arctic regions it almost nightly kindles its unearthly glories.[1] In itself it is lightning diluted and sublimated to the point of harmlessness.[2] Sometimes these electric discharges not only fill the whole heaven with palpitating draperies, but also tip the hills with lambent flame, and cause the very soil on which one stands to prickle with a kind of life.[3]

But after all the glories of the night begin the greater glories of the polar day. Who with any approach to adequacy has ever described a dawn? What poet has not attempted it, and what poet has not failed? But if it be impossible to picture one

[1] A lately published report, speaking of the last winter at one of these circumpolar stations of the far North, says : " Auroræ have been seen here during the winter almost every night, and during all weathers. . . . The auroral forms or types which have appeared have been those generally known, from the grand corona to the modest, pulsating, little luminous cloud ; but as a characteristic feature attending them all, I must mention the absence of stability in the types. Thus only on a few occasions has there been an opportunity to watch the stationary arc, but in general the auroræ have represented wafting draperies and shining streamers with ever-changing position and intensity." — A. S. Steen, " The Norwegian Circumpolar Station," in *Nature*, October 11, 1883, p. 568.

[2] " The electric discharges which take place in the polar regions between the positive electricity of the atmosphere and the negative electricity of the earth are the essential and unique cause of the formation of the polar light." — M. de la Rive in *The Arctic Manual*, p. 742.

[3] "Mr. Lemström concluded that an electric discharge which could only be seen by means of the spectroscope was taking place on the surface of the ground all round him, and that from a distance it would appear as a faint display of Aurora," — a display like " the phenomena of pale and flaming light which is sometimes seen on the top of the Spitzbergen mountains " — *The Arctic Manual*, p. 739. Compare Elias Loomis, *Aurora Borealis*, Smithsonian Report, 1865. H. Fritz, *Das Polarlicht.* Leipsic, 1881.

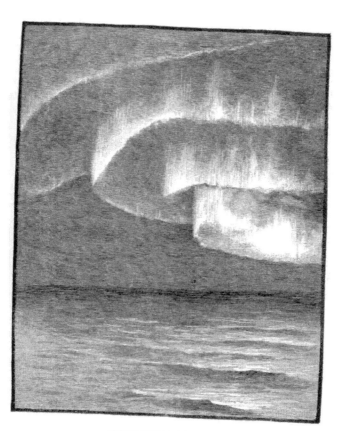

NIGHT SKIES OF EDEN.

An actual Aurora Borealis.

of our brief and evanescent day-dawns, who shall attempt a description of that surpassing spectacle in which all the splendors and loveliness of sixty of our dawns are combined in one. No words can ever portray it. No poet's imagination, even, has ever given us such unearthly scenery.

First of all appears low in the horizon of the night-sky a scarcely visible flush of light. At first it only makes a few stars' light seem a trifle fainter, but after a little it is seen to be increasing, and to be moving laterally along the yet dark horizon. Twenty-four hours later it has made a complete circuit around the observer, and is causing a larger number of stars to pale. Soon the widening light glows with the lustre of "Orient pearl." Onward it moves in its stately rounds, until the pearly whiteness burns into ruddy rose-light, fringed with purple and gold. Day after day, as we measure days, this splendid panorama circles on, and, according as atmospheric conditions and clouds present more or less favorable conditions of reflection, kindles and fades, kindles and fades, — fades only to kindle next time yet more brightly, as the still hidden sun comes nearer and nearer his point of emergence. At length, when for two long months such prophetic displays have been filling the whole heavens with these increscent and revolving splendors, the sun begins to emerge from his long retirement, and to display himself once more to human vision. After one or two circuits, during which his dazzling upper limb grows to a full-orbed disk, he clears all hill-tops of the distant horizon, and for six full months circles around and around the world's great axis in full view, suffering no night to fall upon his favored home-land at the

Pole. Even when at last he sinks again from view he covers his retreat with a repetition of the deepening and fading splendors which filled his long dawning, as if in these pulses of more and more distant light he were signaling back to the forsaken world the promises and prophecies of an early return.

In these prosaic sentences we aim at no description of the indescribable ; we only remind ourselves of the bald facts and conditions which govern the unpicturable transformations of each year-long polar night and day.

Enough, however, has been said for our purpose. Whoever seeks as a probable location for Paradise the heavenliest spot on earth with respect to light and darkness, and with respect to celestial scenery, must be content to seek it at the Arctic Pole. Here is the true City of the Sun. Here is the one and only spot on earth respecting which it would seem as if the Creator had said, as of His own heavenly residence, "There shall be no night there."

CHAPTER III.

THE TESTIMONY OF PHYSIOGRAPHICAL GEOLOGY.

Die arctische Geologie birgt die Schlüssel zu Lösung vieler Räthsel. — PROFESSOR HEER.

An extensive continent occupied this portion of the globe when these strata were deposited. — BARON NORDENSKJÖLD.

OUR hypothesis calls for an antediluvian continent at the Arctic Pole. It is interesting to find that a writer upon the Deluge writing more than forty years ago advanced the same postulate.[1] Is the supposition that there existed such a continent scientifically admissible?

Until very recently too little was known of the geology of the high latitudes to warrant or even to occasion the discussion of such a question. Even now, with all the contemporary interest in Arctic exploration, it is difficult to find any author who has distinctly propounded to himself and discussed the question as to the geologic age of the Arctic Ocean. It will not be strange, therefore, if we have here to content ourselves with showing, first, that geologists

[1] "On peut supposer, et je tâcherai de developper cette idée plus tard, qu'il a existé une periode géologique plus reculée, . . . et qu'à cette époque l'Europe, l'Asie, et l'Amérique septentrionale se joignaient au pole nord de manière à former un continent d'une étendue prodigeuse, se prolongueant vers le pôle sud en trois presqu'îles, savoir: l'Amérique méridionale, l'Afrique, et l'Océanie. C'est des débris de cet ancien continent que des révolutions violentes ont formé les terres actuelles." Frédérik Klee, *Le Déluge*, French ed. Paris, 1847: p. 83. (Danish original, 1842.)

and paleontologists do not think the present distribution of Arctic sea and land to be the primeval
one ; and secondly, that in their opinion, incidentally
expressed, a " continent" once existed within the
Arctic Circle of which at present only vestiges remain.

We will begin with the distinguished Alfred Russel Wallace, who in speaking of the Miocene period
presents us with a very different Northern hemisphere from ours of to-day.   For instance, in his
view Scandinavia was at that time a vast island. He
says: "The distribution of the Eocene and Miocene
formations shows that during a considerable portion
of the Tertiary period an inland sea, more or less occupied by an archipelago of islands, extended across
Central Europe between the Baltic and the Black
and Caspian seas, and thence by narrower channels
southeastward to the valley of the Euphrates and
the Persian Gulf, thus opening a communication
between the North Atlantic and the Indian Ocean.
From the Caspian also a wide arm of the sea extended, during some part of the Tertiary epoch,
northwards to the Arctic Ocean, and there is nothing to show that this sea may not have been in
existence during the whole Tertiary period. Another channel probably existed over Egypt into the
eastern basin of the Mediterranean and the Black
Sea ; while it is probable that there was a communication between the Baltic and the White Sea, leaving Scandinavia as an extensive island.   Turning to
India, we find that an arm of the sea, of great width
and depth, extended from the Bay of Bengal to the
mouths of the Indus ; while the enormous depression
indicated by the presence of marine fossils of Eo-

cene age at a height of 16,500 feet in Western Tibet renders it not improbable that a more direct channel across Afghanistan may have opened a communication between the West Asiatic and Polar seas." [1]

Later, in the same book, Mr. Wallace incidentally shows that the facts of Arctic paleontology call for the supposition of a primitive Eocene continent in the highest latitudes, — a continent which no longer exists. His language is, " The rich and varied fauna which inhabited Europe at the dawn of the Tertiary period — as shown by the abundant remains of mammalia wherever suitable deposits of Eocene age have been discovered — proves that an extensive Palearctic continent then existed." [2]

Another most eminent authority in Arctic paleontology, the late Professor Heer, of Zürich, fully fifteen years ago arrived at and published the conclusion that the facts presented in the Arctic fossils plainly point to the existence in Miocene time of a no longer existing polar continent. Fuller reference to his views will be made in our next chapter.[3]

On another and more lithological line of evidence Baron Nordenskjöld, the eminent Arctic explorer, has arrived at the same conclusion. Speaking of certain rock strata north of the 69th degree of north latitude, he says, " An extensive continent occupied this portion of the globe when these strata were deposited." [4] Elsewhere he speaks of this "ancient polar continent " as something already accepted and universally understood among scientific men. He

---

[1] *Island Life*. London, 1880 : pp. 184, 185.

[2] Ibid., p. 362.

[3] Professor Heer, deceased Sept. 27, 1883. On the preëminence of his authority in this field, see *Nature*, Oct. 25, page 612.

[4] *Expedition to Greenland. Arctic Manual*, London, 1875 : p. 423.

also alludes to the conspiring evidences of its former existence found in different departments of research. "These basalt beds," he remarks, "probably originated from a volcanic chain, active during the Tertiary period, which perhaps limits the ancient polar continent, in the same manner as is now the case with the eastern coast of Asia and the western of America; this confirming the division of land and water in the Tertiary period, which upon totally different grounds has been supposed to have existed." [1]

Another authority in this field, writing of the theory that continuous land once connected Europe and North America at the North, remarks, "In further support of this theory we have the fact that no trace of sea deposit of Eocene age has ever been found in the polar area, all the vestiges of strata remaining showing that these latitudes were then occupied by dry land." [2]

Finally, as our assumption of the early existence of a circumpolar Arctic continent is thus supported by most competent geological authority, so is also our hypothesis that its disappearance was due to a submergence beneath the waters of the Arctic Ocean. On this point what could be more explicit and satisfactory than the following, from one of the greatest of living geologists: "We know very well that . . . within a comparatively recent geological period . . . a wide stretch of Arctic land, of which Novaia Zemlia and Spitzbergen formed a part, has been submerged." [3]

---

[1] *Arctic Manual,* p. 420.

[2] J. Starkie Gardner in *Nature,* London, Dec. 12, 1878: p. 127.

[3] James Geikie, LL. D., F. R. S., *Prehistoric Europe. A Geological Sketch.* London, 1881: p. 41. Compare Louis Faliés, *Études*

As to the natural conditions and forces which may be conceived as having brought about this continental catastrophe, geologists are not so well agreed. The French *savant*, Alfonse-Joseph Adhémar,[1] has advanced a theory that this North-polar deluge was only one of an alternating series, which in age-long periods recur first at the North and then at the South Pole. Flammarion, writing of it, says: "This theory depends on the fact of the unequal length of the seasons in the two hemispheres. Our autumn and winter last 179 days. In the southern hemisphere they last 186 days. This seven days, or 168 hours of difference, increase each year the coldness of the pole. During 10,500 years the ice accumulates at one pole and melts at the other, thereby displacing the earth's centre of gravity. Now a time will arrive when, after the maximum of elevation of temperature on one side, a catastrophe will happen which will bring back the centre of gravity to the centre of the figure, and cause an immense deluge. The deluge of the North Pole was 4,200 years ago; therefore the next will be 6,300 hence."[2]

Another recent theory teaches that the poles are periodically deluged, but simultaneously, not in alternation. The alternative movement is at the equator. The crust of the earth at the equator is all the time rising or sinking in a kind of æonian rhythm.

historiques et philosophiques sur les Civilisations Européenne, Romaine, Greque, etc. Paris, 1874: vol. i., pp. 348–352.

[1] In his *Révolutions de la Mer.* 2 ed., 1860.

[2] Flammarion naturally adds, "It is very obvious to ask on this, *Why* should there be a *catastrophe*, and why should not the centre of gravity return *gradually*, as it was gradually displaced?" *Astronomical Myths*, p. 426. But a gradual displacement would produce a deluge, only a gradual one.

Whenever it sinks beyond the equilibrium figure, due to its actual rate of rotation, lands emerge at the poles; whenever it rises beyond the equilibrium figure, the polar lands sink and are submerged beneath the waters of the ocean. Professor Alexander Winchell thus expounds the view: " It has been shown that one of the actions of tides upon a planetary body tends to diminish its rate of rotation. Correspondingly, its equatorial protuberance will tend to diminish. In the case of a planet still retaining its liquid condition, the equatorial subsidence will keep nearly even pace with the retardation. To whatever extent viscosity exists, the subsidence will *follow* the retardation. There will exist an excess of protuberance beyond the equilibrium figure due to the actual rotation, and this will act as an additional retardative cause. In the case of an incrusted and somewhat rigid planet, the excess of ellipticity would attain its greatest value. It would continue to augment until the strain upon the mass should become sufficient to lower the excessive protuberance to the equilibrium figure. The recovery of this figure might take place convulsively. The equatorial regions would then subside, and the polar would rise. In the case of an incrusted planet extensively covered, like the earth, by a film of water, retarded rotation would be attended by a prompt subsidence of the equatorial waters and rise of the polar waters to about twice the same extent. In other words, the equatorial lands would emerge, and the polar lands would become submerged. The amount of emergence would diminish with increase of distance from the equator, and the amount of submergence would diminish with increase of dis-

tance from the pole. In about the latitude of 30°
the two tendencies would meet and neutralize each
other. Under these conditions, an incrusted and
ocean-covered planet, since it must be undergoing
a process of rotary retardation, must possess the
deepest oceans about the poles and the shallowest
about the equator. The first emergences of land,
accordingly, will take place within the equatorial
zone ; and the highest elevations and greatest land
areas will exist within that zone. The elevation of
equatorial land-masses would interpose new obstruc-
tions to the equatorial ocean current. This would
divert it in new directions, and thus modify all climates within reach of oceanic influences. Changes
of currents would necessitate the migration of marine faunas, and changes of climate would modify
the faunas and floras of the land.

"But the protrusion of the equatorial land-mass
could not increase indefinitely. The same central
force which retains the ocean continually at the equilibrium figure strains the solid mass in the same direction. The strain must at length become greater
than the rigidity of the mass can withstand. The
equatorial land protuberance will subside toward
the level of the ocean. Some parts of the ocean's
bottom must correspondingly rise. Naturally, the
parts about the poles will rise most. Thus some
equatorial lands will become submerged, and some
northern and southern areas may become newly
emergent.

"But these vertical movements would not be ar-
rested precisely at the point of recovery of the equilibrium figure. As suggested by Prof. J. E. Todd,
and less explicitly by Sir Wm. Thomson, the move-

ment would pass the equilibrium figure to an extent proportional to the cumulation of strain. The equatorial region would become too much depressed, and the polar regions too much elevated. The effect of this would be to accelerate the rotation sufficiently to neutralize the ceaseless tidal retardation. The day would be shortened. The ocean would rise still higher along the shores of equatorial lands, and subside along the shores of polar lands. An extension of polar lands would immediately modify the climates of the higher latitudes. They would become subject to greater extremes. A considerable elevation of polar lands would diminish the mean temperature, and the region of perpetual snow would be enlarged. These effects would visit the northern and southern hemispheres simultaneously.

"Such effects would follow from an excessive subsidence of equatorial lands. But the constant retardative action of the tides would cause the equatorial lands again to emerge, and protrude beyond the limits of the equilibrium figure attained in a later age. Thus the former condition would return, and the former events would be repeated. In the nature of force and matter these oscillations should be repeated many times. Professor Todd suggests that the present terrestrial age is one of equatorial land subsidence and of high latitude emergence. Immediately preceding the present, the Champlain epoch was one of northern and probably of south polar subsidence ; while further back, in the Glacial epoch, we have evidence of northern, and perhaps also south latitude elevation." [1]

[1] *World-Life; or Comparative Geology.* Chicago, 1883 : pp. 278–280.

Leibnitz, Deluc, and others, have presented a still different view of the etiology of all deluges, according to which they are the result of a steady shrinkage of the earth in consequence of its secular cooling. According to this theory, after once a solid earth-crust had been formed, the cooling nucleus within it withdrew the support on which the crust had rested, in proportion as it shrank away from beneath it, until, as often as the subterranean voids thus created became too great for the strength of the crust, this of necessity fell in with the force of incomputable tons, carrying the ruined surface to such a depth as to cause it immediately to be overflowed and submerged by the adjacent waters of the ocean. The geologic history of the earth is divided into its strongly marked periods by these successive "collapsions" of the rocky strata which constituted the primitive crust. "Each succeeding cataclysm," says a recent advocate of the view, "considered as a universal catastrophe, must leave the globe a wreck, like the ruin of some immense cathedral whose dome and arches have fallen in. Cornice and frieze, pillar and entablature, broken and dislocated, lie at all angles of inclination and in the utmost confusion. So it is with the ancient rocks and more modern strata. Only to this mighty wreck have been added the outgushings of molten matter into fissures, creating dikes, and the unsparing movements of oceans sweeping loose materials and perishing forms of all sorts from one place to another, partially covering up and disguising the desolation."

Again, the same writer says: "The present surface of the earth is comparatively recent. The last great cataclysm is, geologically speaking, not very ancient. Accumulating evidence compels us to believe that one of those destructive events has occurred since the human race was created. The facts I have presented plainly indicate that another is in the course of preparation. Each of these vast periodical voids between the nucleus and the crust is filled by collapsion of the surface. . . . Thus, if we assume that the globe was one hundred or three hundred miles greater in all its diameters when its crust became hard and was bathed with the earliest seas, and when marine plants and trilobites and mollusca began to appear, the lithological characteristics of the paleozoic ages will be more acceptably deciphered. So successively with the carboniferous periods, whose vast areas have been folded up and overflowed, and whose fields for reproduction have been so numerous and extensive as to convince us that Arctic America, during those remote ages, presented tropical positions to the sun." [1]

Although starting with no such purpose, the author, in expounding this general Leibnitzian theory of all deluges, incidentally explains the submersion of the primeval Arctic continent. In accordance with his theory, he asserts that "the diameter of the earth at the poles must have been at some more ancient epoch very much greater than now. It must have been more than twenty-seven miles greater to permit such equatorial or tropical exposures to the

[1] C. F. Winslow, M. D., *The Cooling Globe, or the Mechanics of Geology.* Boston, 1865 : pp. 50, 51. For the latest presentations and criticisms of this general theory, see Winchell's *World-Life*, 1883, pp. 302–308, and the literature there given. Among the older treatises constructed upon it, none is perhaps of so great interest to the general reader as the work on *The Deluge*, by Frédérik Klee (Danish 1842, German 1843, French 1847).

sun as we know to be necessary for the production of those vegetable forms which abound in the coal measures of Arctic latitudes.[1] If it was fifty or a hundred miles greater during any portion of the carboniferous age, it might have been two hundred during the 'Taconic' period, and perhaps three hundred or more when the life-force began to fashion its primordial and rudimentary organisms upon its waiting surface." He furthermore distinctly asserts that Sir Isaac Newton's supposed demonstration that the oblateness of the earth's figure is due to the centrifugal force generated by its rotation "is an error unworthy of further consideration among geologists." The true explanation, as he regards it, is stated as follows : " The shorter axes of the globe — what at present are our poles — are not the result of flattening by rotation, but by a sudden falling in of surface." [2]

Here, of course, is just that down-sinking of wide *polar* regions, in " comparatively recent " geologic time, demanded by the facts of Arctic geology. It must have been greater than any of those which have occurred in other portions of the globe, for it has permanently modified the originally and naturally spherical figure of the earth. The author is "compelled to believe " that it, or one like it, " occurred since the human race was created." Moreover, this belief is in no wise built upon the Biblical record of the Deluge, for he speaks almost bitterly of " the retarding influence of Jewish legends upon the free expansion of the human intellect," and

[1] Dr. Winslow seems here to forget that the primeval polar continent was of necessity the sunniest of all lands.

[2] Ibid., p. 49.

makes Moses one of the two men whose "declarations and authority, more than the statements of all others, have retarded the advancement of general knowledge." Happily for Moses, the second in this portentous duumvirate is no worse a man than Sir Isaac Newton !

It is by no means necessary to commit ourselves to any one of these theories of deluges, or to seek still other explanations of the recognized subsidence of the basin now occupied by the Arctic Ocean. Enough for the present that upon the authority of eminent physiographic geologists we have shown : —

1. That the present distribution of land and water within the Arctic Circle is, geologically speaking, of very recent origin.

2. That the paleozoic data of the highest explored latitudes demand for their explanation the hypothesis of an extensive circumpolar continent in Miocene time.

3. That lithological authorities affirm that such a continent existed.

4. That physical geography has reached the conclusion that the known islands of the Arctic Ocean, such as Novaia Zemlia and the Spitzbergen, are simply mountain tops still remaining above the surface of the sea which has come in and covered up the primeval continent to which they belonged.

5. And finally, that the problem of the process by which this grand catastrophe was brought about is now sporadically engaging the thoughts of terrestrial physicists and geologists.[1]

[1] See the very interesting paper " On Ice-Age Theories," in *Transactions of the British Association*, 1884, by E. Hill, M. A., F. G. S. Also in the same volume W. F. Stanley's criticism of the theory of Croll.

CHAPTER IV.

THE TESTIMONY OF PREHISTORIC CLIMATOLOGY.

Ver illud erat, ver magnus agebat Orbis. — VERGIL.

One of the most startling and important of the scientific discoveries of the last twenty years has been that of the relics of a luxuriant Miocene flora in various parts of the Arctic regions. It is a discovery which was totally unexpected, and is even now considered by many men of science to be completely unintelligible, but it is so thoroughly established, and it has such an important bearing on the subjects we are discussing in the present volume, that it is necessary to lay a tolerably complete outline of the facts before our readers. — A. R. WALLACE (1880).

THUS far, then, we have found theoretical geogony demanding a location at the Pole for the first country presenting conditions of Eden life ; we have found the requisite astronomical conditions to give it an abundance of light ; we have found the geologists attesting the former existence of such a country ; we must now interrogate Prehistoric Climatology, and ascertain whether this lost land ever enjoyed a temperature which admits of the supposition that here was the primitive abode of man. The answer to our question comes, not from one, but from several sources.[1]

[1] We have no use here for mere fancy sketches, like the following, which appeared on the 10th of May, 1884, in *The Norwood Review and Crystal Palace Reporter* (Eng.), and which looks very much like an unacknowledged loan from Captain Hall, of Arctic fame : "We do not admit that there is ice up to the Pole. No one has been nearer that point than 464 miles. Once inside the great ice-barrier, a new world breaks upon the explorer ; a climate first mild like that of England, and afterwards balmy as that of the Greek Isles, awaits the hardy adventurer who first beholds those wonderful shores. Wonderful, indeed ; for he will be greeted by a branch of the human race

First, geogony gives us an almost irresistible antecedent probability. For if the earth from its earliest consolidation has been steadily cooling, it is hardly possible to conceive of a method by which any region once too hot for human residence can have become at length too cold except by passing through all the intermediate stages of temperature, some of which must have been precisely adapted to human comfort.

Again, paleontological botany shows that in Europe in Tertiary times this hypothetical cooling of the earth was going on, and going on in the steady and regular way postulated by theoretic geogony.[1] But if a telluric process as essentially universal as this was going on in Europe, there is no reason why it should not have been going on in all countries, whether to the north, or to the south, or to the east, or to the west of Europe.

But we are not left to inferences of this sort. It is now admitted by all scientific authorities that at one time the regions within the Arctic Circle enjoyed a tropical or nearly tropical climate. Profes-

cut off from the rest of humanity by that change of climate which came over Northern Europe about 2,000 years ago, but surrounded by a profusion of life bewildering in the extreme."

Speculations or fancies of this sort have ever clustered about this mysterious region of the Pole. As we shall hereafter see, they abounded in remote antiquity. Even the singular fancy known to the public as "Symmes' Hole" antedates Symmes, and may be found in much more attractive form in Klopstock's *Messiah*. (K.'s *Sämmtliche Werke*. Leipsic, 1854: vol. i., pp. 24, 25.)

[1] "L'étude des flores nous démontre que le climat de l'Europe, pendant les temps tertiaires, est toujours allé *en se refroidissant d'une manière continue et regulière*."— *Le Préhistorique. Antiquité de l'Homme*. Par Gabriel de Mortillet, Professeur d'anthropologie préhistorique à l'École d'Anthropologie de Paris. Paris, 1883: p. 113.

sor Nicholson uses the following language : "In the early Tertiary period the climate of the northern hemisphere, as shown by the Eocene animals and plants, was very much hotter than it is at present; partaking, indeed, of a sub-tropical character. In the Middle Tertiary or Miocene period the temperature, though not high, was still much warmer than that now enjoyed by the northern hemisphere ; and we know that the plants of the temperate regions at that time flourished within the Arctic Circle." [1]

Mr. Grant Allen says, "One thing at least is certain, that till a very recent period, geologically speaking, our earth enjoyed a warm and genial climate up to the actual poles themselves, and that all its vegetation was everywhere evergreen, of much the same type as that which now prevails in the modern tropics." [2]

Alluding to those distant ages, M. le Marquis de Nadaillac remarks : "Under these conditions, life spread freely even to the Pole." [3] Similar is the language of Croll : "The Arctic regions, probably up to the North Pole, were not only free from ice, but were covered with a rich and luxuriant vegetation." [4] Keerl holds that at the very Pole it was then warmer than now at the equator.[5] Professor Oswald Heer's calculations would possibly modify Keerl's estimate to a slight degree, but only enough to make the circumpolar climate of that far-off age a

---

[1] *The Life-History of the Globe,* p. 335.

[2] *Knowledge.* London, Nov. 30, 1883 : p. 327.

[3] *Les Premiers Hommes et les Temps Préhistoriques.* Paris, 1881 : tom. ii., p. 391.

[4] *Climate and Time.* Am. ed., 1875 : p. 7.

[5] *Die Schöpfungsgeschichte und Lehre vom Paradies.* Basel, 1861 : Abth. I., p. 634.

little more Edenic than is that of the hottest portions of our present earth.[1]

Sir Charles Lyell, who in the discussion of this subject is characteristically cautious and "uniformitarian," does not hesitate to say, "The result, then, of our examination, in this and in the preceding chapter, of the organic and inorganic evidence as to the state of the climate of former geological periods is in favor of the opinion that the heat was generally in excess of what it now is. In the greater part of the Miocene and preceding Eocene epochs the fauna and flora of Central Europe were sub-tropical, and a vegetation resembling that now seen in Northern Europe extended into the Arctic regions as far as they have yet been explored, and probably reached the Pole itself. In the Mesozoic ages the predominance of reptile life and the general character of the fossil types of that great class of vertebrata indicate a warm climate and an absence of frost between the 40th parallel of latitude and the Pole, a large ichthyosaurus having been found in lat. 77° 16' N."[2]

Averaging the above views and estimates of scientific authorities, we have at the Pole, in the age of the first appearance of the human race, a temperature the most equable and delightful possible; and with this we may well be content.

---

[1] *Flora Fossilis Arctica.* Zurich, 1868: Bd. i., pp. 60–77. See also Alfred Russel Wallace, *Island Life.* London, 1880: ch. ix., pp. 163–202. Well, therefore, sings a rollicking rhymster of the age, —

> "When the sea rolled its fathomless billows
> Across the broad plains of Nebraska;
> When around the North Pole grew bananas and willows,
> And mastodons fought with the great armadillos
> For the pine-apples grown in Alaska."

[2] *Principles of Geology,* eleventh ed., vol. i., p. 231.

CHAPTER V.

THE TESTIMONY OF PALEONTOLOGICAL BOTANY.

Damals, von dort aus — d. h. aus diesem Bildungsherd für die Pflanzen süd- licher Breiten im hohen Norden — hat eine strahlenförmige Verbreitung von Typen stattgehabt. — PROFESSOR HEER.

It is now an established conclusion that the great aggressive faunas and floras of the continents have originated in the North, some of them within the Arctic Circle. — PRINCIPAL DAWSON (1883).

ALL traditions of the primeval Paradise require us to conceive of it as possessed of a tropical flora of the most beautiful and luxuriant sort, — as adorned with "every tree that is pleasant to the sight, or good for food." Any theory, therefore, as to the site of Eden must of necessity present a locality where this condition could have been met. How is it with the hypothesis now under consideration?

To reply that a polar Eden is scientifically admissible in this respect would be to state but a small part of the truth. So much might unhesitatingly be affirmed in view of the facts presented in the last chapter. Given in any country on the face of the globe a long-continued tropical climate, and a tropical vegetation may well be expected. Anything else would be so abnormal as to require explanation.

But the study of Paleontological Botany has just conducted to a new and entirely unanticipated result. The best authorities in this science, both in Europe and America, have lately reached the conclusion that *all the floral types and forms revealed in the oldest fossils of the earth originated in the region of the North Pole, and thence spread first over the northern and then over the southern hemisphere, proceeding from North to South.* This is a conception of the origin and development of the vegetable world which but a few years ago no scientific man had dreamed of, and which, to many intelligent readers of these pages, will be entirely new. Its profound interest, as related to the present discussion, will at once be seen.

Without attempting a chronological history of this remarkable discovery, or in any wise assuming to assign to each pioneer student his share of the credit, we may say that Professor Asa Gray, of America, Professor Oswald Heer, of Switzerland, Sir Joseph Hooker, of England, Otto Kuntze, of Germany, and Count G. de Saporta, of France, have all been more or less prominently associated with the establishment of the new doctrine. Sir Joseph Hooker's studies of the floral types of Tasmania furnished data, before lacking, for a general trans-latitudinal survey of the whole field. He was struck by the fact that in that far-off Southern world "the Scandinavian type asserts his prerogative of ubiquity." Though at that time he seems not to have divined its significance, he clearly saw the paleontological and other vestiges of the great movement by which the far North has slowly clothed the north-temperate, the equatorial, and the southern regions with verdure. In one passage he describes the impression made upon him by the facts in the following graphic language: "When I take a comprehensive view of the vegetation of the Old World, I am struck with the appearance it presents of there having been a continuous current of vegetation, if I may so fancifully express myself, from Scandinavia to Tasmania." [1]

Light on this problem of the far South was soon to come from the far North. In 1868 Professor Oswald Heer, of Zurich, published his truly epoch-making work on the fossil flora of the Arctic regions, in which he modestly yet with much confidence advanced the idea that the *Bildungsherd*, or mother-region, of all the floral types of the more southern latitudes was originally in "a great continuous Miocene continent within the Arctic Circle," and that from this centre the southward spread or dispersion of these types had been in a radial or out-raying manner. [2] His demonstration of the existence in Miocene times of a warm climate and of a rich tropical vegetation in the highest attainable Arctic latitudes was complete and overwhelming. Our latest geologists are still accustomed to speak of his result as "one of the most remarkable geological discoveries of modern times." [3] His theory of a primeval circumpolar mother-region whence all floral types proceeded is also at present so little questioned that to-day among representative scholars in this field the absorbing and only question seems to be, Who first proposed and to whom belongs the chief honor of the verification of so broad and beautiful a generalization? [4]

[1] *The Flora of Australia.* London, 1859: p. 103. On the remarkable qualifications of Dr. Hooker to speak on this subject, see Sir Charles Lyell, *The Antiquity of Man*, pp. 417, 418.

[2] *Flora Arctica Fossilis : Die fossile Flora der Polarländer.* Zurich, 1868: I. Vorwort, pp. iii., iv., and elsewhere.

[3] Archibald Geikie, LL. D., F. R. S., *Textbook of Geology.* London, 1882 : p. 868.

[4] Some twenty-five years ago, in a paper on " The Botany of Japan "

Here, then, is a new and wonderful light just thrown upon the problem of the site of Eden. Theology in some of its representatives had anticipated the geologists in teaching that the earth's vestment of vegetation originally proceeded from one primeval centre, but it is the glory of paleontology to have located that centre and to have given us an evidence scientifically valid. Wherever man originated, the biologist and botanist now know where was the cradle of some of the world's tenants. Whatever the direction of the first human migrations, we are now clear as to the direction of that "great invasion of

(*Memoirs of the American Academy of Science*, 1857, vol. vi., pp. 377–458), Professor Asa Gray suggested the possibility of the common origination in high northern latitudes of various related species now widely separated in different portions of the north-temperate zone. In 1872, four years after the publication of Heer's work, in treating of "The Sequoia and its History," in an address (see *Journal of the Am. Ass. for the Advancement of Science*, 1872), he renewed in a clearer and stronger manner his advocacy of the idea. In the same year, and also in 1876, Count Saporta, with due acknowledgment of the work of Professor Heer, gave currency to the theory in the scientific circles of France. Alluding to this, the Count has recently written, "Asa Gray was not the only botanist who had the idea of explaining the presence of disjoined species and genera dispersed across the boreal temperate zone and the two continents, by means of emigrations from the pole as the mother-region whence these vegetable races had radiated in one or several directions. This had been *parallèlement* conceived and developed in France upon the occasion of the remarkable works of Professor O. Heer." *Am. Journal of Science*, May, 1883, p. 394. The annotation appended to this by Professor Gray may be seen on the same page. For a German acknowledgment see Engler, *Entwickelungsgeschichte der Pflanzenwelt*, Th. i., S. 23; for an English, see *Nature*, London, 1881, p. 446; for an American, J. W. Dawson, "The Genesis and Migration of Plants," in *The Princeton Review*, 1879, p. 277. But Dr. Dawson, referring to Saporta's *Ancienne Végétation Polaire*, Hooker's *Presidential Address* of 1878, Thistleton Dyer's *Lecture on Plant Distribution*, and J. Starkie Gardner's *Letters* in *Nature*, 1878, well remarks that "the basis of most of these brochures is to be found in Heer's *Flora Fossilis Arctica*."

Arctic plants and animals which in the beginning of Quaternary ages came southward into Europe." [1]

But it may be that the testimony of Paleontological Botany is not yet exhausted. What if it should at length appear that along with the plants prehistoric men — and civilized men at that — must have descended from the mother-region of plants to the place where history finds them ? Without any reference to or apparent recognition of the great anthropological interest of such a question, at least one botanist of Germany, reasoning from botanical facts and postulates alone, has reached precisely this conclusion.

This *savant* is Professor Otto Kuntze, who has made special studies of the cultivated tropical plants. What other botanists had found true of the wild flora in continents separated by wide oceans he finds true of domesticated plants. But the problem of the spread of these plants from continent to con-

---

[1] Geikie, *Textbook of Geology*, p. 874. Compare Wallace : "We have now only to notice the singular want of reciprocity in the migrations of northern and southern types of vegetation. In return for the vast number of European plants which have reached Australia, not one single Australian plant has entered any part of the north temperate zone, and the same may be said of the typical southern vegetation in general, whether developed in the Antarctic lands, New Zealand, South America, or South Africa." *Island-Life.* London, 1880: p. 486. In like manner Sir Joseph Hooker affirms : "Geographically speaking, there is no Antarctic flora except a few lichens and seaweeds." *Nature*, 1881: p. 447. Possibly, however, the progress of research may bring to light evidences of a second and less powerful polar *Bildungsherd* of primitive flora forms in the Antarctic region. Some of the discoveries of F. P. Moreno look in that direction. See "*Patagonia, resto de un antiguo continente hoy sumerjido.*" *Anales de la sociedad cientifica Argentina.* T. xiv., Entrégua III., p. 97. Also, "*La faune éocène de la Patagonie australe et le grande continent antarctique.*" Par M. E. L. Trouessart. *Revue Scientifique*, Paris, xxxii., pp. 588 ss. (Nov. 10. 1883). Also Samuel Haughton in last lecture of *Physical Geography.* Dublin, 1880.

tinent raises peculiar and most interesting questions.
Taking the banana-plantain, which was cultivated in
America before the arrival of Europeans in 1492,
Professor Kuntze asks, "In what way was this plant,
which cannot stand a voyage through the temperate
zone, carried to America?" The difficulty is that
the banana is seedless, and can be propagated in a
new country only by carrying thither a living root
and planting it in a suitable soil. Its very seedless-
ness is evidence of the enormous length of time that
it has been cared for by man. As the Professor
says, "A cultivated plant which does not possess
seeds must have been under culture for a very long
period, — we have not in Europe a single exclusively
seedless, berry-bearing cultivated plant, — and hence
it is perhaps fair to infer that these plants were cultivated as early as the middle of the diluvial period."
But now as to its transportation from the Old World
to the New, or *vice versa.* "It must be remembered," he says, "that the plantain is a tree-like,
herbaceous plant, possessing no easily transportable
bulbs, like the potato or the dahlia, nor propagable
by cuttings, like the willow or the poplar. It has
only a perennial root, which, once planted, needs
hardly any care." After discussing the subject in
all aspects, he reaches the twofold conclusion, first,
that civilized man must have brought the roots of
the plant into any new regions into which it has
ever come; and secondly, that its appearance in
America can only be accounted for on the supposition that it was carried thither by way of the north-
polar countries at a time when a tropical climate
prevailed at the North Pole.[1]

[1] Pflanzen als Beweis der Einwanderung der Amerikaner aus Asien
in präglazialer Zeit. Published in *Ausland*, 1878, pp. 197, 198.

CHAPTER VI.

THE TESTIMONY OF PALEONTOLOGICAL ZOÖLOGY.

All the evidence at our command points to the Northern hemisphere as the birth-place of the class, Mammalia, and probably of all the orders. — ALFRED RUSSEL WALLACE.

C'est à des émigrations venues, sinon du pôle, du moins des contrées attenantes au cercle polaire, qu'il faut attribuer la présence constatée dans les deux mondes de beaucoup d'animaux propres à l'hémisphère boréal. — COUNT SAPORTA.

BUT in settling the site of Eden the animal kingdom must also have a voice. According to the Hebrew story, the representatives of this kingdom were an earlier creation than Adam, and in Eden was the world-fest of their christening. Evidently the lost cradle of humanity must be fixed in time posterior to the beginnings of animal life, and in space so located that from that spot as a centre all the multitudinous species, and genera, and orders, and families of the whole animal creation might have radiated forth to the various habitats in which they are respectively found.

Now it is one of the striking facts connected with Zoölogy that if we pass around the globe on any isothermal line, at the equator, or in any latitude south of it, or in any latitude north of it, — *until we come to the confines of the Arctic zone,* — we find, as we pass from land to land, that the animals we encounter are specifically unlike. Everywhere we find, along with like climatic and telluric conditions, different animals. The moment, however, we reach the Arctic zone, and there make the circuit of the globe, we are everywhere surrounded by the same species.

On the other hand, if we take great circles of the earth's longitude, and pass from the Arctic region down along the continental masses of the New World to the South Pole, thence returning up a meridian which crosses Africa and Europe, or Australia and Asia, we shall find in the descent abundant fossil evidence that we are moving forward on the pathway along which the prehistoric migrations of the animal world proceeded; while on our return on the other side of the planet we shall find that we are no longer following in the track of ancient migrations, but are advancing counter to their obvious movement. All this is as true of the flora of the world as it is of the fauna. Hence the language of the late Professor Orton : "Only around the shores of the Arctic Sea are the same animals and plants found through every meridian, and in passing southward along the three principal lines of land specific identities give way to mere identity of genera ; these are replaced by family resemblances, and at last even the families become in a measure distinct, not only on the great continents, but also on the islands, till every little rock in the ocean has its peculiar inhabitants." [1]

Another well-known naturalist says : "It should also be observed that in the beginning of things the continents were built up from North to South, — such has been, at least, the history of the North and South American and the Europeo-Asiatic and the African continents ; and thus it would appear that north of

---

[1] *Comparative Zoölogy.* New York, 1876 : p. 384.

the equator, at least, animals slowly migrated southward, keeping pace as it were with the growth
and southward extension of the grand land-masses
which appeared above the sea in the Paleozoic ages.
Hence, scanty as is the Arctic and Temperate region
of the earth at the present time, in former ages
these regions were as prolific in life as the tropics
now are, the latter regions, now so vast, having
through all the Tertiary and Quaternary ages been
undisturbed by great geological revolutions, and
meanwhile been colonized by emigrants driven down
by the incoming cold of the glacial period."[1]

As long ago as 1876 Mr. Alfred Russel Wallace
wrote, "All the chief types of animal life appear
to have originated in the great north temperate or
northern continents, while the southern continents
have been more or less completely isolated during
long periods, both from the northern continent and
from each other."[2]   And again, speaking of mammalia, he said, "All the evidence at our command
points to the Northern Hemisphere as the birth-
place of the class, and probably of all the orders."[3]

From all the facts but one conclusion is possible,
and that is that like as the Arctic Pole is the mother-
region of all plants, so it is the mother-region of all
animals, — the region where, in the beginning, God
created every beast of the earth after his kind, and

---

[1] A. S. Packard, *Zoölogy.* New York, 2d ed., 1880 : p. 665. — In his
Elements of Geology, New York, 1877, p. 159, Le Conte gives a graphical representation of the polocentric zones of the earth's flora and
fauna (Fig. 131), which ought to have suggested the true genetic connection of the whole.

[2] *The Geographical Distribution of Animals.* New York ed., vol. i.,
p. 173.

[3] Ibid., vol. ii., p. 544.

cattle after their kind, and everything that creepeth on the earth after his kind. And this is the conclusion now being reached and announced by all comparative zoölogists who busy themselves with the problem of the origin and prehistoric distribution of the animal world. But to believe that Professor Heer's " Miocene Arctic Continent " was the cradle of all floral types and the cradle of all faunal forms, and yet deny that it was also the cradle of the human race, is what few philosophical minds are likely long to do.

CHAPTER VII.

THE TESTIMONY OF PALEONTOLOGICAL ANTHROPOL-
OGY AND ETHNOLOGY.

Quittons donc pour un instant les jardins d'Armide, et, nouveaux Argonautes, parcourons les régions hyperborées ; cherchons-y, armés de patience et surtout de scepticism, l'origine de la plupart des nations et des langues modernes, celle même des habitans de l'Attique, et des autres peuples de la Grèce, objets de notre savante idolatrie. — CHARLES POUGENS (A. D. 1799).

Telle est la théorie qui s'accord le mieux avec la marche présumée des races humaines. — COUNT SAPORTA (A. D. 1883).

MAN is the one traveler who has certainly been in the cradle of the human race. He has come from the land we are seeking. Could we but follow back the trail of his journeyings it would assuredly take us to the garden of pleasantness from which we are exiled. Unfortunately the traveler has lost whole volumes of his itinerary, and what remains is in many of its passages not easy of decipherment.

What says anthropologic and ethnic Paleontology — or what some French writers are beginning to call *Paléoethnique* Science — respecting the hypothesis of a Polar Eden?

At the time when the present writer began his university lectures on this subject the teachings of professed anthropologists were in the chaotic and contradictory condition indicated in Part First. One of the strongest proofs he could then find that a new light was about to dawn on this field was in the there cited work of Quatrefages, entitled "The

7

Human Species." [1] Accordingly, in discussing the probable verdict of this science upon the admissibility of the new theory of human distribution, the lecturer presented the following paragraph, and there rested the case : —

"Anthropology as represented by Quatrefages seems to be actually feeling its way to the same hypothesis. This writer first argues that in the present state of knowledge we should be led to place the cradle of the race in the great region 'bounded on the south and southwest by the Himalayas, on the west by the Bolor mountains, on the northwest by the Ala-Tau, on the north by the Altai range and its offshoots, and on the east by the Kingkhan, on the south and southeast by the Felina and Kwen-lun.' Later on, however, he says that paleontological studies have very recently led to results which are 'capable of modifying these primary conclusions.' And after briefly stating these results, he starts the question whether or no the first centre of human appearance may not have been 'considerably to the north of the region' just mentioned, even ' *in polar Asia.*' Without deciding, he adds, ' Perhaps prehistoric archeology or paleontology will some day confirm or confute this conjecture.' "

The cautious anticipation here expressed was quickly fulfilled. At the concluding lecture of the same first course it was possible to present the following as the ripe conclusion of a fellow countryman of Quatrefages, one of the foremost savants of

---

[1] New York edition, pp. 175, 177, 178. See M. Zaborowski's support of Quatrefages' conjecture in the *Revue Scientifique*, Paris, 1883, p. 496.

Europe, Count Saporta :[1] " We are inclined to remove to the circumpolar regions of the North the
probable cradle of primitive humanity. From there
only could it have radiated as from a centre to
spread into the several continents at once, and to
give rise to successive emigrations toward the South.
*This theory best agrees with the presumed march of
the human races.*"[2]

---

[1] The following note appeared in the *Boston Daily Advertiser* of
May 25, 1883 : —

THE CRADLE OF THE RACE.

A few years ago, about the time of the appearance of the first edition of Dr. Winchell's *Preadamites*, in a letter addressed to its
learned author, I expressed my belief that the Garden of Eden, the
first abode of man, was to be sought in a now submerged country, situate at the North Pole. More than a year ago, in a printed essay
on *Ancient Cosmology*, I made the statement that " all ethnic traditions point us thither for the cradle of the race." Early last January I began a course of lectures in the post-graduate department
of the university, setting forth my view and the astonishing mass of
cosmological, historic, mythologic, paleontologic, paleoethnic, and
other evidences which conspire to its support. Last Monday after-
noon, about twenty minutes before I was to give the concluding lecture
of the course, I opened the fresh-cut leaves of the *Revue des Deux
Mondes*, the number for the first of this month. In it my eye quickly fell
upon *Un Essai de Synthèse Paléoethnique*, in which M. le Marquis G.
de Saporta sums up and sets forth the latest results of paleontological
research, so far as they bear upon ethnology. Judge of my gratification to find some twenty pages devoted to the question of the cradle
of the human race in the light of the latest science, and to read as the
conclusion of this learned savant that this cradle must have been
" within the Arctic Circle."

As Count Saporta has lately shown a little anxiety that American
scholarship should not receive too exclusive credit for first proposing
a closely related doctrine which he holds in common with our Professor Gray, and with Switzerland's Professor Heer (see *American
Journal of Science*, May, 1883, p. 396, footnote), he will doubtless
pardon the public statement of this, to me, most interesting coincidence. WILLIAM F. WARREN.

Boston, May 24, 1883.

[2] See APPENDIX, Sect. II. : " How the Earth was Peopled."

In the foregoing we have more than a demonstration of the bare admissibility of our hypothesis. We have in it the latest word of anthropological science respecting the birth-place of the human race. To make it a complete confirmation of our theory, so far as this field of knowledge is concerned, but one thing is lacking, and that is a clearer recognition of the great natural revolution or catastrophe which destroyed man's primitive home and occasioned the world-wide post-diluvian dispersion. This lack, however, is abundantly supplied by the foremost German ethnographers, and even by such as represent the most radical Darwinian views. Thus Professor Friedrich Müller, of Vienna, and Dr. Moritz Wagner, both of whom place the probable cradle of the race *in some high latitude* in Europe or Asia, lay the utmost stress upon the mighty climatic revolution which came in with the glacial age, ascribing to it the most stupendous and transforming influences that have ever affected mankind.[1] In our view the deterioration of natural environment reduced the

---

[1] " Es muss dort, wo der Mensch aus dem Zustand, den er mit den Thieren gemeinsam hat, sich entwickelte, ein gewaltiger Wechsel der Naturkräfte und seiner Umgebung stattgefunden haben. Nichts ist natürlicher als an die Eiszeit des Endes der Pleiocänen und der Diluvial-Periode, welche durch eine Reihe schlagender geologischer Thatsachen für das nördliche Europa, Asien und America bestätigt wird, zu denken. Damals, wo das Paradies des in der Befriedigung leiblicher Bedürfnisse einzig und allein dahinlebenden, unschuldigen, Gutes und Böses noch nicht unterscheidenden Menschen mit eisiger Hand zertrümmert wurde, damals fing der Mensch den eigentlichen Kampf ums Dasein an, und stieg durch Anspannung aller seiner Kräfte zum Herrn der Natur empor." As the tree no more bore fruit the " climber " was forced to " become a runner ; " this differentiated the foot from the hand, modified the leg, and in time changed the pithecoid ancestors of humanity into men. Friedrich Müller, *Allgemeine Ethnographie.* Wien, 1873 : p. 36.

vigor and longevity of the race ; in theirs it changed one of the tribes of the animal world into men ! Which of these views is the more rational may safely be left to the reader's judgment. Few will be disposed to accept the doctrine that man is simply a judiciously-iced pithecoid.

CHAPTER VIII.

CONCLUSION OF PART THIRD.

We must now be prepared to admit that God can plant an Eden even in Spitz-bergen ; that the present state of the world is by no means the best possible in re-lation to climate and vegetation ; that there have been and might be again condi-tions which could convert the ice-clad Arctic regions into blooming Paradises. —
PRINCIPAL J. W. DAWSON.

WE are at the end of the first series of tests, and with what results?

1. Scientific Cosmology, searching for the place where the physical conditions of Eden-life first appeared on our globe, is brought to the very spot where we have located the cradle of our race.

2. Contrary to all ordinary impressions, we have found this same spot the most favored on the globe, not only as respects the glories of night, but also in respect to prevalence of daylight.

3. In its geology we have found scientific evidence of the vast cataclysm which destroyed the antedilu-vian world and permanently transferred to lower latitudes the habitat of humanity.

4. We have found scientifically accepted evidence that at the time of the advent of man the climate at the Arctic Pole was all that the most poetic leg-ends of Eden could demand.

5. From Paleontological Botany we have learned that this locality was the cradle of the floral life-forms of the whole known earth.

6. By Paleontological Zoölogy we have been as-

sured that here too originated, and from this centre eradiated, the fauna of the prehistoric world.

7. And lastly, we have found the latest ethnographers and anthropologists slowly but surely gravitating toward the same Arctic Eden as the only centre from which the migrations of the human race can be intelligibly interpreted.

We asked of these sciences simply, "Is our hypothesis admissible?" Their answer is more than an affirmative; it is an unanticipated and pronounced confirmation.

Some months after the foregoing chapters had been written and delivered in lectures before classes of students in the University, a very interesting reinforcement of the views therein advanced appeared in a little work by Mr. G. Hilton Scribner, of New York, entitled "Where did Life Begin?"[1] As Mr. Scribner was conducted to a belief in the north polar origin of all races of living creatures by considerations quite independent of those mythological and historical ones which first led the present writer to the same opinion, the reader of these pages will find in the following extracts a special incentive to procure and read the entire treatise from which they are taken. That two minds starting with such entirely different data should have reached so nearly simultaneously one and the same conclusion touching so difficult and many-sided a problem is surely not without significance.

[1] Published by Charles Scribner's Sons, New York. 12mo, pp. 64. Ex-Chancellor Winchell (anonymously) reviews the work with much respect in *Science*, March 7, 1884, p. 292. For courteous permission to quote from the treatise without restriction I publicly return the author my thanks.

Our first extract is from pp. 21–23, where the following summary of previous reasonings and conclusions is given : " We may therefore safely conclude, if the code of natural laws has been uniformly in force, —

" First, — That life commenced on those parts of the earth which were first prepared to maintain it ; at any rate, that it never could have commenced elsewhere.

" Second, — As the whole earth was at one time too hot to maintain life, so those parts were probably first prepared to maintain it which cooled first.

" Third, — That those parts which received the least heat from the sun, and which radiated heat most rapidly into space, in proportion to mass, and had the thinnest mass to cool, cooled first.

" Fourth, — That those parts of the earth's surface, and those only, answering to these conditions are the Arctic and Antarctic zones.

" Fifth, — That as these zones were at one time too hot, and certain parts thereof are now too cold, for such life as inhabits the warmer parts of the earth, these now colder parts, in passing from the extreme of heat to the extreme of cold, must have passed slowly through temperatures exactly suited to all plants and all animals in severalty which now live or ever lived on the earth.

" Sixth, — If the concurrent conditions which have usually followed lowering temperature followed the climatic changes in this case, life did commence on the earth within one or both of certain zones surrounding the poles, and sufficiently removed therefrom to receive the least amount of sunlight necessary for vegetal and animal life.

"It seems almost superfluous to say that those parts of the earth which first became cool enough to maintain life had a climate warmer at that time than that which we now call torrid. It was for an epoch, and probably a very long one, as hot as it could be and maintain life.

"It is also quite obvious, in the light of the foregoing considerations, that as the temperate zones have always received more heat from the sun, and have had more mass per square foot to cool, in proportion to radiating surface, than the polar zones, so, on the other hand, they have always received less heat from the sun and have had less mass to cool, in proportion to radiating surface, than the torrid zone; and so when the arctic zones cooled from a tropical to what we now call a temperate climate, the temperate zones had cooled down to that temperature which we now call a torrid climate, while the equatorial belt was still too hot for any form of life. Thus the lowering of temperature, climatic change, and that life which made its advent in these zones surrounding the poles have crept thence slowly along, *pari passu*, from these polar regions to the equator."

Farther on (pp. 26, 27) he claims that the progressive cooling of the region at the Pole is all-sufficient, as a natural cause, to account for that dispersion of life, vegetable and animal, which proceeded from the Arctic centre southward: "As might be readily supposed, these Arctic regions which first became cool enough to maintain life would from the same causes be the first to become too cold for the same purpose. And this cold would occur first as a temperate climate near and around the pole; at any rate,

in the centre of a zone just sufficiently removed
from the pole to combine the influence of the sun
with its own cooling temperature, so as to become
the first fit habitation of life.

"This central cold creating a temperate climate
would thus have become the first and all-sufficient
cause of a dispersion and distribution of both the
tropical plants and animals over another zone next
south, next further removed from the pole, and next
sufficiently cool to maintain such life. Moreover,
this cooler climate occurring in the centre would
have driven out and dispersed such life equally, in
all possible directions. So, if the first habitable zone
included the northernmost land of all the great continents which converge around the North Pole, this
dispersion from an increasing cold to the north of
each of them would have sent southward plants and
animals from a common origin and ancestry, to people and to plant all the continents of the earth, with
the possible exception of Australia, whose flora and
fauna are certainly anomalous and possibly indigenous."

In section fourth (pp. 28–34) the author briefly
touches upon some of the surface features of the
globe peculiarly favorable to the southward migration of plants and animals : " Let us now see how
admirably the earth is adapted, by its surface formation and topography, for a southern migration from
a zone surrounding the North Pole. In the first
place, nearly the whole of the earth's surface (and
all the northern hemisphere) is corrugated north and
south with alternate continents and deep sea channels almost from pole to pole. Both the eastern and
western continents extend with unbroken land con-

nections from the Arctic zone through the northern temperate, the torrid, and through the southern temperate, almost to the Antarctic zone. Between these great continents lie the deep oceans, whose channels run north and south through as many degrees of latitude. The great air and ocean currents run north or south ; all the mountain ranges of the western continent and many of the eastern continents run mainly north and south. Nearly all the great rivers of the northern hemisphere run north or south. To a southern migration — in other words, a migration from the Arctic region toward the equator — these peculiarities of topography, these great corrugations and mountain ranges, these channels and currents, are roads and vehicles, guides and helps ; while to an east and west migration the same features are not only obstacles and hindrances, but in the main barriers insuperable.

"The impassability of mountain ranges for most plants is shown by the fact that strongly marked varieties in great numbers and many distinct species occur upon the eastern slopes of the Rocky Mountains, the Sierra Nevadas, the Alleghanies, and even lower ranges, which are not found at all upon their western sides, and *vice versa.* Such a condition of things, incompatible as it is with an eastern and western migration, is quite consistent, however, with a north and south movement. For all the climatic conditions, especially that of rainfall, are so different on the opposite sides of all long mountain ranges that the same variety, split and separated by the northern extremities of these ranges, would, in moving southward along their eastern and western sides, and encountering such diverse conditions, have become in the course of time, under the laws of adaptation, distinct varieties, and probably different species.

"It may be well now to examine some of the conditions assisting this movement. Hot air being lighter than cold, the heated air of the northern equatorial belt has always risen and passed mainly toward the North Pole in an upper current, while the cooler and heavier currents from the north have swept southward, hugging the surface of the continents, laded with pollen, minute germs and spores, and all the winged seeds of plants, bending grass and shrubs and trees constantly to the southward, and so, by small yearly increments, moving the whole vegetal kingdom through valleys and along the sides of mountain ranges, down the great continents, always moving with, and never across, these great surface corrugations. It is unnecessary to add that all insects and herbivorous animals would follow the plants, or that the birds and carnivorous animals would follow the herbivorous animals and the insects. So, too, the currents of the ocean have been established in obedience to similar laws: as hot water is lighter than cold, great surface currents have been formed in both the Atlantic and Pacific oceans, flowing from the equator to the Arctic regions; while the cooler and heavier currents from the Arctic have swept the floor of both oceans from shore to shore to the southward, carrying all kinds of marine life from the pole toward the equator with them.

"It may be well in this connection to allude to another fact seriously affecting the bottom currents from the pole toward the equator of both air and ocean. By reason of the revolution of the earth upon its axis, a given point upon its surface 1,000 miles south of the North Pole moves to the eastward at the rate of about 260 miles an hour, while another point in the same meridian at the equator would be moving to the eastward a little more than 1,000 miles an hour; so every cubic yard of air and water which starts in a bottom current from the polar regions for the equator must, before reaching the equator, acquire an eastward motion of about 750 miles an hour. The tendency, therefore, of all bottom currents of air and ocean moving to the south is to press to the westward every obstacle met with in its course, and the result, both as to the currents and all movable things they come in contact with, would be to give them a southwestern course and movement.

" Now it is a strange coincidence, if nothing more, that the eastern coasts of all the continents have a southwestern trend, are full of bays, inlets, and shoal water, as though the floor of the ocean was being constantly swept up against them; while the western coasts are more abrupt, straight, and touch deeper water, as though the sweepings from the land were being constantly rolled into the sea along their entire lines.

" Notwithstanding all these indications of a southern or southwestern movement, ever since the migration of plants and animals first attracted attention, students of natural science, careful and conscientious observers, able and discriminating investigators, have, almost with one accord, been looking east and west across these great north and south corrugations and natural barriers for the paths of

their journeyings ; searching along every parallel of
latitude, across lofty mountain ranges, broad continents, deep and wide oceans, and ocean currents,
to and fro; and if perchance they looked north or
south it was only in search of some ferry or ford
south of the ice-fields by which to pass the flora and
fauna from one continent to another, and thus account for what is very evident, namely, that many
widely distributed species and varieties have come
from the same locality and had a common ancestry
and origin.   Is it not evident that the very plants
and animals (in a tribal sense) whose migrations
they have been engaged in unraveling were as
much older than ice and snow on the earth as it
would require in time to lower the average temperature over a vast area from a tropical to a frigid climate ?"

The portion of the little treatise least satisfactory,
even to its author, is the part which relates to man
(pp. 52–54). By making the human race the descendants (or, as on Darwinist principles we ought
rather to say, the *ascendants*) of one or more pairs
of lower animals, and assuming that our animal ancestry had already been driven from the polar region
before they were blessed with this unanticipated
progeny, the author suggests a possible manner in
which "the absence on the earth of our immediate
predecessor," the missing link, might be accounted
for. He says, "If it is true that, in common with
many existing plants and animals, the ancestry of
man — some animal with a thumb, and so having
the possibility of all things — shared this northern
home, this common and immensely remote origin,
earlier by long epochs than the glacial period, it

would afford a possible ground for the claim of the unity of the origin of man, and also a reason for the absence on earth of his immediate predecessor. His arboreal progenitor in the pioneer ranks of this great southern movement, ages before the Quaternary (during all of which period man has probably inhabited the earth), was possibly driven naked by the ever-following, merciless cold, thus keeping him within the southward-moving tropical climate, down the eastern and western continents alike, until it and he, arriving in the lapse of ages at the equatorial belt, and being always at the head and still rising in the scale of being by this movement, discipline, and process, became sufficiently advanced by slow degrees to build fires, clothe himself, make implements, and, possibly, domesticate animals, — at least the first and most useful to primitive man, the dog, — and so prepared for conflict and for all climates, turned backward to the verge of everlasting ice, subduing, slaying, and exterminating, first his own ancestry, his nearest but now weak rival, which by lingering behind and struggling for life in a climate of increasing cold, would have become extremely degenerated and so easily disposed of, if not actually exterminated by the climate itself ; thus leaving as the nearest in resemblance to man, and yet the remotest in actual relationship both to him and to his ancestry, the later tribes of anthropoid apes since developed, nearer to the equator, from the next lower animals which accompanied him in his southward march."

In this speculation, it will be observed, the place of the origin of the human race is entirely indeterminate. When its far-off arboreal ancestor left the

Pole his only prophetic endowment was "a thumb." But possessing this, he "had the possibility of all things." In his successors, ages afterward, the real transition from the plane of animal to that of human life seems to be represented as having taken place "at the equatorial belt." Unfortunately, however, for the theory, the claim of the new men to the virtue and name of humanity was now poorer than before the change, for their first act was to turn fiercely upon those who brought them into being, "subduing, slaying, and exterminating their own ancestry" in a frenzy worse than brutal. The shock to the feelings of the near but younger relatives of the massacred victims — the mild-mannered apes — must have been violent in the extreme. In fact, among all the tens of thousands of their descendants not one, from that day to this, has ever been seen to smile.

But in justice to our author it should be stated that he attaches little, if any, weight to this Darwinistic episode. He frankly says, "This last proposition, however, is but a vague and very deductive supposition, for which nothing is claimed beyond a possibility or bare probability." It is possible that he is only slyly indulging in a bit of quiet pleasantry at the expense of the new-school anthropogonists. Whether so or not, he hastens without further words to return from it to the impregnable positions of his main argument, and to reinforce them by a fresh study of the power and function of heat in the cosmic unfoldment and distribution of life.

The next two divisions of the present work will show us that the birth-memories of mankind conduct us, not to "the equatorial belt," but to the polar world, and that in Mr. Scribner's answer to the question, "Where did Life begin ?" human as well as floral and faunal life should be included. After examining these fresh lines of evidence it is believed that the reader will find more impressive than ever the words with which our author concludes his charming tractate : —

"Thus the Arctic zone, which was earliest in cooling down to the first and highest heat degree in the great life-gamut, was also first to become fertile, first to bear life, and first to send forth her progeny over the earth. So, too, in obedience to the universal order of things, she was first to reach maturity, first to pass all the subdivisions of life-bearing climate and finally the lowest heat degree in the great life-range, and so the first to reach sterility, old age, degeneration, and death. And now, cold and lifeless, wrapped in her snowy winding sheet, the once fair mother of us all rests in the frozen embrace of an ice-bound and everlasting sepulchre."

PART FOURTH.

THE HYPOTHESIS CONFIRMED BY ETHNIC TRADITION.

All these things happened in the North; and afterward, when men were created, they were created in the North; but as the people multiplied they moved toward the South, the Earth growing larger also, and extending itself in the same direction. — H. H. BANCROFT, *Native Races*, vol. iii., p. 162.

Il y a donc beaucoup d'apparence que les peuples du Nord, en descendant vers le Midi, y portent les emblêms relatifs au physique de leur climat ; et ces emblêms sont devenus des fables, puis des personnages, puis des Dieux, dans des imaginations vives et prêtes à tout animer, comme celles des Orientaux. — JEAN SYLVAIN BAILLY.

CHAPTER I.

ANCIENT COSMOLOGY AND MYTHICAL GEOGRAPHY.

Not enough credit has been given to the ancient astronomers. For instance, there is no time within the scope of history when it was not known that the earth is a sphere, and that the direction DOWN at different points is toward the same point at the earth's centre. Current teaching in the text-books as to the knowledge of astronomy by the ancients is at fault.[1] — SIMON NEWCOMB, LL. D.

Hic vertex nobis semper sublimis, at illum
Sub pedibus Styx atra videt manesque profundi.
VERGIL.

BACK of every mythological account of Paradise lies some conception of the world at large, and especially of the world of men. Rightly to understand and interpret the myths, we must first understand the world-conception to which they were adjusted. Unfortunately, the cosmology of the ancients has been totally misconceived by modern scholars. All our maps of " The World according to Homer" represent the earth as flat, and as surrounded by a level, flowing ocean stream. "There can be no doubt," says Bunbury, " that Homer, in common with all his successors down to the time of Hecatæus, believed the earth to be a plane of circular form."[2] As to the sky, we are generally taught that the early Greeks believed it to be a solid metallic vault.[3] Pro-

[1] Lowell Lecture. *Boston Daily Advertiser*, Nov. 29, 1881.

[2] E. H. Bunbury, *History of Ancient Geography among the Greeks and Romans.* London, 1879: vol. i., p. 79. Professor Bunbury was a leading contributor to Smith's *Dictionary of Ancient Greek and Roman Geography.* Compare Friedreich, *Die Realien in der Ilias und Odysee.* 1856, § 19. Buchholz, *Die Homerische Realien.* Leipsic, 1871 : Bd. i., 48.

[3] See Voss, Ukert, Bunbury, Buchholz, and the others.

fessor F. A. Paley aids the imagination of his readers as follows: "We might familiarly illustrate the Hesiodic notion of the flat circular earth and the convex overarching sky by a circular plate with a hemispherical dish-cover of metal placed over it and concealing it. Above the cover (which is supposed to rotate on an axis, πόλος) live the gods. Round the inner concavity is the path of the sun, giving light to the earth below." [1]

That all writers upon Greek mythology, including even the latest,[2] should proceed upon the same assumptions as the professed Homeric interpreters and geographers building upon their foundations is only natural. And that the current conceptions of the cosmology of the ancient Greeks should profoundly affect current interpretations of the cosmological and geographical data of other ancient peoples is also precisely what the history and inner relationships of modern archæological studies would lead one to expect. It is not surprising, therefore, that the earth of the Ancient Hebrews, Egyptians, Indo-Aryans, and other ancient peoples has been assumed to correspond to the supposed flat earth of the Greeks.[3]

---

[1] *The Epics of Hesiod, with an English Commentary.* London, 1861 : p. 172.

[2] See, for example, Sir George W. Cox: *An Introduction to the Science of Comparative Mythology and Folk-Lore.* London and New York, 1881 : p. 244. Decharme, *Mythologie de la Grèce Antique.* Paris, 1879: p. 11.

[3] It is true that Heinrich Zimmer remarks, "Die Anschauung die sich bei Griechen und Nordgermanen findet, dass die Erde eine Scheibe sei, um die sich das Meer schlingt, begegnet in den vedischen Samhitā nirgends." *Altindisches Leben.* Berlin, 1879: p. 359. But even he does not advance from this negative assertion to an exposition of the true Vedic cosmology. Compare M. Fontane : "Leur cosmog-

A protracted study of the subject has convinced the present writer that this modern assumption, as to the form of the Homeric earth is entirely baseless and misleading. He has, furthermore, satisfied himself that the Egyptians, Akkadians, Assyrians, Babylonians, Phœnicians, Hebrews, Greeks, Iranians, Indo-Aryans, Chinese, Japanese, — in fine, all the most ancient historic peoples, — possessed in their earliest traceable periods a cosmology essentially identical, and one of a far more advanced type than has been attributed to them. The purpose of this chapter is to set forth and illustrate this oldest known conception of the universe and of its parts.

In ancient thought, the grand divisions of the world are four, to wit : the abode of the gods, the abode of living men, the abode of the dead, and, finally, the abode of demons. To locate these in right mutual relations, one must begin by representing to himself the earth as a sphere or spheroid, and as situated within, and concentric with, the starry sphere, *each having its axis perpendicular, and its north pole at the top.* The pole-star is thus in the true zenith, and the heavenly heights centring about it are the abode of the supreme god or gods. According to the same conception, the upper or northern hemisphere of the earth is the proper home of living men ; the under or southern hemisphere of the earth, the abode of disembodied spirits and rulers of the dead ; and, finally, the undermost region of all, that centring around the southern pole of the

raphie est embryonaire. La terre est pour l'Arya ronde et plate comme un disque. Le firmament védique, concave, vien se souder à la terre, circulairement, à l'horizon." *Inde Védique.* Paris, 1881 : p. 94. With this agrees Bergaine, *La Religion Védique.* Paris, 1878 : p. 1.

heavens, the lowest hell.[1] The two hemispheres of
the earth were furthermore conceived of as separated
from each other by an equatorial ocean or oceanic
current.

To illustrate this conception of the world, let the
two circles of the diagram which constitutes the
frontispiece of this work represent respectively the
earth-sphere and the outermost of the revolving
starry spheres. A is the north pole of the heavens,
so placed as to be in the zenith. B is the south pole
of the heavens in the nadir. The line A B is the
axis of the apparent revolution of the starry heavens
in a perpendicular position. C is the north pole of
the earth; D its south pole; the line C D the axis
of the earth in perpendicular position, and coincident with the corresponding portion of the axis of
the starry heavens. The space 1 1 1 1 is the abode
of the supreme god or gods; 2, Europe; 3, Asia; 4,
Libya, or the known portion of Africa; 5 5 5, the
ocean, or "ocean stream;" 6 6 6, the abode of disembodied spirits and rulers of the dead; 7 7 7 7,
the lowest hell.[2]

---

[1] It is worthy of notice that the sight of portions of the south-
polar heavens, especially the starless region known as "the black Coal
Sack," is to this day capable of suggesting the associations of the
bottomless pit. Thus in a recent traveler's letter of the ordinary kind
we read, "Every clear evening we could see the Magellan Clouds,
soft and fleece-like, floating airily among the far-off constellations.
These mysterious bodies look like star-spray, or borrowed bits of the
Milky Way. Then, too, our eyes would seek out, as by some strange
fascination, those still more mysterious 'chambers of the South,' the
black Coal Sack, with its retreating depths of darkness, wherein no
star shines. These irregular spaces, emptinesses, as it were, in the
heavens, impress one with a sense of *something uncanny, as though
these were, indeed, the 'blackness of darkness forever.'*" — *The Sunday
School Times.* Philadelphia, 1883: p. 581.

[2] The reception accorded to the foregoing "True Key" is illustrated in the APPENDIX, Sect. III.

Now, to make this key a graphic illustration of
Homeric cosmology, it is only necessary to write in
place of 1 1 1 1 "LOFTY OLYMPOS;" in place of
5 5 5, "THE OCEAN STREAM;" in place of 6 6 6,
"HOUSE OF AÏDES" (Hades); and in place of 7 7 7 7,
"GLOOMY TARTAROS." Imagine, then, the light as
falling from the upper heavens, — the lower terrestrial hemisphere, therefore, as forever in the shade;
imagine the Tartarean abyss as filled with Stygian
gloom and blackness, — fit dungeon-house for de-
throned gods and powers of evil; imagine the "men-
illuminating" sun, the "well-tressed" moon, the
"splendid" stars, silently wheeling round the central
upright axis of the lighted hemispheres, — and suddenly the confusions and supposed contradictions of
classic cosmology disappear. We are in the very
world in which immortal Homer lived and sang.[1] It
is no longer an obscure crag in Thessaly, from which
heaven-shaking Zeus proposes to suspend the whole
earth and ocean. The eye measures for itself the
nine days' fall of Hesiod's brazen anvil from heaven
to earth, from earth to Tartarus. The Hyperboreans
are now a possibility. Now a *descensus ad inferos*
can be made by voyagers in the black ship. Un-
numbered commentators upon Homer have professed their despair of ever being able to harmonize
the passages in which Hades is represented as "beyond the ocean" with those in which it is represented as "subterranean." Conceive of man's dwell-
ing-place, of Hades, and the ocean, as in this key,
and the notable difficulty instantaneously vanishes.
Interpreters of the Odyssey have found it impossible to understand how the westward and north-

[1] See cut in APPENDIX, Sect. VI.: "Homer's Abode of the Dead."

ward sailing voyager could suddenly be found in
waters and amid islands unequivocally associated
with the East. The present key explains it perfectly, showing what no one seems heretofore to
have suspected, that the voyage of Odysseus is a
poetical account of an imaginary *circumnavigation
of the mythical earth in the upper or northern hemisphere, including a trip to the southern or under hemisphere and a visit to the* ὀμφαλὸς θαλάσσης, *or North
Pole.*

In this cosmological conception the upright axis
of the world is often poetically conceived of as a
majestic pillar, supporting the heavens and furnish-
ing the pivot on which they revolve. Euripides [1] and
Aristotle [2] unmistakably identify the Pillar of Atlas
with this world-axis. How interesting a feature this
pillar became in ancient mythologies will be seen
below in chapter third of this part, in chapter second of part six, and elsewhere in this volume.

Again, according to this view the highest part of
the earth, its true summit, would of course be at the
North Pole. And since the whole of the upper or
northern hemisphere would in this case be conceived of as rising on all sides from the equatorial
ocean toward that summit, nothing would be more
natural than to view the entire upper half of the earth
as itself a vast mountain, the mother and support of
all lesser mountains. [3] Moreover, as the abode of the
supreme God or gods was thought to be directly
over this summit of the earth, it would be extremely
easy for the imagination to carry the summit of so

---

[1] *Peirithous*, 597, 3-5, ed. Nauck.
[2] *De Anim. Motione*, c. 3.
[3] See *Bundahish*, chaps. viii., xii., etc.

stupendous a mountain into and far above the clouds, and even to extend it to such a height that the gods of heaven might be conceived of as having their abode upon its top. This is precisely what came to pass, and hence in the cosmology of the ancient Egyptians, Akkadians, Assyrians, Babylonians, Persians, Indians, Chinese, and others we find, under various names, but always easily recognizable, this *Weltberg,* or "Mountain of the World," situated at the North Pole of the earth, supporting or otherwise connect-

ing with the city of the gods, and serving as the axis around which sun, moon, and stars revolve. Often we also find evidence that the under hemisphere was in like manner conceived of as an inverted mountain, antipodal to the mountain of the gods, and connecting at its apex with the abode of demons.[1] The adjoining figure may illustrate this conception of the earth, the upper protuberance be-

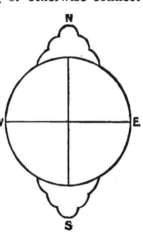

The Antipodal Polar Mountains.

ing the "Mount of the Gods," the lower the inverted "Mount of Demons."

A clear view of the first of these remarkable

[1] " Dans les conceptions de la cosmogonie mythique des Indiens on oppose au Sou-Merou ' le bon Merou,' du Nord, un Kou-Merou mauvais et funeste, qui y fait exactement pendant et en est l'antithèse. De même les Chaldéens opposaient à la divine et bienheureuse montagne de l'Orient accadien *'garsag-babbarra* = assyrien *šad çit šamši,* une montagne funeste et ténébreuse . . . accadien, *'garsag-gigga* = assyrien *šad erib šamši,* située dans les parties basses de la terre."— Lenormant, *Origines de l'Histoire,* tom. ii. 1, p. 134.

World-Mountains is so essential to any right understanding of mythical geography and of the mythical
terrestrial Paradise that a more extended examination of the subject seems a necessity.

Beginning with the Egyptians we may note this
remarkable fact; that notwithstanding his sharing
the common and mistaken modern assumption that
the Egyptians conceived of the earth as flat, Brugsch,
confessedly the foremost authority in ancient Egyptian geography, places the highest and most sacred
part of the Egyptians' earth at the North, *making
the land there to rise until in actual contact with
heaven.* He also places at the farthest southern
extremity of the earth another lofty mountain, *Ap-
en-to* or *Tap-en-to*, literally "the horn of the world."[1]
Now, while several professed Egyptologists have recently come to the conviction that the earth of the
Egyptians was a sphere, no one has brought out the
fact that these two heights are two antipodal polar
projections of the spherical earth, the upper or celestial one being the mount of the gods, and the lower
or infernal one the mount of demons. Of the former the following passage in the "Book of Hades"
may naturally be understood to speak : —

"Draw me [the nocturnal sun], infernal ones ! . . .

"Retreat towards the eastern heavens, toward the
dwellings which support Sar, that mysterious mountain that spreads light among the gods [or, that I
may spread light among the gods ?], who receive me
when I go forth from amongst you, from the retreat."[2]

[1] *Geographische Inschriften altægyptischer Denkmäler.* Leipsic,
1858 : vol. ii., p. 37.

[2] *Records of the Past*, vol. x., p. 103. I understand this to refer to
the (northward and southward) *annual*, and not to the diurnal, movement of the sun.

To the inverted infernal mountain seem to apply the expressions in chapter one hundred and fifty of the "Book of the Dead:" —

"Oh, the very tall Hill in Hades! The heaven rests upon it. There is a snake or dragon upon it: Sati is his name," etc.[1]

In another chapter of the same book a place is spoken of as "the inverted precinct," which place is Hades.[2] Moreover, the translator of another text, called the "Book of Hades," describes a "pendant mountain" as a curious feature in the vignette illustrations of the original. This can hardly be anything other than *Ap-en-to,* the inverted mountain of Hades.[3]

[1] The mention of the starry serpent or dragon completes the parallelism between the North Polar and South Polar mountains. "Mr. Procter has remarked that when the North Pole Star was *Alpha Draconis,* the Southern was most probably the star *Eta Hydri,* and certain to have been in the constellation Hydra. . . . The encircling Serpent, the symbol of eternal going round, was figured at both Poles, the two centres of the total starry revolution." Massey, *The Natural Genesis,* vol. i., p. 345. In our discussion of the Pillar of Atlas we have spoken of the identity of *Draco* with the dragon which assisted the nymphs in watching the golden apples in the North Polar Gardens of the Hesperides. See Depuis, *Origines des Constellations,* p. 147. The same parallelism is alluded to in the following: "The hypocephalus in question is divided into four compartments, two of which are opposed to the two others as if to indicate the two celestial hemispheres; the upper one above the terrestrial world and the lower one below it." *Proceedings of the Society of Biblical Archaeology,* March 4, 1884. London, 1884: p. 126. See also *Revue Archéologique.* Paris, 1862: vi., p. 129.

[2] Bunsen, *Egypt's Place in Universal History,* vol. v., p. 208.

[3] *Records of the Past,* vol. x., p. 88. Two years after the above was written I met with the following: "The god advancing in a reversed position" (in a certain New Zealand legend) "is the sun in the Underworld. The image exactly accords with an Egyptian scene of the sun passing through Hades, where we see the twelve gods of the earth, or the lower domain of night, marching towards a mountain

The Akkadians, who antedated even the most ancient empires of the Tigro-Euphrates valley, had in like manner a "Mountain of the World," which was unlike all other mountains in that it was a support on which the heavens rested and around which they revolved. It was called Kharsak Kurra. It was so rich with gold and silver and precious stones as to be dazzling to the sight. An ancient Akkadian hymn respecting it uses this language : —

"O mighty mountain of Bel, Im-Kharsak, whose head rivals heaven, whose root is in the holy deep!

"Among the mountains like a strong wild bull it lieth down.

"Its horn like the brilliance of the sun is bright.

"Like the star of heaven it is filled with sheen."[1]

In another hymn, apparently of great antiquity, we find the goddess Istar addressed as "Queen of this Mountain of the World," which is further located and identified by its connection with "the axis of heaven," and with "the four rivers" of the Akkadian Paradise.[2]

---

turned upside down, and two typical personages are also turned upside down. This is an illustration of the passage of the sun through the Underworld. The *reversed* on the same monument are the dead. Thus the Osirified deceased, who has attained the second life, in the Ritual says exultingly, '*I do not walk upon my head.*' The dead, as the Akhu, are the spirits, and the Atua [of the New Zealand legend] is a spirit who comes walking upside down." Massey, *The Natural Genesis.* London, 1883 : vol. i., p. 529. (The italics are Massey's.) The passage is the more remarkable from the fact that Massey elsewhere states that the earth "was considered flat by the first myth-makers," who in his scheme appear to have been the Egyptians. Ibid., vol. i., p. 465.

[1] *Records of the Past.* London, vol. xi., pp. 131, 132. Lenormant, *Chaldæan Magic*, p. 168. Lenormant's latest revised translation may be seen in *Les Origines de l'Histoire*, tom. ii. 1, pp. 127, 128.

[2] George Smith, *Assyrian Discoveries*, pp. 392, 393. Mr. G. Mas-

Lenormant places this mountain in the North (but sometimes incorrectly in the East or Northeast), and makes it the "*lieu de l'assemblée des dieux;*" but when he locates the corresponding antipodal mountain of Hades in the West, instead of in the South, he seems to have gone entirely beyond the evidence. At least, Dr. Friedrich Delitzsch affirms that in the cuneiform literature thus far known he has discovered no trace of such a location.[1] But on this question of the site of these mountains more will be said in chapter sixth of the present division.

The Assyrians and Babylonians inherited the Akkadian conception. One of the titles of the supreme divinity of the Assyrians related to the sacred mount. An invocation to him opens thus: "Assur, the mighty god, who dwells in the temple of Kharsak Kurra."[2] An Assyrian hymn speaks of the

> "feasts of the silver mountain,
> The heavenly courts," —

and the translator makes the expression refer to this "Assyrian Olympos."[3] Sayce finds in the following a plain reference to the same : —

"I am lord of the steep mountains, which tremble whilst their summits reach to the firmament.

sey remarks, "In an Akkadian hymn to Ishtar, the goddess is addressed as the 'Queen of the Mountain of the World' and 'Queen of the land of the four rivers of Erech;' that is, as the goddess of the mythical Mount of the Pole and the four rivers of the four quarters, which arose in Paradise. The Mountain of the World was the Mount of the North." *The Natural Genesis*, vol. ii., p. 21.

[1] *Wo lag das Paradies?* Leipsic, 1881 : p. 121.

[2] *Cuneiform Inscriptions of Western Asia.* London : vol. i., pp. 44, 45. Translated by Mr. Sayce in *Records of the Past*, vol. xi., p. 5.

[3] *Records of the Past*, vol. iii., p. 133.

"The mountain of alabaster, lapis, and onyx, in my hand I possess it."[1]

How current the idea must have been among the Babylonians is shown by the rhetorical use made of it by the prophet Isaiah. Rebuking the arrogance of the king of Babylon and pre-announcing to him his doom, the prophet beholds his fall as already accomplished, and in a passage of wonderful pictorial power and beauty exclaims, "How art thou fallen from heaven, O Lucifer, son of the morning! how art thou cut down to the ground, which didst weaken the nations! For thou hast said in thine heart, I will ascend into heaven, I will exalt my throne above the stars of God: I will sit also upon the mount of the congregation in the sides of the North (or more correctly in the uttermost parts of the North, in the extreme northern regions), I will ascend above the heights of the clouds; I will be like (or equal to) the Most High. Yet thou shalt be brought down to Sheol, to the sides (or regions) of the pit."[2]

Since the publication of Gesenius's commentary on this passage and his excursus upon the "*Götterberg im Norden*" appended to it, no question has remained in the minds of scholars as to the character of the *Har Moed*, the "mount of the congregation," in the far-off North.

Among the Chinese we find a similar celestial mount, the mythical Kwen-lun. It is often called simply "The Pearl Mountain." On its top is Paradise, with a living fountain from which flow in opposite directions the four great rivers of the world.[3]

---

[1] *Records of the Past*, vol. iii., p. 126.   [2] Isaiah xiv. 12–15.

[3] Stollberg, *Mémoires concernant les Chinois*, t. i., p. 101, cited in Keerl, *Lehre vom Paradies.* Basle, 1861 : p. 796.

Around it revolve the visible heavens ; and the stars nearest to it, that is nearest to the Pole, are supposed to be the abodes of the inferior gods and genii. To this day, the Tauists speak of the first person of their trinity as residing in "the metropolis of Pearl Mountain," and in addressing him turn their faces to the northern sky.[1]

A striking parallel to the Egyptian and Akkadian idea of two opposed polar mountains, an arctic and an antarctic, — the one celestial and the other infernal, — is found among the ancient inhabitants of India. The celestial mountain they called Su-Meru, the infernal one Ku-Meru.[2] In the Hindu Puranas the size and splendors of the former are presented in the wildest exaggerations of Oriental fancy. Its height, according to some accounts, is not less than eight hundred and forty thousand miles, its diameter at the summit three hundred and twenty thousand. Four enormous buttress mountains, situated at mutually opposite points of the horizon, surround it. One account makes the eastern side of Meru of the color of the ruby, its southern that of the lotus, its western that of gold, its northern that of coral. On its summit is the vast city of Brahma, fourteen thousand leagues in extent.[3] Around it, in the cardinal

[1] Joseph Edkins, *Religion in China.* 2d ed., 1878 : p. 151. The Ainos of Japan, although declared to be "ausserordentlich arm an Sagen," have nevertheless their corresponding mythical Gold-mountain, Kogane-yama. Dr. B. Scheube, *Die Ainos.* Yokohama, 1882 : p. 24.

[2] "Meru, in Sanskrit, signifies an *axis* or *pivot.*" Wilford in *Asiatic Researches.* London, 1808 : vol. viii., p. 285. The prefix "Su" signifies "beautiful."

[3] In Brugsch's *Astronomische Inschriften,* p. 177, we read, "Es gab ein himmliches *Anu* or *Òn,* Heliopolis, dessen *östliche Lichtseite* und *westliche Lichtseite* öfters erwähnt werden." Was this perhaps the

9

points and the intermediate quarters, are situated the magnificent cities of Indra and the other regents of the spheres. The city of Brahma in the centre of the eight is surrounded by a moat of sweet flowing celestial waters, a kind of river of the water of life (Gangâ), which after encircling the city divides into four mighty rivers flowing towards four opposite points of the horizon, and descending into the equatorial ocean which engirdles the earth.[1]

Sometimes Mount Meru is represented as planted so firmly and deeply in the globe that the antarctic or infernal mountain is only a projection of its lower end. Thus the Sûrya Siddhânta says: " A collection of manifold jewels, a mountain of gold, is Meru, passing through the middle of the earth-globe (*bhugola*), and protruding on either side. At its upper end are stationed along with Indra the gods and the Great Sages (*maharishis*) ; at its lower end, in like manner, the demons have their abode, — each [class] the enemy of the other. Surrounding it on every side is fixed, next, this great ocean, like a girdle about the earth, separating the two hemispheres of the gods and of the demons."

Conceiving of Meru in this way, as a kind of core extending through the earth and projecting at each pole, one can easily understand the following passage, in which two pole-stars are spoken of instead of one: " In both [*i. e.*, the two opposite] directions from Meru are two pole-stars fixed in the midst of the sky." As these mark the two opposite poles of

---

Vorbild and Egyptian counterpart of the city of Brahma, the city of Sakra, and all the other Asiatic *Götterstädte* in the celestial pole? It would be very interesting to know.

[1] See APPENDIX, Sect. IV. : " The Earth of the Hindus."

the heavens, it is correctly added that " to those who are situated in places of no latitude [*i. e.*, on the equator] both these pole-stars have their place in the horizon." Farther on in the same treatise the common designation used for the northern hemisphere is the hemisphere of the gods, and for the southern the hemisphere of the *asuras*, or demons.[1]

A picture of " the Earth of the Hindus," showing the exact position of Meru and its buttress-mounts, will be given below in chapter fourth of the present Part (p. 152).

That the cosmology of ancient India should have been retained and propagated in its main features by all the followers of Buddha was only natural. Accordingly, in their teachings our earth, and every other, has its Sumeru, around which everything centres.[2] Its top, according to the Nyâyânousâra Shaster, is four-square, and on it are situated the three and thirty (Trayastriñshas) heavens. Each face of the summit measures 80,000 yôjanas. Each of the four corners of the mountain-top has a peak seven hundred yôjanas high. These, of course, are simply the four buttress-mountains of the Hindu Meru lifted to the summit and made the culminating

---

[1] Chapter xii., sections 45–74. On the origin and age of this treatise see the notes of the translator, Rev. Ebenezer Burgess, in the *Journal of the American Oriental Society*, vol. vi. New Haven, 1860 : pp. 140–480.

[2] Its name, in Japanese, is written *Sxi-meru ;* in Chinese, *Si-mi-liu*, or *Siu-mi ;* in Tibetan, *Rirap*, or *Ri-rap-hlumpo ;* in Mongolian (Kalmuck), *Sümmer Sola*, or *Sjumer Sula ;* in Burmese, *Miem-mo.* C. F. Koeppen, *Die Religion des Buddhas.* Berlin, 1857 : vol. i., p. 232. See, also, A. Bastian, *Die Völker des östlichen Asiens*, Bd. iii., S. 352, 353; vi., 567, 568, 578, 580, 587, 589, 590. Spence Hardy, *Manual of Buddhism*, pp. 1–35. The same, *Legends of the Buddhists.* London, 1866 : pp. xxix., 42, 81, 101, 176, etc.

peaks. They are ornamented, we are told, with the seven precious substances, — gold, silver, lapis-lazuli, crystal, cornelian, coral, and ruby. One of the cities on the summit is called Sudarsana, or Belle-vue. It is 10,000 yôjanas in circuit. The storied gates are 1½ yôjanas high, and there are 1,000 of these gates, fully adorned. Each gate has 500 blue-clad celestial guards, fully armed. In its centre is a kind of inner city called the Golden City of King Sakra, whose pavilion is 1,000 yôjanas in circuit, and its floor is of pure gold, inlaid with every kind of gem. This royal residence has 500 gates, and on each of the four sides are 100 towers, within each of which there are 1,700 chambers, each of which chambers has within it seven Devîs, and each Devî is attended by seven handmaidens. All these Devîs are consorts of King Sakra, with whom he has intercourse in different forms and personations, according to his pleasure. The length and breadth of the thirty-three heavens is 60,000 yôjanas. They are surrounded by a sevenfold city wall, a sevenfold ornamental railing, a sevenfold row of tinkling curtains, and beyond these a sevenfold row of Talas-trees. All these encircle one another, and are of every color of the rainbow, intermingled and composed of every precious substance. Within, every sort of enjoyment and every enchanting pleasure is provided for the occupants.

Outside this wonderful city of the gods, there is on each of its four sides a park of ravishing beauty. In each park there is a sacred tower erected over personal relics of Buddha. Each park has also a magic lake, filled with water possessing eight peculiar excellences. Thus beauties are heaped upon beauties, splendors upon splendors, marvels upon marvels, until in sheer despair the wearied and exhausted imagination abandons all further effort at definite mental representation.[1]

It is worthy of note that, while most scholars have supposed the Sumeru of Buddhism to be simply a development of the Indian idea, Mr. Beal, a high authority, has, in one of his latest publications, claimed for it an independent and coördinate, if not primitive, character.[2] Other peculiarities in Buddhist cosmography, especially the detachment of Uttara-kuru and of Jambu-dwîpa from Mount Meru, — in both of which particulars the Buddhist cosmos differs from the Puranic, — lend some apparent confirmation to this claim.

In ancient Iranian thought this same celestial mountain presents itself to the student. Its name is Harâ-berezaiti, the mythical Albordj,[3] — "the seat of the genii : around it revolve sun, moon, and stars ; over it leads the path of the blessed to heaven."[4]

---

[1] See Beal, *Catena of Buddhist Scriptures*, pp. 75–81. Comp. Beal, *Lectures on Buddhist Literature in China*, pp. 146–159.

[2] "I cannot doubt that the Buddhist myth about Sume or Sumeru is distinct from the later Brahmanical account of it, and allied with the universal belief in and adoration of the highest." — *Buddhist Literature in China*. London, 1882 : p. xv.

[3] "Das erste Vorkommen des Namens im Zend ist im Gebet an Mithra (invoco, celebro supremum umbilicum aquarum, nach Duperrons Uebersetzung) welches E. Burnouf wortgetreuer übersetzt : 'Ich preise den hohen göttlichen Berggipfel, die Quelle der Wasser, und das Wasser des Ormuzd,' wo die Bezeichnung eine ganz allgemeine ist. Vom Adjectiv *berezat*, d. i. 'erhaben' in der Parsen Uebersetzung, stammt erst der '*Bordj*,' d. i. *der Erhabene*. Als Berg aus dem die Wasser hervortreten, wird er im Zend '*Nafedrô*' (*Nabhi* im Sanskrit.) d. i. '*der Nabel*' genannt, als Erhöhung welche Wasser giebt ; und als Berg der das befruchtende Princip enthält zum Genius der Frauen erhoben." — Ritter, *Erdkunde*, viii. 47.

[4] Spiegel, *Erânische Alterthumskunde*. Leipsic, 1871 : Bd. i., S. 463. *The Venîdâd.* Fargard xxi., *et passim*. See references in Index

The following description of it in one of the invocations of Rashnu in the Rashn Yasht forcibly reminds one of the Odyssean description of the heavenly Olympos : " Whether thou, O holy Rashnu, art on the Harâ-berezaiti, the bright mountain around which the many stars revolve, where come neither night nor darkness, no cold wind and no hot wind, no deathful sickness, no uncleanness made by the Daêvas, and the clouds cannot reach up to the Haraiti Bareza ; we invoke, we bless Rashnu." [1]

The following description is from Lenormant : " Like the Meru of the Indians, Harâ-berezaiti is the Pole, the centre of the world, the fixed point around which the sun and the planets perform their revolutions.   Analogously to the Gangâ of the Brahmans, it possesses the celestial fountain Ardvî-Sûra, the mother of all terrestrial waters and the source of all good things.   In the midst of the lake formed by the waters of the sacred source grows a single miraculous tree, similar to the Jambu of the Indian myth, or else two trees, corresponding exactly to those of the Biblical Gan-Eden. . . . There is the garden of Ahuramazda, like that of Brahma on Meru. Thence the waters descend toward the four cardinal points in four large streams, which symbolize the four horses attached to the car of the goddess of the sacred source, Ardvî - Sûra - Anâhita.   These four horses recall the four animals placed at the source of the paradisaic rivers in the Indian conception." [2]

to *Pahlevi Texts*, translated by E. W. West.   Vol. v. of *Sacred Books of the East*.   Also Haug, *Religion of the Parsees*.   2d ed., Boston, 1878 : pp. 5, 190, 197, 203-205, 216, 255, 286, 316, 337, 361, 381, 387, 390.

[1] Darmesteter, *The Zend-Avesta*, ii. 174.

[2] " Ararat and Eden." *The Contemporary Review*, September, 1881,

The Hellenic and Roman myths concerning the "World-mountain" were numerous, but in later times not a little confused, as Ideler has learnedly shown.[1] By some, as for example Aristotle, it was identified with the Caucasus, and it was asserted that its height was so prodigious that after sunset its head was illuminated a third part of the night, and again a third part before the rising of the sun in the morning. This identification explains the later legend, according to which, in order to prove his rightful lordship of the world, Alexander the Great plucked "the shadowless lance" (the earth's axis) out of the topmost peak of the Taurus Mountains.[2] More commonly the mount is called Atlas, or the Atlantic mountain. Proclus, quoting Heraclitus, says of it, "Its magnitude is such that it touches the ether and casts a shadow of five thousand stadia in length. From the ninth hour of the day the sun is concealed by it, even to his perfect demersion under

Am. ed., p. 41. Compare the following : " L'Albordj des Perses correspond parfaitement au Merou des Hindous ; de même que la tradition de ceux-ce divise la terre en sept Dwipas ou isles, de même les livres zends et pehlvis reconnaissent sept *Keschvars* ou contrées groupées également autour de la montagne sainte," etc. — *Religions de l'Antiquité.* Creuzer, trad. Guigniaut. Tom. I., pt. ii., p. 702, note.

[1] On the Homeric and Hesiodic Olympos, see below, part sixth, chapter second.

[2] " Auch in den Alexandersagen des Mittelalters ist die Erinnerung an das Naturcentrum im Nordpol erhalten, und zwar in merkwürdiger Uebereinstimmung der morgen- und abendländischer Dichter. In dem altenglischen Gedicht von Alisaunder (bei Jacobs und Uckert, S. 461) findet Alexander der Grosse auf dem höchsten Gipfel des Taurus eine schattenlose Lanze, von welcher geweissagt war, wer sie aus dem Boden reissen könne, werde Herr der Welt werden. Alexander aber riss sie heraus. Die Lanze ist ein Sinnbild der Weltachse. Sie weist vom höchsten Berge auf den Nordpol hin, und ist schattenlos weil von dort ursprünglich alles Licht ausging." — Menzel, *Die vorchristliche Unsterblichkeitslehre*, Bd. i., S. 86.

the earth." [1] Strabo's account of it is full of the legendary features characteristic of an earthly Paradise. The olive - trees were of extraordinary excellence, and there were there seven varieties of refreshing wine. He informs us that the grape clusters were a cubit in length, and the vine-trunks sometimes so thick that two men could scarcely clasp round one of them. Herodotus describes the mountain as "very tapering and round ; so lofty, moreover, that the top (they say) cannot be seen, the clouds never quitting it either summer or winter. The natives call this mountain ' *The Pillar of Heaven,*' and they themselves take their name from it, being called Atlantes. They are reported not to eat any living thing and never to have any dreams." [2] Equally strange is the story told by Maximus Tyrius, according to which the waves of the ocean at high water stopped short before the sacred mount, "standing up like a wall around its base, though unrestrained by any earthly barrier." " Nothing but the air and the sacred thicket prevent the water from reaching the mountain." According to other ancient legends, a river of milk descended from this marvelous height. Noticing such curious stories, Pliny well describes the mountain as *fabulosissimum.* [3]

[1] See Taylor's *Notes on Pausanias*, vol. iii., p. 264.

[2] Herodotus, Bk. iv. 184.

[3] "When Cleanthes asserted that the earth was in the shape of a cone, this, in my opinion, is to be understood only of this mountain, called Meru in India. Anaximenes said that this column was plain and of stone : exactly like the *Meru-pargwette* of the inhabitants of Ceylon, according to Mr. Joinville in the seventh volume of the *Asiatic Researches*. This mountain, says he, is entirely of stone, 68,000 yôjanas high, and 10,000 in circumference from top to bottom. The divines of Tibet say it is square, and like an inverted pyramid. Some

Everywhere, therefore, in the most ancient ethnic thought, — in the Egyptian, Akkadian, Assyrian, Babylonian, Indian, Persian, Chinese, and Greek, — everywhere is encountered this conception of what, looked at with respect to its base and magnitude, is called the "Mountain of the World," but looked at with respect to its glorious summit and its celestial inhabitants is styled the "Mountain of the Gods." We need not pursue the investigation further. Enough has been said to warrant the assertion of Dr. Samuel Beal: "It is plain that this idea of a lofty central primeval mountain belonged to the undivided human race." [1] Elsewhere the same learned sinologue has said, "I have no doubt — I can have none — that the idea of a central mountain, and of the rivers flowing from it, and the abode of the gods upon its summit, is a primitive myth derived from the earliest traditions of our race." [2]

The ideas of the ancients respecting the Underworld, that is the southern hemisphere of the earth beyond the equatorial ocean, are sufficiently set forth in the writer's essay on "Homer's Abode of the Dead," printed in the Appendix of the present work.[3]

In all these studies one important caution has too often been overlooked. In interpreting the cosmological and geographical references of ancient religious writings it should never be forgotten that the ideas expressed are often poetical and symbolical, —

---

of the followers of Buddha in India insist that it is like a drum, with a swell in the middle, like drums in India ; and formerly in the West, Leucippus said the same thing." — F. Wilford, in *Asiatic Researches,* vol. viii., p. 273.

[1] *Buddhist Literature in China,* p. 147.

[2] Ibid., p. xiv.

[3] See APPENDIX, Sect. VI.

religious ideas, hallowed in sacred song and story. If, some thousands of years hence, one of Macaulay's archæologists of New Zealand were to try to ascertain and set forth the geographical knowledge of the Christian England of to-day by a study of a few fragments of English hymns of our period, critically examining every expression about a certain wonderful mountain, located sometimes on earth and sometimes in heaven, and bearing the varying name of "Sion" or "Zion;" then making a microscopical study of all the references to the strange river, which according to the same texts would seem to be variously represented as "dark," and as possessed of "stormy banks," and as "rolling between" the singer living in England and the abode of the dead located in Western Asia, and called "Canaan,"—a river sometimes addressed and represented as so miraculously discriminating as to know for whom to divide itself, letting them cross over "dry shod,"—surely, under such a process of interpretation, even the England of the nineteenth century would make in geographical science a very sorry showing. Or again, if some Schliemann of a far-off future were to excavate the site of one of the dozen American villages known by the name of "Eden," and, finding unequivocal monumental evidence that it was thus called, were thereupon to conclude and teach that the Americans of the date of that village *believed* its site to be the true site of the Eden of Sacred History, and that here the race of man originated, this would be a grave mistake, but it would be a mistake precisely similar to many an one which has been committed by *our* archæologists in interpreting and reconstructing the geography of the ancients.

In concluding this sketch of ancient cosmology one further question naturally and inevitably thrusts itself upon us. It is this : How are the rise and the so wide diffusion of this singular world-view to be explained ? In other words, how came it to pass that the ancestors of the oldest historic races and peoples agreed to regard the North Pole as the true summit of the earth and the circumpolar sky as the true heaven ? Why were Hades and the lowest hell adjusted to a south polar nadir ? The one and sole satisfactory explanation is found in the hypothesis of a primitive north polar Eden. *Studied from that standpoint*, the appearances of the universe would be exactly adapted to produce this curious cosmological conception. Thus the very system of ancient thought respecting the world betrays the point of view from which the world was first contemplated. This, though an indirect evidence of the truth of our hypothesis, is for this very reason all the more convincing.

CHAPTER II.

THE CRADLE OF THE RACE IN ANCIENT JAPANESE THOUGHT.

According to the most ancient texts Japan is the centre of the earth. — W. E. GRIFFIS.

ACCORDING to the earliest cosmogony of the Japanese, as given in their most ancient book, the Ko-ji-ki,[1] the creators and first inhabitants of our world were a god and goddess, Izanagi and Izanani by name. These, in the beginning, — we quote from Sir Edward Reed, — "standing on the bridge of heaven, pushed down a spear into the green plain of the sea, and stirred it round and round. When they drew it up the drops which fell from its end consolidated and became an island. The sun-born pair descended on to the island, and planting a spear in the ground, point downwards, built a palace round it, taking that for the central roof-pillar. The spear

[1] Speaking of this work, M. Léon de Rosny calls it l'un des monuments les plus authentiques de la vieille littérature japonaise, and says, "Nous devons non seulement à cet ouvrage la connaissance de l'histoire du Nippon antérieure au vii. siècle de notre ère, mais l'exposé le plus autorisé de l'antique mythologie sintauïste. Il y a même ce fait remarquable, que les dieux primordiaux du panthéon japonais, mentionnés dans ce livre, ne figurent déjà plus au commencement du *Yamato bumi*, qui est postérieur seulement de quelques années à la publication du *Ko ji ki*. Ces dieux primordiaux paraissent oubliés, ou tout au moins négligés, dans les ouvrages indigènes qui ont paru par la suite." *Questions d'Archéologie Japonaise.* Paris, 1882 : p. 3. An English translation of the Ko-ji-ki, by B. H. Chamberlain, has just appeared in *Transactions of the Asiatic Society of Japan*, vol. v.

became *the axis of the earth,* which had been caused to revolve by the stirring round." [1]

This island, however, was the Japanese Eden. Here originated the human race. Its name was Onogorojima, "The Island of the Congealed Drop." Its first roof-pillar, as we have seen, was the axis of the earth. Over it was "the pivot of the vault of heaven." [2] Mr. Reed, who has no theory on the subject to maintain, says, "The island must have been situated at the Pole of the earth." [3] In like manner, with no idea of the vast anthropological significance and value of the datum, Mr. Griffis remarks, "The island formed by the congealed drops was once at the North Pole, but has since been taken to its present position in the Inland Sea." [4]

Here, then, is the testimony of the most ancient

---

[1] Sir Edward J. Reed, *Japan,* vol. i., 31.

[2] Léon Metchnikoff, *L'Empire Japonais.* Genève, 1881 : p. 265.

[3] Ibid. — Our interpretation of ancient cosmology and of the true Eden location at once brings light into the whole system of Japanese mythology. In the following, extracted from Mr. Griffis, no one has ever before known what to make of "*the Pillar of Heaven and Earth,*" "*the Bridge of Heaven,*" the position of primitive Japan "*on the top of the globe,*" and at the same time at "*the centre of the Earth :*" — "The first series of children born were the islands of Japan. . . . Japan lies on the top of the globe. . . . At this time heaven and earth were very close to each other, and the goddess Amaterazu being a rare and beautiful child, whose body shone brilliantly, Izanagi sent her up the Pillar that united heaven and earth, and bade her rule over the high plain of heaven. . . . As the earth-gods and evil deities multiplied, confusion and discord reigned, which the sun goddess (Amaterazu), seeing, resolved to correct by sending her grandson Ninigi to earth to rule over it. Accompanied by a great retinue of deities, he descended by means of the floating Bridge of Heaven, on which the divine first pair had stood, to Mount Kirishima. After his descent, heaven and earth, which had already separated to a considerable distance, receded utterly, and further communication ceased. . . . According to the most ancient texts Japan is the centre of the earth."

[4] McClintock and Strong, *Cyclopædia,* vol. ix., p. 688. Art. "Shinto."

Japanese tradition. Nothing could be more un-equivocal. Izanagi's divinely precious spear of jade,[1] like the transverse jade-tube of the ancient Shû King,[2] is an imperishable index, not only to the astronomical attainments of prehistoric humanity, but also to humanity's prehistoric abode.

In Part fifth, chapter fourth, further illustration of the Japanese conception of the origin of their race will be given.

[1] Émile Burnouf, " La pique céleste de jade rouge." — *La Mythologie des Japonais d'après le Kokŭ-si-Ryakŭ.* Paris, 1875 : p. 6.

[2] " He examined the pearl-adorned turning sphere, with its transverse tube of jade, and reduced to a harmonious system the movements of the Seven Directors." Legge's Translation in *The Sacred Books of the East*, vol. iii., p. 38. Professor Legge once examined this passage in my presence, and found unexpected corroboration of the interpretation which identifies " the transverse tube of jade " with the axis of heaven.

CHAPTER III.

THE CRADLE OF THE RACE IN CHINESE THOUGHT.

The rationalistic genius of the matter-of-fact Chinese is apparent even in the way in which they conceived their primitive history ; and in this respect, as in many others, it brings them into nearer relations with the best modern science than belong to the other Oriental races. — SAMUEL JOHNSON (of Salem).

It is through this wonderfully pure seer [Lao-tse], as it appears to me, that we ascend to the primitive revelation of truth given to this ancient people. — WILLIAM HENRY CHANNING.

APPROACHING this theme, a reviewer of the *Shin Seën Tung Kcën* — a " General Account of the Gods and Genii," in twenty-two volumes — offers the following observations : " All nations have some tradition of a Paradise, a place of primeval happiness, a state of innocence and delight. The Tauists [1] are by no means behind in referring to an abode of lasting bliss, which, however, still exists on earth. It is called Kwen-lun." [2]

In another article, by a student of Chinese sources, it is stated, " This locality, being the abode of the gods, is Paradise ; it is round in form, and like Eden it is ' the mount of assembly.' " [3]

Like the Gan-Eden of Genesis it is described as a

---

[1] " Die Secte der Tao-sse hat die Sagen und religiösen Gebräuche des alten China's noch am Meisten aufbewahrt." Lüken, *Traditionen des Menschengeschlechtes*, p. 77. " Lao-tse abounds in sentences out of some ancient lore, of which we have no knowledge but from him." Samuel Johnson, *Oriental Religions — China.* Boston, 1877: p. 861.

[2] *The Chinese Repository*, vol. vii., p. 519.

[3] *The Chinese Recorder and Missionary Journal*, vol. iv., p. 94. Compare Isaiah xiv. 13, 14.

garden, with a marvelous tree in the midst ; also with a fountain of immortality, from which proceed four rivers, which flow in opposite directions toward the four quarters of the earth.[1]

In the language of the writer first quoted in this chapter, "Sparkling fountains and purling streams contain the far-famed ambrosia.   One may there rest on flowery carpeted swards, listening to the melodious warbling of birds, or feasting upon the delicious fruits, at once fragrant and luscious, which hang from the branches of the luxuriant groves. Whatever there is beautiful in landscape or grand in nature may also be found there in the highest state of perfection.   All is charming, all enchanting, and whilst Nature smiles the company of genii delights the ravished visitor." [2]

Where, now, is this Paradise mountain located ? At the North Pole.

The sentence before those last quoted reads as follows : " Here is the great pillar that sustains the world, no less than 300,000 miles high."

This world-pillar, or axis of the earth, is sometimes conceived of as slender enough for the use of a climber.   Thus we read, " One of the Chinese kings, anxious to become acquainted with the delightful spot, set out in search of it.   After much wandering he perceived the immense column spoken of, but, trying to ascend it, he found it so slippery that he had to abandon all hopes of gaining his end, and to endeavor by some mountain road which was rugged in the extreme to find his way to Paradise. When almost fainting with fatigue, some friendly

[1] Lüken, *Traditionen des Menschengeschlechtes*, p. 72.
[2] *The Chinese Repository*, vol. vii., p. 519.

nymphs, who had all the time from an eminence compassionated the weary wanderer, lent him an assisting hand. He arrived there, and immediately began to examine the famous spot."[1]

Such a pillar connecting the earth with an upper Paradise, and affording a means of access thereto, necessarily recalls to mind the analogous conception set forth in the Talmud : "There is an upper and a lower Paradise. And between them, upright, is fixed a pillar ; and by this they are joined together ; and 't is called 'The Strength of the Hill of Sion.' And by this Pillar on every Sabbath and Festival the righteous climb up and feed themselves with a glance of the Divine majesty till the end of the Sabbath or Festival, when they slide down and return into the lower Paradise."[2]

In this conception we have a twofold Paradise, one celestial and one terrestrial. Among the Chinese

---

[1] *The Chinese Repository*, vol. vii., p. 520.

[2] Eisenmenger, *Entdecktes Judenthum*, Bd. ii., p. 318. (English translation, vol. ii., p. 25.) Compare Schulthess, *Das Paradies*, p. 354. Also the story of Er, the Pamphylian, in which we have the same "*column, brighter than the rainbow, extending right through the whole heaven and through the earth ;*" here also the spirits visiting the earth are allowed seven days before ascending. Plato, *Republic*, 616. Also the Chaldæo-Assyrian conception of "the celestial and terrestrial Paradises, supposed to be united by means of the Paradisaic Mount itself." *The Oriental and Biblical Journal.* Chicago, 1880 : p. 173. Also the Greek idea : "Sehr merkwürdig ist, was Pindar (Olymp., ii., 56 f.) von den Seligen sagt. Wenn sie nämlich auf der Insel der Seligen sich befinden, steigen sie zum *Thurme des Chronos* empor. Dieser Höhentendenz entspricht nun die alte Vorstellung vom Naturcentrum am Nordpol und so führen uns denn auch die griechischen Dichter auf einem langen Umwege doch zuletzt nach Nysa, wo uns die griechischen Künstler alle Wonnen des dionysischen Himmels aufthun." Menzel, *Die vorchristliche Unsterblichkeitslehre*, ii., p. 10. Finally, the Japanese idea in Griffis, *The Mikado's Empire*, p. 44.

we find the same. The upper is situated in the centre or pole of heaven, the lower directly under it, at the centre or pole of the northern terrestrial hemisphere. The Pillar connecting them is of course the axis of the heavenly vault.

We quote : " Within the seas, in the valleys of Kwen-lun, at the northwest is Shang-te's *Lower* Recreation Palace. It is eight hundred *le* square, and eighty thousand feet high. In front there are nine walls, inclosed by a fence of precious stones. At the sides there are nine doors, through which the light streams, and it is guarded by beasts. Shang-te's wife also dwells in this region, immediately over which is Shang-te's Heavenly Palace, which is situated in the centre of the heavens [the celestial pole], as his earthly one is in the centre of the earth [the terrestrial pole]." [1]

There can be no mistaking this use of the term "centre" for pole, for the Chinese astronomers expressly state, " The Polar star is the centre of heaven." [2]

Elsewhere, instead of Kwen-lun being a World-pillar in the " valleys," or " plain," or "mound" of the terrestrial Paradise, we find it described as a stupendous heaven-sustaining mountain, marking the centre or pole of the earth : " The four quarters of the earth incline downwards. . . . On this vast plain or mount, surrounded on all sides by the four seas, arise the mountains of Kwen-lun, the highest in the world according to the Chinese geographers : ' Kwen-

---

[1] *The Chinese Recorder*, vol. iv., p. 95.

[2] *The Chinese Repository*, vol. iv., p. 194. Compare Menzel : " Der Polarstern heisst Palast der Mitte." *Unsterblichkeitslehre*, Bd. i., p. 44.

lun is the name of a mountain ; it is situated at the northwest, fifty thousand *le* from the Sung-Kaou mountains, and is *the centre of the earth.* It is eleven thousand *le* in height ' (Kang-he)." [1]

The significance of the foregoing as respects the location of Paradise cannot be doubtful. But compare further the sixth head under chapter third of Part fifth ; also chapter fourth of the same Part.

[1] *The Chinese Recorder*, vol. iv., p. 94.

CHAPTER IV.

THE CRADLE OF THE RACE IN EAST ARYAN OR HINDU THOUGHT.

The reader cannot have failed to be struck, as the first explorers of Sanskrit literature have been, with the close analogy, we might even say the perfect identity, of all the essential features of the typical description of Mount Meru in the Puranas with the topography of Eden in the second chapter of Genesis. The garden of Eden (gan-Eden), the garden of God (gan-Elohim, Ezek. xxviii. 13), which is guarded by the anointed and protecting Kerub (Ezek. xxviii. 14, 16), is placed, like the garden of delight of the gods of India, on the summit of a mountain, the holy mountain of God (har qodesh Elohim (Ezek. xxviii. 14, 16), all sparkling with precious stones (Ibid.).[1] — LENORMANT.

IN what kind of a world lived the ancient Brahman? And what was his conception of the location of the cradle of the race?

One of the oldest of the elaborate geographical treatises of India is the Vishnu Purana. Taking this as a guide, let us place ourselves alongside one of the ancients of the country, and look about us.

First, we will look to the South, far down the Indian Ocean. What was supposed to lie in that

---

[1] The continuation of the passage is as follows: "The Jehovistic writer does not say so in Genesis, but the prophets are express in this respect. The tree of life grows 'in the midst of the garden' (*bethoch haggan*) with the tree of the knowledge of good and evil (Gen. ii. 9; iii. 3), exactly like the tree Jambu, in the centre of the delightful plateau which crowns the height of Meru. A river goes out of Eden to water the garden, and from thence it divides and forms four arms (Gen. ii. 10). This corresponds in the most precise manner with the way in which the spring Gangâ, after having watered the Celestial Land, or the Land of Joy at the summit of Meru, forms four lakes on the four counterforts of this holy mountain, whence it afterwards flows out in four large rivers toward the four cardinal points."

direction? To begin with their distribution of the different quarters of the world among the gods, this is the quarter belonging to Yama, the god of the dead : —

> "May he whose hands the thunder wield
> Be in the East thy guard and shield ;
> May Yama's care the South befriend,
> And Varun's arm the West defend ;
> And let Kuvera, lord of gold,
> The North with firm protection hold." [1]

In precise accordance with our Key to Ancient Cosmology, it is the direction of descent. North is upwards (*uttarāt*), south is downwards (*adharāt*).[2] Hence the abode and kingdom of Yama is not only to the south, but also below the level of India, *i. e.*, on the under hemisphere, or, as Monier Williams locates it, in "the lower world." [3] All Hindu literature is full of similar references. The exact time required for the soul's journey was supposed to be four hours and forty minutes.[4]

In this direction, evidently, we shall vainly seek a paradise. Let us turn to the North and "ascend."

---

[1] Griffiths, *Ramayana*, ii. 20.

[2] Zimmer, *Altindisches Leben.* Berlin, 1879 : p. 359.

[3] Yama: "one of the eight guardians of the world as regent of the South quarter, in which direction in some region of the lower world is his abode called Yama-pura ; thither a soul, when it leaves the body, is said to repair, and there, after the recorder, Citra-gupta, has read an account of its actions, kept in a book called Agra-Sandānī, receives a just sentence, either ascending to heaven, or to the world of the Pitris, or being driven down to one of the twenty-one hells." — Williams, *Sanskrit Dictionary*, sub. "Yama."

[4] "The soul is believed to reach Yama's abode in four hours and forty minutes ; consequently a dead body cannot be burned until that time has passed after death." — W. J. Wilkins, *Hindu Mythology, Vedic and Puranic.* London, 1882 : Art. "Yama." See, also, Muir, *Sanskrit Texts*, v. 284-327, and our references in "Homer's Abode of the Dead."

First, of course, we come to the Himalaya range, the *Himavat* of Indian geography. All that portion of the earth lying between this mountain range and the great ocean to the South constitutes one of the seven, or nine, "varshas," or divisions of the habitable (upper) hemisphere. Its name is Bhârata. If now our ancient Hindu could proceed due North and cross the Himavat, — which he does not think possible to mortals, — he would find himself in Kimpurusha, an equally extensive but more elevated and beautiful varsha, extending northward till bounded by a second range of incredibly lofty mountains, the Himakuta. Still "ascending," or going North, until he had crossed this division and passed the Himakuta, he would enter Harivarsha, a still loftier and diviner country. This extends, in turn, to another boundary range, the Nishadha, crossing which one would come to Ilâvrita, the central varsha of all, which occupies the top as well as the centre of the world. To the adequate description of the beauty and glory and preciousness of this country no tongue is equal. In its centre is situated the mount of the gods, "Beautiful Meru," described in chapter first of the present Part. It is at the Pole, and around it revolve all constellations of heaven. It is the centre of the habitable world.

Continuing our imaginary journey across this divine country of Ilâvrita, crossing of course this colossal central mountain, we should now begin to descend on the meridian opposite to that on which we ascended on the India side of the globe. The boundary of the central region on that side is the Nila range, then comes the varsha of Rumyâka ; its farther boundary is the Sweta range, beyond which is the varsha of Hiranmâya. Still descending, we cross this and the range which bounds it on the farther side, the Sringin, and we are in Uttarakuru, the last of the seven grand divisions of the earth, the one corresponding, in distance from Meru, to Bhârata, or our starting-point. It, of course, is on the equatorial ocean, and here too we have only to cross this ocean in order to reach the underworld.

The way in which the varshas are made to number "nine" is by subdividing the great central cross-section of the hemispherical surface, leaving Ilâvrita a perfect square on the top of the globe, the land descending eastward to the sea being called Bhadrâsva, and the corresponding country to the West being called Ketumâlâ.

To assist the reader to a clearer conception of this sacred geography we give herewith two cuts, one of which presents in outline the side-aspect of the Puranic earth, and the other a flat polocentric projection of its upper hemisphere.[1]

Having now answered our first question, and showed in what kind of a world the ancient Hindu lived, we pass to the second : "What was his conception of the location of the cradle of the race?"

The question is answered the moment we say that in the Hindu conception and tradition man proceeded from Meru. His Eden-land was Ilâvrita. It was therefore at the Pole.

How strange that Lenormant could have written the following, and still have imagined that the true primeval Eden of the Hindu was anywhere else than at the terrestrial Pole! He says, " In all the leg-

[1] See also APPENDIX, Sect. IV., "The Earth and the World of the Hindus."

ends of India the origin of mankind is placed on Mount Meru, the residence of the gods, a column which unites the sky to the earth. . . . At first sight, on reading the description of Mount Meru furnished by the Puranas, it appears overcharged with so many purely mythological features that one hesi-

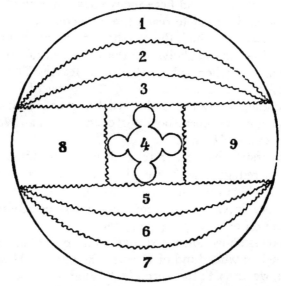

The Earth of the Hindus, viewed from above.

1. Uttarakuru. 5. Harivarsha.
2. Hiranmâya. 6. Kimpurusha.
3. Ramyâka. 7. Bhârata (India).
8. Ketumâlâ. 9. Bhadrâsva.
4 Su-meru in Ilâvrita.

tates to believe that it has any basis in reality. To realize these descriptions one must represent one's self in the centre of a vast level and very elevated surface, surrounded by various mountain-ranges, a gigantic block, *the axis of the world*, raising its head to the highest point of the heavens, whence there

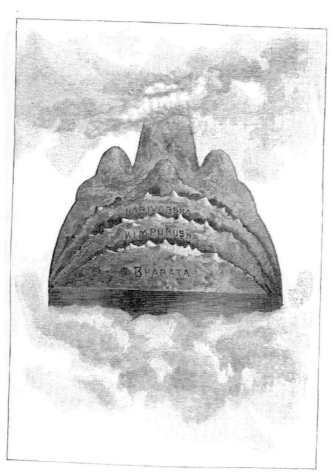

THE EARTH OF THE HINDUS

Side View of Upper Hemisphere.

falls upon its summit, *on the North Pole,* the divine
Gangâ, the source of all rivers, which there discharges itself into an ideal lake, the Mânasa-Sâro-
vara. . . . Meru, then, is at one and the same time
the highest part of the terrestrial world and the central point of the visible heaven, — the two having
been confounded through ignorance [1] of the real
constitution of the universe: it is also, at one and
the same time, *the north pole and the centre of the
habitable earth,* Jambu-dwîpa, — literally of the continent of the tree Jambu, the tree of life. Leaving
the higher basin of the mountain in which its waters have at first collected the source, Gangâ travels
seven times round the Meru in descending from the
abode of the seven Rishis of the Great Bear, to
empty itself afterward into four lakes placed on four
summits adjacent to this vast pyramid, and serving
as buttresses on its four sides. . . . Fed by the
waters of the celestial Gangâ the four lakes in
their turn feed four terrestrial rivers which flow out
through the mouths of four symbolical animals.
These four great rivers water as many distinct regions, . . . and discharge themselves into four opposite seas, to the east, south, west, and north of the
central Meru. . . . The four lakes, the four rivers,
and the four oceans are composed of different liq-
uids, corresponding to the four castes, and these
latter, with which are connected all the nations of
the human race, are reputed to have set out from
the four sides of Meru to people the whole earth." [2]

[1] Lenormant here follows the misleading arguments of Wilford in
Asiatic Researches, vol. viii., pp. 312, 313.

[2] *The Contemporary Review,* Sept., 1881 : Am. ed., p. 39. Also
Les Origines de l'Histoire, tom. ii. 1, ch. i. Compare *Essai de Com-
mentaire des Fragments Cosmogoniques de Bérose.* Paris, 1871 : pp.

A similar illustration of the power of a wrong prepossession is given us in the illustrious Carl Ritter, who after expressly declaring that "the numberless Puranas and their most diverse interpretations by the Pundits teach that *Meru is the middle of the earth,* and itself literally designates its *centre and axis,*" [1] thereupon in the coolest manner imaginable proceeds to identify the same sacred height with the mountains of Central Asia. Still worse is the procedure of Mr. Massey, who after locating the Garden of Eden on Mount Meru, and saying explicitly, " *The Pole, or polar region, is Meru,*" and again, " *Meru is the garden of the Tree of Life,*" nevertheless tells us that in equatorial Africa beasts first grew into men. [2] Happier is the inconsistency of Mr. Lillie, who, despite his adhesion to the flat-earth theory of Hindu cosmology, still incidentally speaks of "the blissful Garden" as "at the Pole." [3]

300–328. Also Muir, *Sanskrit Texts,* vol. ii., p. 139. "In his *Indische Studien,* vol. i., p. 165, Weber speaks of the Aryan Indians being *driven by a deluge* from their home, and coming from the North, not from the West (as Lassen, i., 515 will have it), into India."

[1] "Die zahllosen Puranas und ihre verschiedenartigsten Auslegungen durch die Pundits lehren, dass Meru die Mitte der Erde sei, und selbst wörtlich auch das Centrum, die Axe, bezeichne." — *Erdkunde,* Bd. ii., p. 7.

[2] *The Natural Genesis,* vol. ii., pp. 28, 162.

[3] *Buddha and Early Buddhism.* London, 1882 : p. 8.

CHAPTER V.

THE CRADLE OF THE RACE IN IRANIAN, OR OLD-PERSIAN, THOUGHT.

Aus den Angaben über die Paradiesströme und den Lauf derselben erhellt nun auch, wo wir das Paradies selbst zu suchen haben, nämlich im äussersten Norden.— FR. SPIEGEL.

ACCORDING to the sacred books of the ancient Persians all the five-and-twenty races of men which people the seven "keshvares" of the earth descended from one primitive pair, whose names were Mâshyoi and Mâshya. The abode of this primitive pair was in the keshvare Kvanîras, the central and the fairest of the seven.[1] Let us see if we can determine its location.

As a key to the old Iranian conception of the world let us investigate the nature and location of the "Chinvat bridge." This, like the Bifröst of the Northmen and the Al Sirat of Islam, is the bridge on which the souls of the dead, the evil as well as the good, leave this world to enter the unseen.[2] The investigation is in itself and for its own sake full of interest, for no writer on the ideas and faith of the

---

[1] *Bundahish*, ch. xv., 1–30.

[2] "This," says Professor Rawlinson, "is evidently the original of Mohammed's famous 'way extended over the middle of hell, which is sharper than a sword and finer than a hair, over which all must pass.'" *Ancient Monarchies*, vol. ii., p. 339 n. Compare Sale's *Koran*, Prelim. Discourse, Sect. iv. Professor Tiele thinks "it was borrowed from the old Aryan mythology," and that it "was probably originally the rainbow." *History of Religion*. London and Boston, 1877 : p. 177.

Mazdaeans has ever professed to be able to tell either the origin or true meaning of the myth. Most interpreters have either carefully abstained from all attempts at explanation, or have suggested that it probably refers to the rainbow or to the Milky Way, or to both.[1] To dispose of these suggestions, let us raise a few questions : —

1. Do we find in any part of the Avestan literature any evidence that the Chinvat Bridge possessed a curvilinear form ?

None.

2. Straight, or curved as a whole, were its two ends conceived of as on a common level?

No, for motion upon it in one direction is described as upward, and in the opposite direction as downward.

3. Where was the upper end ?

In the heaven of Ahura Mazda, the Supreme God, to whose abode the bridge conducts good souls.

4. But where is this abode ?

At the Northern Pole of the sky, as elsewhere shown.

5. Where is the earthward end ?

It rests upon "the Daitîk peak."

6. Is this peak in Persia ?

No ; it is part of a sacred mountain in Aîrân-vej, the Eden of Iranian tradition.

7. And where is Aîrân-vej ?

"In the middle of the world."

---

1 "The Bridge of Souls cannot be always the Milky Way. . . . Supposing the myths which once belonged to the Milky Way to have been passed on to the Rainbow, the name of the former might also have been inherited by the latter." C. F. Keary, *Primitive Belief.* Lond., 1882 : p. 292. Comp. pp. 286–294, 347. Also Justi, *Handbuch der Zendsprache.* Leipsic, 1864 : p. 111, *sub voce* "Cinvañt."

8. In what keshvare?

In Kvanîras, the central of the seven divisions of the earth, and the one in which men and the good religion were first created.

9. And in what direction from Persia was Aîrân-vej supposed to lie?

Far to the North.

10. What natural "centre of the earth" is situated in that direction?

The North Pole.

11. What other evidence is there that the Daitîk peak is at the North Pole?

The fact that the mountain of which this is simply "the peak of judgment" is Harâ-berezaiti, around which the heavenly bodies revolve, and which, as all allow, answers to the north polar Su-Meru of the Hindus.[1]

12. Then the Chinvat bridge extends from the North Pole of the heavens to the North Pole of the earth: what is its shape?

It is "*beam-shaped.*" To quote the sacred book: "That bridge is like a beam, of many sides, of whose edges there are some which are broad, and there are some which are thin and sharp; its broad sides are so large that its width is twenty-seven reeds, and its sharp sides are so contracted that in thinness it is just like the edge of a razor. And when the souls of the righteous and wicked arrive, it turns to them that side which is suitable to their necessities."[2]

[1] "Like the Meru of the Indians, Harâ-berezaiti is the pole and centre of the world, the fixed point around which the sun and the planets perform their revolutions." — Lenormant, "Ararat and Eden," in the *Contemporary Review*, September, 1881. Am. ed., p. 41.

[2] *Dâdistân-î-Dînîk*, ch. xxi., 2–9. West, *Pahlavi Texts*, ii., pp. 47–49. It is a curious coincidence that in Polynesian mythology Buataranga,

The Chinvat bridge, then, is simply the axis of the
northern heavens, the Pillar of Atlas, the Talmudic
" Strength of the Hill of Sion," the column which in
the Chinese legend the emperor vainly sought to
climb! In solving this long-standing problem we
have at the same time unlocked the mystery which
has hitherto attached to Bifröst and Al Sirat.[1]

But in locating our bridge we have located the
Persian Eden. And the location is unquestionably
at the North Pole. More than this, we have made
clear the fact that in the mythical or sacred geography of this ancient people the world of living men
was originally the northern circumpolar hemisphere.
The arrangement of the keshvares now becomes
entirely clear.[2] Like the divinely beautiful Ilâvrita
varsha of the Hindus, "illustrious Kvanîras" holds
the central position. In its centre, as in the centre

"guardian of the road to the invisible world," is wife to Ru, "the
supporter of the heavens." Gill, *Myths and Songs of the South Pacific.* London, 1876: p. 51. So if Heimdallr's true station were at
the top of the rainbow, his title "son of nine mothers" (Vigfusson
and Powell, *Corpus Poeticum Boreale*, London, 1883, ii. 465) would
have no such obvious significance as our interpretation gives.

[1] One of the etymologies of Chinvat makes it the "Bridge of the
Judge." (Haug, *Essays*, 2d ed., p. 165 n.) As among the ancient
Assyrians, and some other peoples, the pole star has been styled
"the judge of heaven," it is possible that we have here at once the
origin of the name and a new identification of the position of the
mythical "beam-shaped" bridge. It is interesting to note in this
connection that Heimdallr, the Norse god who stands at the top of
Bifröst, is also, etymologically considered, the "World-judge" or
"World-divider." Menzel, *Unsterblichkeitslehre*, i. 134. In Plato
(*Repub.*, 614 ff.) the judge stands at the bottom of the column. — For
grotesque survivals of the Bridge of Souls in folklore, see Tylor,
Primitive Culture, Index.

[2] The diagram attempted by Windischmann, *Zoroastrische Studien*,
p. 67, is inconsistent with the *Bundahish*, ch. v., 9. So must be every
attempt to arrange the keshvares on a flat earth.

of Ilâvrita, is the holiest mount in the world. Directly over it is the true heaven. In this central polar country North and South and East and West would have no application; but speaking from their own geographical standpoint as south of Aîrân-vej, the Persians located to the east of this holy central Kvanîras the keshvare Savah, to the west Arzah, to the south the keshvares Fradadafsh and Vidadafsh, and to the north Vôrûbarst and Vôrûgarst.[1] This gives a map of the northern hemisphere which in a

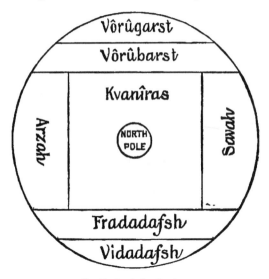

The Earth of the Persians.

[1] Darmesteter transliterates the names as follows: "The earth is divided into seven Karshvares, separated from one another by seas and mountains impassable to men. Arezahi and Savahi are the western and eastern Karshvare; Fradadhafshu and Vidadhafshu are in the south; Vourubaresti and Vourugaresti are in the north; *Hvani*-ratha (Kvanîras) is the central Karshvare. *Hvani*ratha is the only Karshvare inhabited by man (*Bundahish*, xi. 3)." — Darmesteter, *The Zend-Avesta*, vol. ii., p. 123 n.

plane polocentric projection may be represented as on the foregoing page, the polar centre of course being occupied by Harâ-berezaiti.

It would be a fascinating task to reinterpret the whole Avestan literature and mythology in the new light of this recovered geography and cosmology, but this would require a book of itself. It is worthy of remark that the Venidad expressly calls the earth "round," and apparently recognizes the existence of its two far-separated poles.[1] As we have seen, its Chinvat bridge or beam, which is also an idea so ancient as to be found in the Avesta itself (Farg., xix., 30, *et passim*), is the axis of the world, conducting good souls by an upward "flight" into the north polar heaven of Ahura Mazda, but the evil by a fall "headforemost" into the south polar hell.[2] Aîrân-vej, or "Old Iran," was the most natural name in the world for the Iranians to give to the traditional birth-place of their race.[3] But all attempts to find it "on the banks of the Aras" or "in the far-off lands

---

[1] *The Avesta* (Darmesteter), i., p. 205 ; ii., pp. 143, 144. Compare Windischmann's version of the Farvardin Yasht, i. 3 : "die beiden Enden des Himmels." *Studien*, p. 313.

[2] Apparently through the passage forced through the earth by Aharman (Ahriman). See *Zâd Sparam*, ch. ii., 3, 4, 5. West, *Pahlavi Texts*, vol. i., p. 161. Also *Bundahish*, iii. 13. Rhode, *Die heilige Sage des Zendvolks*, p. 235. Windischmann's translation of *Bundahish*, ch. xxxi. (in Darmesteter numbered xxx.), seems especially to support this idea : "Ahriman und die Schlange werden durch die Kraft der Lobgesänge geschlagen und hülflos und schwach gemacht. Auf jener Brücke des Himmels, auf welcher er herbeilief, wird er in die tiefste Finsterniss zurücklaufen. . . . Auch dies ist gesagt : Diese Erde wird rein und eben sein : ausser dem Berg Cakat-Cinvar wird ein Aufsteigen und ein Hinabtragen nicht sein." *Zoroastrische Studien*, p. 117. Compare Plato's "chasms," with ways leading hellward and heavenward. *Republic*, 614.

[3] F. C. Cook, *Origins of Religion and Language.* London, 1884 : p. 187.

of the rising sun "[1] are entirely useless. Equally mistaken is the gloss which merely makes it "primitively" the mythic land where the disembodied "souls of the righteous" are assembled by Ahura Mazda.[2] The same must be said of the assertion that "the real site of the Aîrân-vej in its ancient and original conception is to the east of the Caspian Sea and of Lake Aral."[3] By every particular of its description it is identified with the Daitîk peak, with Harâ-berezaiti, with the polar "river," the polar "tree," the polar "centre" of the upper hemisphere. It is simply the Arctic Eden of humanity remembered as it was before the Evil One entered, and "by his witchcraft counter-created winter and the worst of plagues."[4] This being the case we need not wonder that in a paper on "The Aryan Birth-place," read in January, 1884, before the Royal Society of Literature, Mr. C. J. Stone expressed his strong doubt of the current doctrine that the cradle of the Aryans was the upper valleys of the Oxus.[5] The

[1] Darmesteter, *The Avesta*, i., p. 3.

[2] Ibid., i., p. 15.

[3] Lenormant, *The Contemporary Review*, Sept., 1881 (Am. ed.), p. 41.—Pietrement, *Les Aryas*, locates it just east of Lake Balkach, in lat. 45°–47°. Grill is so bewildered by the number of attempted identifications that he pronounces the land a purely mythical one, and denies to the name all historic or geographic reality. *Erzväter*, i. 218, 219.

[4] *Fargard*, i. 3. The passage continues, "There are (now) ten winter months there, two summer months; and those are cold for the waters, cold for the earth, and cold for the trees." This reminiscence of the on-coming of the Glacial Age at the Pole also appears in the Flood legend of the American aborigines, particularly the Lenni-Lenapi, or Delaware Indians. Rafinesque, *The American Nations*. Phila., 1836: Song III.

[5] See also Dr. O. Schrader, *Sprachvergleichung und Urgeschichte. Linguistisch-historische Beiträge zur Erforschung des indogermanischen Alterthums.* Jena, 1883. Dr. S. formerly adhered to the

cradle of the whole Aryan family will at last be found
to be in "Aîrân, the Ancient," — and this in the
Arctic birth-place of man.

theory of a Mid-Asian Aryan birth-land, but has been led to abandon
it. Still more positive and emphatic is Karl Penka, who boldly locates the original home of the Aryans in Scandinavia. See his
*Origines Ariacæ. Linguistisch-ethnologische Untersuchungen zur äl-
testen Geschichte der Arischen Völker und Sprachen.* Vienna, 1883.
Mr. John Gibb argues in the same direction, "The Original Home
of the Aryans," in *The British Quart. Review,* Oct., 1884.

CHAPTER VI.

THE CRADLE OF THE RACE IN ANCIENT AKKADIAN, ASSYRIAN, AND BABYLONIAN THOUGHT.

We have here, even to the most minute details, an exact reproduction of the Aryan conception of Mount Meru, or Albordj, with its accessories. Here is the abode of the heavenly hierarchy, located on the summit of the Kharsak, or sacred mount which penetrates the heavens exactly in the region of the Pole star. —Rev. O. D. Miller.

We have already seen that the prehistoric inhabitants of the Tigro-Euphrates basin, called by some Akkadians, by others Sumerians, by yet others Akkado-Sumerians, had like other Asiatic peoples their Mountain of the World, on whose top was the celestial Paradise, and around which sun, moon, and stars revolved. Our present task is to locate this mountain more exactly, and to consider its significance for our hypothesis respecting the site of Eden.

That the earth, as conceived of by this ancient people, was spherical is not at the present day questioned. With their ideas probably no archæologist was more familiar than the late François Lenormant, and he expresses himself as follows: "'The Chaldees,' says Diodorus Siculus (lib. ii., 31), 'have quite an opinion of their own about the shape of the earth; they imagine it to have the form of a boat turned upside down, and to be hollow underneath.' This opinion remained to the last in the Chaldæan sacerdotal schools; their astronomers believed in it, and tried, according to Diodorus, to support it by scientific arguments. *It is of very ancient origin, a remnant of the ideas of the purely Akkadian period.* . . . Let us imagine, then, a boat, turned over; not such an one as we are in the habit of seeing, but a round skiff, like those which are still used under the name of *Kufa* on the shores of the lower Tigris and Euphrates, and of which there are many representations in the historical sculptures of the Assyrian palaces; the sides of this round skiff bend upwards from the point of the greatest width, so that they are shaped like a hollow sphere deprived of two thirds of its height [?], and showing a circular opening at the point of division. Such was the form of the earth according to the authors of the Akkadian magical formulæ and the Chaldæan astrologers of after years. We should express the same idea in the present day by comparing it to an orange of which the top had been cut off, leaving the orange upright upon the flat surface thus produced. The upper and convex surface constituted the earth properly so called, the inhabitable earth (*ki*) or terraqueous surface (*ki-a*), to which the collective name *kalama*, or the countries, is also given." [1]

It is well known that in minor details Diodorus is often found not altogether trustworthy. He was not a critical reporter. While, therefore, in the above quotation he has undoubtedly preserved to us one of the ancient Chaldæan similes,[2] by the use of which the true figure of the earth was taught, I can but think that the statement as to the hollowness of the

[1] *Chaldæan Magic*, p. 150.

[2] The figure was also used by the Egyptians, and other ancient nations. See Wilford, in *Asiatic Researches*, vol. viii., p. 274. Also articles and works on " The Ark " and " Arkite Symbols."

earth underneath is an unauthorized inference, suggested by the hollow boat, and made by the comparatively uninstructed Greek solely upon his own responsibility. It is true that, in the same work from which the above extract is taken, Lenormant endeavors to adjust Akkadian cosmology to such a notion of a hollow sphere, saying, "The interior concavity opening from underneath was the terrestrial abyss, *ge*, where the dead found a home (*kur-nu-de, ki-gal, aralli*). The central point in it was the nadir, or, as it was called, 'the root,' *uru*, the foundation of the whole structure of the world; this gloomy region witnessed the nocturnal journey of the sun."[1] But nothing can be more evident on examination than that this attempt involves the writer in at least three inconsistencies: First, if the sun visits the interior of the earth at night, its proper orbit cannot be round and round the Mountain of the World to the northeast of Babylonia, as our author elsewhere represents. Second, if *aralli*, the abode of the dead, is in the interior of the hollow earth, it cannot be to the northeast of Babylonia, as it is represented to be in the context. Third, if the earth was conceived of as hollow, of course its whole central portion was empty space; but according to this presentation its central point "was called 'the root,' *uru*, the foundation of the whole structure of the world." Surely the foundation of the world can scarcely have been supposed to be mere emptiness. To a layman in these studies this *uru* would much rather suggest

---

[1] Ibid., p. 150. — It is worthy of note that the expression "*root*" of the world, or "root-land," is applied to the same subterranean region of darkness in Japanese mythology. See "Shintoism," by Griffis in McClintock and Strong's *Cyclopædia*, vol. ix., p. 688.

the antarctic *Tap-en-to* mountain of ancient Egyptian thought, the *Ku-Meru* of ancient India.

But it is time to return to the Akkadian, or Akkado-Sumerian, mountain of the gods. Again we quote Lenormant: "Above the earth extended the sky (*ana*), spangled with its fixed stars (*mul*), and revolving round the Mountain of the East (*Kharsak Kurra*), the column which joins the heavens and the earth, and serves as an axis to the celestial vault. The culminating point in the heavens, the zenith (*nuzku*),[1] was not this axis or pole ; on the contrary, it was situated immediately above the country of Akkadia, which was regarded as the centre of the inhabited lands, whilst the mountain which acted as a pivot to the starry heavens was to the northeast of this country. Beyond the mountain, and also to the northeast, extended the land of *aralli*, which was very rich in gold, and was inhabited by the gods and blessed spirits." [2]

Here we have the "Mountain of the East" located, not in the east, but in the northeast. Elsewhere our author recognizes most fully the identity of this mount with the *Har-Moed* of Isaiah xiv. 14, and the difficulty of placing it anywhere but at the North Pole.[3] He adduces from the cuneiform texts no evidence whatever for a location to the "northeast," and seems to fix upon that direction only as a compromise of his own. "*Nous devons conclure*" is his language. His only reason for thinking of any other position than one due north appears to be a cuneiform expression which seems to make Kharsak Kurra at the same time "the mountain of the

---

[1] *Paku* in the French edition.   [2] *Chaldæan Magic*, p. 150.
[3] *Fragments de Bérose*, pp. 392, 393.

sunrise." [1]   This, in reality, instead of being a reason for searching among the mountains to the east of Assyria or Babylonia, is, when rightly understood, precisely an additional reason for looking to the north. [2]

One other statement in the extract calls for notice. The writer seems to have anticipated that his readers would inevitably locate a mountain, described as "the column which joins the heavens and the earth, and serves as an axis to the celestial vault," under the celestial pole ; and believing that the cuneiform texts which locate the celestial pole directly over Akkad (or Akkadia), "the centre of the inhabited lands," to be inconsistent with such a location, he introduces the remark that "the culminating point in the heavens" was "not the axis or pole; on the contrary, it was situated immediately over the country of Akkadia, which was regarded as the centre of the inhabited lands, whilst the mountain which acted as a pivot to the starry heavens was to the northeast of this country."

---

[1] The following from his latest account of the mountain will be valued : " La 'montagne des pays' est le lieu où résident les dieux. . . . Elle est située au nord, vient de nous dire Yescha' yâhoû ; à l'est disent les documents cunéiformes, où l'expression accadienne '*garsag babbara* == assyriene *šad çit šamši*, ' la montagne du levant,' apparaît comme synonyme de l'accadien '*garsag kurkurra* == assyrien *šad* matâti ; d'où nous devons conclure que c'est au nord-est du bassin de l'Euphrate et du Tigre qu'on la supposait placée. C'est elle qui vaut à l'orient, son nom accadien de *mer kurra* et son nom assyrien de *šadû* signifiant tous les deux ' le point cardinal de la montagne.' Et le sens de ce terme est bien précisé par la variante accadienne *mer* '*garsag*, où ce mot, dont le sens ' la montagne' est incontestable, se substitue à son synonyme *kur*, dont la signification eût pu être douteuse." — *Les Origines de l'Histoire*, vol. ii., 1, p. 126.

[2] See Menzel, *Die vorchristliche Unsterblichkeitslehre*, Bd. i., chapter entitled "Der Sonnengarten am Nordpol," pp. 87–93.

From so eminent an authority one naturally hesitates to differ ; but inasmuch as M. Joachim Ménard, in a work as recent as the one from which we have quoted, while agreeing with M. Lenormant in making Akkad the traditional " centre of the earth," differs from him in locating *precisely in this central country* " the mountain on whose apex the heaven of the fixed stars is pivoted," [1] we cannot avoid the conclusion that Lenormant's distinction between the zenith of Akkad and the celestial pole is based upon a misapprehension, and is productive only of confusion. The solution of all difficulties is found the moment the mythological Akkad is made a circumpolar mother-country, after which the Akkad of the Tigro-Euphrates valley was commemoratively named.[2] This supposition is made all the easier by three noteworthy facts : (1) that both the names Akkad and Sumir are not Assyrio-Babylonian, but loan - words from an older prehistoric tongue ; [3] (2) that the etymological signification and appellatives of Akkad thoroughly identify it with the lofty country at the north polar summit of the earth ; [4]

[1] " Le pays d'Akkad est regardé, d'après les plus antiques traditions, comme le centre de la terre ; c'est là que s'élève la montagne sur la cîme de laquelle pivote le ciel des étoiles fixes." — *Babylone et la Chaldée*. Paris, 1875: p. 46.

[2] Compare the primitive name of Babylon, *Tin-tir-ki*, " Place of the Tree of Life." Lenormant, *Beginnings of History*, p. 85.

[3] " Il est certain que les mots Sumir et Akkad n'appartiennent pas à la langue assyro-chaldéenne. Ils sont propres à une langue antérieure ; et nous savons, par les explications mêmes des Assyriens, que Akkad veut dire ' montagne.' " — Ménant, *Babylone et la Chaldée*. Paris, 1875 : p. 47.

[4] " Akkad is bovendien zeker een hoog land, geen lage vlakte bij de zee, zooals ook een glosse het door *tilla*, hoogte, verklaart." C. P. Tiele, *Is Sumer en Akkad hetzelfde als Makan en Melucha ?* Amsterdam, 1883: p. 6. Compare last preceding note : Akkad = " mon-

and (3) that recently discovered tablets are compelling the Assyriologists to recognize two Akkads, one in the Tigro-Euphrates valley and one much farther to the North, though as yet none of these scholars have looked as far in that direction as to the Pole.[1]

If further proof were needed that the Kharsak Kurra of the earliest inhabitants of Mesopotamia was identical with the north polar World-mountain of Egypt and the surrounding Asiatic nations, it would be found on investigating their conceptions of the region of the disembodied dead and their notion of a mountain of the rulers of the dead *antipodal* to the mount of the gods. The Akkadians, like the ancients generally, conceived of the realm of the dead as located to the South. Their underworld being simply the under or southern hemisphere of the earth, they could not place it in any other direction. In naming the cardinal points the Akkadians therefore called the South "the *funereal* point."[2] In this quarter was located the mount of the rulers of the

tagne." Also Smith, *The Phonetic Values of the Cuneiform Characters.* London, 1871 : p. 17.

[1] See *Proceedings of the Society of Biblical Archæology.* London, Nov.–Dec., 1881. "Mr. Pinches, in a further communication on the Paris Tablet [in cuneiform characters, but supposed to be Cappadocian in origin], observes : 'The question of the original home of the Akkadians is affected thereby. . . . As it seems that the country *north of Assyria* was also called Akkad, as well as the northern part of Babylonia, the neighborhood of Cappadocia as the home of the Akkadian race may be regarded as a very possible explanation, etc.' " Brown, *Myth of Kirkê.* London, 1883 : p. 87. Finzi, in his *Carta del Mondo conosciuto dagli Assiri tracciata secondo le inscrizioni cuneiformi,* does not venture to locate either Akkad or Kharsak Kurra.

[2] *Chaldæan Magic,* Eng. ed., p. 168, 169. Compare F. Finzi, *Ricerche per lo Studio dell' Antichità Assira.* Turin, 1872 : p. 109 note 18.

dead. It was the under or south polar projection of the earth. It corresponded with the south polar mount of demons in Hindu and in Egyptian thought. Even Lenormant, whose mistake in locating the mount of the gods in the East, logically leads to the mistake of locating this mount of the rulers of the dead in the West, still unconsciously gives evidence as to the true location by stating that it is "situated in the low-down portions of the earth." [1] And elsewhere he has told us that in the Akkadian language to descend and to go southward were synonymous expressions.[2]

With Professor Friedrich Delitzsch, then, we locate the Akkadian Kharsak Kurra at the North.[3] Once make the *primæval* Akkad the equivalent of Ilâvrita in Hindu, or of Kvanîras in Iranian, mythology, and all is perfectly plain and self-consistent. The primitive Akkad is now "the centre of all lands" in the same sense in which Ilâvrita and Kvanîras are in their respective systems. As in both these systems the mount of the gods is in the centre of this central country, so is Kharsak Kurra. Su-Meru and Harâ-berezaiti and Kwen-lun are each exactly under the Pole-star, having it in their zenith; the same is true of Kharsak Kurra. As every splendor of a divine abode crowns the top of all the former, so is the summit of Kharsak resplendent beyond description. As the sun, moon, and stars revolve around the Hindu and Iranian and Chinese mounts, so is Kharsak the point "on which

---

[1] "Située dans les parties basses de la terre." — *Origines*, tom. ii. I, p. 134.

[2] *The Beginnings of History*, p. 313 n. 4.

[3] *Wo lag das Paradies?* p. 121.

the heaven of the fixed stars is pivoted." Moreover from its top flows that Eden river, which, like Gungâ and Ardvî-Sûra, waters the whole earth.[1]

Under these circumstances the candid reader will probably be prepared to agree with the statement of Mr. Miller which we have made the motto to this chapter, and to say with Gerald Massey, only with better understanding than his, "The cradle of the Akkadian race was the 'Mountain of the World,' that 'Mount of the Congregation in the thighs of the North.' . . . The first mount of mythology was the Mount of the Seven Stars, Seven Steps, Seven Stages, Seven Caves, which represented the celestial North as the birth-place of the initial motion and the beginning of time. This starting-point in heaven above is the one original for the many copies found on the earth below. . . . The Akkadians date from Urdhu, the district of the northern Mountain of the World." [2]

---

[1] Of this celestial source Lenormant speaks as follows: " . . . et la fontaine divine Ghetim-kour-koû de la montagne des pays des Chaldéens. Cette dernière fontaine, dont le nom est accadien et veut dir 'las ource qui enveloppe la montagne sainte,' est dite 'fille de l'Océan,' *marat apsi*, et invoquée comme une déesse douée d'une personalité vivante, pareille à celle que revêt chez les Iraniens Ardvîçourâ-Anâhitâ. L'existence chez les Chaldéens de la croyance à un cours d'eau mythique d'où procèdent tous les fleuves de la terre semble attestée par la mention d'une rivière (dont le nom est malheureusement en partie détruit sur la tablette qui contient ce reseignement) laquelle est qualifiée d'*umme* nâ'rï 'la mère des fleuves.' " *Origines*, tom. ii. 1, p. 133. Compare Siouffi, *La Religion des Soubbhas ou Sabéens*, Paris, 1880, p. 7 n., where the Euphrates is represented as rising in a celestial Paradise (Olmi Danhouro) under the throne of Avatha, whose throne is under the Pole star.

[2] *A Book of Beginnings.* London, 1881 : vol. ii., p. 520.

CHAPTER VII.

THE CRADLE OF THE RACE IN ANCIENT EGYPTIAN THOUGHT.

According to the Kamite legend related by Diodorus, Osiris and Isis lived together in Nysa, or Paradise. Here there was a garden wherein the deathless dwelt. Here they lived in perfect happiness until Osiris was seized with the desire to drink the water of immortality. Then he went forth in search of it, and fell. . . . But an earlier couple than Osiris and Isis was Sevekh and Ta-urt, who as the two constellations of the seven stars revolving round the Tree, or Pole, were the primeval pair in Paradise. — The Natural Genesis.

THE mythical geography of the ancient Egyptians is as yet too little known to allow us to hope for much light from this quarter on the question of the site of Eden. Even their cosmology is little understood, and their scientific attainments are by many inexcusably underestimated. So good a scholar as Mr. Villiers Stuart could recently write, "The Egyptians had not attained to a sufficiently advanced point in science to solve the problem of how the sun in his daily course, having sunk behind the western horizon, returned to rise at the opposite quarter of the heavens." [1] Nevertheless, as we desire to test our hypothesis as far as possible by all most ancient traditions and myths, whether favorable or unfavorable, we must inquire whether anything can be ascertained as to the ideas of the ancient Egyptians touch-

[1] *Nile Gleanings.* London, 1879: p. 262. This is as bad as the declaration of Lauer: "Und so glaube ich dass auch Homer nie daran gedacht hat, wie die Sonne wieder aus dem Westen in den Osten gelange." *Nachlass.* Berlin, 1851: vol. i., p. 317.

ing the form of the earth and the theatre of man's first history.

The leading features of Egyptian cosmology, as interpreted by the present writer, are in perfect accord with the cosmological ideas of other ancient nations as described in chapter first of the present division. They may be briefly expressed in the six following theses : —

1. That in ancient Egyptian thought the earth was conceived of as a sphere, with its axis perpendicular and its North Pole at the top.

2. That in the earliest time *Amenti* was conceived of neither as a cavern in the bowels of the earth, nor as a region of the earth to the West, on the same general plane as the land of Egypt, but was simply the under or southern hemisphere of the earth, conceived of as just described.

3. That the *Tat* pillar symbolized the axis of the world (heaven and earth) upright in space.

4. That *Ta nuter*, whatever its later applications, originally signified the extreme northern or topmost point of the globe, where earth and heaven were fabled to meet.

5. That *Cher-nuter* was the inferior celestial hemisphere underarching Amenti.

6. That *Hes* and *Nebt-ha* (Isis and Nephthys) were respectively goddesses of the North and South poles, or of the northern and southern heavens.[1]

Assuming now, with Chabas, Lieblein, Lefèvre, and Ebers, that the earth of the ancient Egyptians,

---

[1] In a brief communication published in *The Independent*, New York, Feb. 8, 1883, the critical attention of Egyptologists was respectfully invited to these theses. Since that time much new evidence of their correctness has come to light. See, for example, the new *Thesaurus Inscriptionum* of Brugsch, pp. 176, 177, *et passim*.

like that of the ancient Asiatic nations, was spherical,
what was their conception of its northern terminus?
In chapter first of this Part, some indication has
been already given. But our present investigation
demands a fuller answer to this question. Turning
to the great work of Brugsch on the "Geographical
Inscriptions of the Old-Egyptian Monuments," we
find that the Egyptians considered the farthest limit
in the North to be "the four pillars or supports of
heaven."[1] The fact that these four supports of
heaven, instead of being situated in four opposite
directions from Egypt, are *all in the farthest North,*
is very significant. It shows that though the people
might speak of heaven as supported on four pillars,
it is not to be inferred therefrom that they conceived
of the earth as flat, and of the sky as a flat Oriental
roof one story above it.[2] Brugsch himself, though
writing upon the supposition that the Egyptians'
earth was flat, avoids this mistake. His inference,
coming from one who had a traditional wrong theory
to support, is most interesting and valuable. He
says, "Inasmuch as these 'four supports of heaven,'
the northern limit of the earth as known to the
Egyptians, nowhere else occur as name of people,
land, or river, it seems to me most probable that we
have herein the designation of a high mountain
which was perhaps characterized by four peaks, or

---

[1] "Die Ansicht von den Enden der Welt ist eine uralte und vielen
Völkern gemeinsame. . . . Als die äusserste Grenze im Süden galt
den Egyptern das Meer ('*Sar*) und der Berg *ap-en-to* oder *tap-en-to,*
wörtlich ' das Horn der Welt; ' als die äusserste Grenze im Norden
dagegen ' die vier Stützen des Himmels.' " *Geographische Inschriften,*
Bd. ii., p. 35. Compare Taylor's *Pausanias,* vol. iii., 255, bot.

[2] Maspéro, *Les Contes Populaires de l'Egypte Ancienne.* Paris,
1882 : pp. lxi.–lxiii.

which consisted of four ranges, from which peculiarity it received its name. Like all peoples of antiquity, — at least all those whose literature has come down to us, — the Egyptians conceived of the earth as rising toward the North, so that at last at its northernmost point it joined the sky and supported it." [1]

In the Buddhist conception of Meru, as given in chapter first of this Part, we have precisely the four-peaked, heaven-supporting mountain which Brugsch here describes : " Each of the four corners of the mountain-top has a peak seven hundred yôjanas high." It is not impossible that in the four dwarfs which support the dome of the modern Buddhist temple we have a far-off survival of ancient Egypt's "four supports of heaven." Certainly the Buddhist temple-roofs symbolize the circumpolar heaven,[2] and a recent author, touching upon the latter's mythological support, writes as follows : " This prop passing through the earth and the heavens at the pole, indicated as we have seen by the Alpha of Draco, became the 'nail' of the old astronomers, the point round which all nature revolved. Between earth and the celestial pole the prop idea was again brought forward as the central column of a huge conical mountain, Mount Meru, guarded at each cardinal point by a mighty king. The four dwarfs propping up some of the columns in the old Buddhist temples are evidently these four kings. . . . When the prop pierced the highest heaven it was a spire called the ' *tee*,' and in Nepal it is confessedly

---

[1] *Geographische Inschriften*, Bd. ii., p. 37.
[2] Koeppen, *Die Religion des Buddhas*, ii. 262.

in all the temples the symbol of Adi Buddha, the supreme, in his heavenly garden, Nandana grove."[1]

But returning from this merely curious question, we remind ourselves that we have seen reason to believe that the ancient Egyptians conceived of the earth as a sphere, with a heaven-supporting mountain in the extreme North. In the extreme South was another mountain, "The Horn of the World," represented as of incredible height (eight *atur* or stadia).[2] This corresponds so perfectly with the earth of the Puranas, with its Su-Meru and Ku-Meru, that we are irresistibly impelled to inquire whether the parallelism extends any farther.

We take the question of the direction of the abode of the dead. All agree that in Indian thought the abode of the dead is in the South. So was it in the thought of the ancient Egyptian. The recently discovered epitaph of Queen Isis-em-Kheb, mother-in-law of Shishak, king of Assyria (*circa* 1000 B. C.), thus reads : " She is seated all beautiful in her place enthroned, among the *gods of the South* she is crowned with flowers. She is seated in her beauty in the arms of Khonsou, her father, fulfilling his desires. He is in Amenti, the place of departed spirits."[3]

Again, in the mythological earth of India, the abode of the dead, being the southern or under hemisphere, is looked upon as inverted. Viewed from the standpoint of gods and men, it is bottom upward, and its inhabitants move about head down-

---

[1] Lillie, *Buddha and Early Buddhism,* p. 50.

[2] See first quotation from Brugsch above.

[3] Villiers Stuart, *The Funeral Tent of an Egyptian Queen.* London, 1882 : p. 34. See also " Homer's Abode of the Dead " in the APPENDIX, Sect. VI.

ward.[1] The same is true of Amenti, the Egyptian underworld, and of its inhabitants.[2]

Again, in Hindu thought all deadly influences proceed from the South, the abode of death; all beneficent and life-giving influences from the North. The same is true in ancient Egyptian thought. "It is curious," says the English editor of Lenormant's "Chaldæan Magic,"[3] — "it is curious that in Egypt all good and healing and life proceeded from the West, the land of the setting sun, and all evil from the East the land of its rising." The statement is "curiously" incorrect. The North is the sacred quarter, and from the North come life and blessing. The North wind is the very breath of God. It "proceeds from the nostrils of Knum and enlivens all creatures."[4] It is one of the high prerogatives of the blessed dead to "breathe the delicious air of the North wind."[5] That they may breathe it is

---

[1] "The gods in heaven are beheld by the inhabitants of hell as they move with their heads inverted." — Garrett, *Classical Dictionary of India:* Art. "Naraka."

[2] See Brugsch, *Hieroglyphisches Demotisches Wörterbuch*, S. 1331, *sub v.* "Set," "Set-mati." Also chapter first of the present division.

[3] Page 51. — Undoubtedly there are Egyptian texts in which the sun-god Ra is represented as going into "the land of life" at his setting (see Brugsch, *Thesaurus Inscriptionum Ægyptiacarum*, 1ste Abth., Leipsic, 1883: p. 29), but this is made quite intelligible by Menzel's "Sonnengarten am Nordpol" in his *Vorchristliche Unsterblichkeitslehre.*

[4] *Records of the Past*, vol. iv., p. 67.

[5] Ibid., p. 3. Compare the expression, "Give the sweet breath of the North wind to the Osiris," *Book of the Dead* (Birch), p. 170; also 311, 312. Gerald Massey remarks, "In Egyptian the *Meh* is the North, the quarter of the waters, and the name of the cool wind that breathed new life." *The Natural Genesis*, vol. ii., p. 168. The following very curious passage from the apocryphal *Book of Adam*, translated from the Ethiopic by Dillmann, shows that this ancient Egyptian idea survived to a very late period: "Als der Herr den

the prayer of bereaved affection.[1]   The " Fields of Peace" are at the North of the fields of Sanchem-u.[2] There is the proper home of the great god of whom the Nile poet sang:—

> " There is no building that can contain him !
> " There is no counselor in thy heart !
> " Thy youth delight in thee, thy children ;
> " Thou directest them as King.
> " Thy law is established in the whole land,
> " In the presence of thy servants *in the North*."

Of the same god it is said : —

> " He createth all works therein,
> " All writings, all sacred words,
> " All his implements, in the North." [3]

As yet no texts have been discovered which represent the earliest Egyptian ideas of the origin of man and the location of his birth-place.   One proof, however, that man was conceived of as having proceeded from the " Land of the Gods" in the North appears in connection with the myth of the reign of Râ.   In Egyptian mythology, the reign of Râ was like the primeval reign of Kronos; the myth of it was a reminiscence of the sinless Golden Age.[4]   But

Adam austrieb, wollte er ihn auf der Südgrenze des Gartens nicht wohnen lassen, *weil der Nordwind, wann er darin bläset, den süssen Geruch der Bäume des Gartens nach der Südgegend hinführt ;* und Adam sollte nicht die süssen Gerüche der Bäume riechen, und die Uebertretung vergessen, und sich über das was er gethan trösten, und durch den Geruch der Bäume befriedigt die Busse für die Uebertretung unterlassen.   Vielmehr liess der barmherzige Gott den Adam in der Gegend westlich vom Garten wohnen."   Dillmann, S. 13.

[1] " Dans le papyre Boulak No. 3, 4, 16, on souhait à un défunt : ' les agréables vents du Nord dans la ÂMIIÎ.' " — Brugsch, *Dictionnaire Géographique.*   Leipsic, 1879 : p. 37.

[2] *Records of the Past*, vol. iv., p. 122.

[3] Ibid., p. 101.

[4] Maspéro, *Histoire Ancienne des Peuples de l'Orient*, p. 38.

in those primeval and perfect days men still dwelt in the country of the gods, which country, as we have seen, was in the highest North. And because they still occupied the heaven - touching mountain, the rebellion by which they forfeited their estate of blessedness is expressly described as "on the mountain,"[1]—an object not easily found in Egypt.

The same teaching is further supported by the language of certain scholars, who, without any particular theory as to the location of Eden, have held that the hieroglyph used in Egyptian texts as the determinative prefix to names designating civilized lands, ⊕, is simply a pictorial symbol of primitive Eden divided by its fourfold river.[2] A writer in the Edinburgh Review, said to be Mr. Walter Wilkins, remarks: " The Buddhists and Brahmans, who together constitute nearly half the population of the world, tell us that the decussated figure of the cross, whether in a simple or complex form, symbolizes the traditional happy abode of their primeval ancestors, — the Paradise of Eden toward the East, as we find it expressed in the Hebrew. And, let us ask, what better picture or more significant characters,

---

[1] "Während er, der Gott der das Sein selber ist, seines Königthums waltete, da waren die Menschen und die Götter zusammen vereint." Brugsch, *Die neue Weltordnung nach Vertilgung des sündigen Menschengeschlechts.* Berlin, 1881 : p. 20. Naville, The Destruction of Mankind by Râ. *Records of the Past*, vol. vi., pp. 103 *seq.*

[2] Sometimes this hieroglyph is accompanied by the character signifying "God" or "divine." In such connection Brugsch renders it "heilige Wohnstätte." On other renderings, however, see the *Zeitschrift für ägyptische Sprache.* 1880 : p. 25. See also *Ceramic Art in Remote Ages ; with Essays on the Symbols of the Circle, the Cross and Circle, the Circle and Ray Ornament, the Fylfot, and the Serpent, showing their relation to the primitive forms of Solar and Nature Worship.* By John B. Waring. London, 1874 : Plates 33-37.

in the complicated alphabet of symbolism, could have been selected for the purpose than a circle and a cross? — the one to denote a region of absolute purity and perpetual felicity, the other those four perennial streams that divided and watered the several quarters of it." [1] Mr. Wilkins claims that in the Egyptian hieroglyph above given we have the same symbol as in the Indian *Swastika.* It was therefore primeval Paradise which was commemorated by "the sacred circular cakes of the Egyptians, composed of the richest materials, — of flour, of honey, of milk, — and with which the serpent and bull, as well as the other reptiles and beasts consecrated to the service of Isis and their higher divinities, were daily fed, and which upon certain festivals were eaten with extraordinary ceremony by the people and their priests." He continues, " 'The cross-cake,' says Sir Gardiner Wilkinson, 'was their hieroglyph for civilized land,' — obviously a land superior to their own, as it was, indeed, to all mundane territories ; for it was that distant, traditional country of sempiternal contentment and repose, of exquisite delight and serenity, where Nature, unassisted by man, produces all that is necessary for his sustentation."

"This," says Donnelly, though arguing in favor of a mid-Atlantic island-Eden, — " this was the Garden of Eden of our race. . . . In the midst of it was a sacred and glorious eminence, — the *umbilicus orbis terrarum,* — 'toward which the heathen in all parts

[1] "The Pre-Christian Cross." *Edinburgh Review*, January, 1870, p. 254. Zöckler did not think the primitive character of this symbolism well established (*The Cross of Christ*, p. 35) ; but the moment Eden is identified with the "middle country" of the Pole the naturalness and primitiveness of the symbol become most easy of belief.

of the world, and in all ages, turned a wistful gaze in every act of devotion, and to which they hoped to be admitted, or rather to be restored, at the close of this transitory scene.' " [1]

In Part fifth, chapter fourth, it will be shown that the *umbilicus orbis terrarum* is indisputably the terrestrial pole.

Finally, if, as Plato represents, the story of lost Atlantis was received from Egypt, and constituted a part of the priestly teaching of the dwellers upon the Nile, our next chapter will present us further evidence that the Eden and the antediluvian world of ancient Egyptian tradition were precisely where the tradition of other ancient peoples placed them, to wit, in the land of sacred memories in the far-off, faerie North.

[1] Donnelly, *Atlantis*, p. 322.

CHAPTER VIII.

THE CRADLE OF THE RACE IN ANCIENT GREEK THOUGHT.

In the Centre of the Sea is the White Isle of great Zeus,
There is Mount Ida, and our race's Cradle.
                            ÆNEAS.

All that is beautiful and rare seems to come from the North. — HERODOTUS.

When transactions are of such antiquity it is not wonderful if the history should prove obscure. — PLUTARCH.

The writings that narrate these fables, not being delivered as inventions of the writers, but as things before believed and received, appear like a soft whisper from the traditions of more ancient nations, conveyed through the flutes of the Grecians. — BACON.

RESPECTING the origin of men there were among Greek writers, as Preller states, "very different opinions." Part of this diversity he ascribes to a difference in the natural environment of the first inhabitants : some, residing in the woody hills, would naturally think the first men came from these ; others, inhabiting a valley, would more naturally think of their ancestors as having come out of the water. The Asiatic-Greek belief that the first of the human race were made out of trees he calls "quite peculiar." [1] What if it should be found that all these notions were merely fragments of an old, old faith, according to which man originated on the mountain of all mountains, by the source of all waters, and under the tree of all trees !

However this may be, it is certainly very interest-

[1] *Griechische Mythologie*, i., pp. 56, 57.

ing to note that in the Greek myth of Meropia, or
Meropis, Renan, Lenormant, and others recognize
the old Asiatic Meru. They hold that "the sacred
expression μέροπες ἄνθρωποι originally meant 'the men
sprung from Meru.'" [1] Stephanus has the same rendering in his "Thesaurus."

In an advance chapter of his " Origines de l'Histoire," Lenormant expressed himself on this point
as follows : " I have stated above, in agreement
with M. Renan, that the sacred expression μέροπες,
as used among the Greeks to designate mankind,
could not have originally been applied to them on
account of their possessing the gift of articulate
speech, as is pretended in the etymology of grammarians of late date, but as having proceeded from
Meru. Such an explanation, the consequence of
which is to carry back this name of the sacred
mountain, the abode of the gods and the birth-place
of mankind, to the most ancient period of Aryan
unity, is corroborated, in a manner to my mind quite
decisive, by the existence of myths which make the
Meropes to be a special and autochthonic population, of a date far back in the most ancient times,
who lead a life of innocence and happiness, marked
by extraordinary longevity (a feature in common with
the Indian legends concerning Uttara-Kuru), under
the government of a king, Merops, who is sometimes
represented as preserving them from the Deluge in
the same way as the Yima of the Iranians, and as-
sembling them around him to shelter them from the
Flood, from which they alone escape. This myth
is usually localized in the island of Kos, which receives the name of Meropêis, Meropis, or Meropê.

[1] Lenormant, *Origines*, ii. 1, p. 56.

But the island of Siphnos is also reputed to have been called Meropia in virtue of a similar tradition, and Strabo speaks of a fabulous region of the name of Meropis, which was described by Theopompus, and which seems to have been placed near the country of the Hyperboreans. Merops is also given as a king of the Ethiopians; the most pious and most virtuous of men, the husband of Klymenê the mother of Phaëthon, and consequently anterior to the catastrophe of the conflagration of the universe, by which the first human race, that of the Golden Age, is often said to have been destroyed. Or else the same name is given to a prophet king of Rhyndakos, in Mysia, who also receives the very significant appellation of Makar, or Makareus, 'the happy.' All this shows that the paradisaic myth of the Meropes was not peculiar to the island of Kos, but was current elsewhere in the Greek world, and had undergone more than one localization there." [1]

Plato's story of lost Atlantis, the island which the ocean-god Poseidon prepared for his son Atlas to rule over, is a fascinating picture of the antediluvian world. Whether originating in Egypt, as claimed by Plato,[2] or inherited as a part of the legendary wealth of the Hellenes, it is of special interest to us in the present discussion; and this for three reasons : —

---

[1] "Ararat and Eden." *The Contemporary Review*, Sept., 1881, Am. ed., p. 44. Compare Bryant, *Analysis of Ancient Mythology.* London, 1807 : vol. v., pp. 75–92. Also Samuel Beal: "It can hardly be questioned that the Buddhist cosmic arrangement is allied with Greek tradition as embodied in Homer." *Buddhist Literature in China.* London, 1882 : p. xv.

[2] "But, O Socrates, you can easily invent Egyptians or anything else ! " — *Phædrus,* 275 B.

First, we have elsewhere shown that in oldest Greek thought Atlas belongs at the North Pole, and it is only reasonable to locate the kingdom of Atlas in the same locality.

Secondly, some authorities have unconsciously placed Atlantis in just this polar position by identifying its inhabitants with the " Hyperboreans." [1]

Thirdly, Apollodorus and Theopompus expressly call the lost land Meropia, and its inhabitants Meropes ; *i. e.*, according to the above authorities, "issued from Meru." [2]

The fabled country further resembles Eden in the difficulties which scholarship of every kind has found in giving it a location in harmony with all the data. These difficulties are so great that some learned writers have located it as far to the West as America, others as far to the East as in the Sea of Azof, or in Persia. Even of those who have sought a place for it in the mid-Atlantic, some have pushed it up and some down, until one of the latest writers says, "All hypotheses are permissible." [3] His illus-

---

[1] Lüken, *Die Traditionen des Menschengeschlechtes*, p. 73. Bryant, *Analysis of Ancient Mythology*, vol. v., p. 157 : " Pindar manifestly makes them [the Hyperboreans] the same as the Atlantians."

[2] " It was a common practice with the Greeks to disguise their own ignorance of the purport of a foreign word by supplying a word of a similar sound and inventing a story to agree with it : thus Meru, or the North Pole, the supposed abode of the *Devatas*, being considered as the birth-place of the god, gave rise to the fable that Bacchus's second birth was from the thigh of Jupiter, because Meros, a Greek word approaching Meru in sound, signifies thigh in that language." — J. D. Paterson, " Origin of the Hindu Religion," in *Asiatic Researches*. London, 1808 : vol. viii., p. 51.

[3] Reference is had to M. le Marquis de Nadaillac, who, being himself uncertain, says, " Que l'Atlantide ait été située vers le Nord, que ses limites aient été reculées vers le Sud, il est difficile de rien préciser et tous les hypothèses sont permises." *L'Amérique Préhis-*

trious countryman, Monsieur J. S. Bailly, a century ago, came nearer the truth, when, in view of the perplexities attending all other locations, he correctly placed his lost Atlantis in the Paleo-Arctic Ocean.

Again, the antediluvian world was, of course, in the vicinity of lost Eden. But it is to be observed that in Hellenic tradition Deukalion is not a Greek, but an inhabitant of a country in the high North, a Scythian. Moreover the Scythians, as we know from Justin, were considered a very much more ancient people than the Greeks ; indeed, as the very oldest in the world.[1] Moreover, Scythia, like polar Meru and Harâ-berezaiti, was conceived of as a lofty region from which all the rivers of the earth descend.[2] All of which obviously connects the ante-

torique. Paris, 1883 : p. 566. See Unger, *Die versunkene Insel Atlantis.* Vienna, 1860. Donnelly, *Atlantis: the Antediluvian World.* New York, 1882. A "conjectural map" is given in Bory de Saint Vincent, *l'Homme, Essai Zoölogique sur le genre humain.* The *Última Teoría sobre la Atlántida,* by D. Pedro de Novo y Colson, appended to the author's *Viajes Apócrifos de Juan de Fuca,* Madrid, 1881, pp. 191–223, has no independent value, being based on the *Studies* of M. Gaffarel. An extended essay by E. F. Berlioux, is entitled "Les Atlantes : Histoire de l'Atlantis et de l'Atlas primitif," appearing in the just issued *Annuaire de la Faculté de Lyon.* Paris, 1884, Première Année, Fasc. i., pp. 1–170.

[1] "Scytharum gentem semper habitam fuisse antiquissimam."

[2] "The geographical indications of the great epic poem of the Mahâbhârata represent Meru rather as a vast and highly elevated region than as a distinct mountain, and make it supply all the rivers of the world with water. This system is pretty much in conformity with that which Justin has borrowed from Trogus Pompeius, and according to which Scythia, the country of the most ancient of mankind, without having, properly speaking, any mountains, is higher than the rest of the earth in such a way as to be the starting-point of all the rivers, *editiorem omnibus terris esse, ut cuncta flumina ibi nata.*" — Lenormant, *The Contemporary Review,* Sept., 1881 (Am. ed.), p. 40.

diluvian Deukalion with the primitive country at the Arctic summit of the globe.

Finally, in Greek tradition, the first men lived under the beneficent rule of Kronos, father of Zeus, enjoying the blessedness of the Golden Age. But it is clear from Strabo and others that the seat of Kronos' kingdom was in the farthest North.[1] Menzel begins his chapter on "The Isles of Kronos" with these words : "The oldest of the Greek gods, Kronos, we must conceive of as enthroned at the North Pole."[2]

We have now interrogated not only natural and ethnological science, but also the history, the traditions and myths of the eldest nations of the world. Nowhere have we found our hypothesis inadmissible; everywhere has it found remarkable confirmatory evidence. The aggregate of this evidence coming from such unexpected and entirely different sources is very great. It is so convincing that an advocate might well be content to leave the argument at this point, — at least until some advocate of a different location shall have made out a better case than any one has yet done. Before leaving the subject, however, we deem it wise to glance back to chapter sec-

---

[1] Pherecydes describes Kronos as dwelling in that part of heaven which is "nearest the earth," *i. e.,* the northern. Strabo, vii., 143, places him in "*the home of Boreas.*" It agrees herewith that Sanchoniathon, as preserved in the Greek version by Philo of Byblos, places the seat of his power "in the *middle* of the lands," ... in "a place *near springs and rivers,* where henceforth the worship of heaven was established." Lenormant, *Beginnings of History,* p. 531. Compare *infra,* Part fifth, chapters fourth and fifth : "The Navel of the Earth," and "The Quadrifurcate River."

[2] *Unsterblichkeitslehre,* i., p. 93.

ond of Part second, and inquire whether the various points there hypothetically set forth as of necessity " marked and memorable features " of a north polar Paradise, if such an one ever existed, are capable of any not yet alleged confirmation from the fields of history and science. The results of this inquiry will appear in the Part next following.

PART FIFTH.

FURTHER VERIFICATIONS BASED UPON THE PECULIARITIES OF A POLAR PARADISE.

When the Sun the East forgets,
When the Star no longer sets,
When the sacred Rishis seven
Wheel all night in highest heaven,
When the sky-descending Sea
Waters but a single Tree,
When each Year is but a Day, —
What shall all these portents say?

CHAPTER I.

THE EDEN STARS.

E vidi stelle
Non viste mai, for che alla prima gente.
                                    DANTE.

WE have already reminded the reader that in an
Eden situated at the North Pole the stars, instead of
seeming to rise and set as with us, would have had
a horizontal motion from left to right round and
round the observer. This appearance of the heavenly bodies could of course be found nowhere but at
the Pole. If, therefore, we could anywhere in the
world of ancient tradition find any statement of a
belief that at the beginning of the world the movements of the heavenly bodies were different from
their present movements, and particularly if we
should be able to find trace of a belief that the primeval motion of the stars was in orbits apparently
horizontal, this would certainly be a most striking
and cogent and unexpected evidence that human
observation of the starry heavens began at the Pole.

Now it so happens that we have traces of just
such a belief. In the tantalizing fragments of ancient lore, preserved to us in the pages of Diogenes
Laërtius, we find ascribed to the illustrious Greek
astronomer Anaxagoras this remarkable teaching:

"*In the beginning* the stars revolved in *a tholiform
manner.*"

Now to revolve in a tholiform manner is to revolve in a horizontal plane, like the θόλος, or "dome," of an astronomical observatory. Anaxagoras himself defined the motion more fully when he said that it was a motion, not ὑπὸ, underneath, but περὶ, around the earth.[1]

Anaximenes would seem to have had the same idea, for he is reported to have likened the primitive revolution of the sky to the rotating of a man's hat upon his head. Another explanatory expression (whether originating with Anaxagoras or with his reporter we do not know) is this: "At first *the Pole star*, which is continually visible, *always appeared in the zenith*, but afterward it acquired a certain declination." [2]

Here, then, we have as a doctrine of the ancient astronomers the singular notion that, in the beginning of the world, the celestial Pole was in the ze-

---

[1] See "Des Écrits et de la Doctrine d'Anaxagore" in *Histoire de l'Académie des Sciences et Belles Lettres de Berlin.* Berlin, 1755: vol. ix., pp. 378 ff.

[2] Diogenes Laërtius, ii., 9: Τὰ δ'ἄστρα κατ' ἀρχὰς μὲν θολοειδῶς ἐνεχθῆναι, ὥστε κατὰ κορυφὴν τῆς γῆς τὸν ἀεὶ φαινόμενον εἶναι πόλον, ὕστερον δὲ τὴν ἔγκλισιν λαβεῖν. Letronne (*Des Opinions Cosmographiques des Pères de l'Église rapprochées des Doctrines Philosophiques de la Grèce*) says that the opinion cannot have been limited to the school of Anaximenes and Zenophanes. "Elle a dû faire partie de la doctrine physique de plusieurs des sects anciennes." *Revue des Deux Mondes.* Paris, 1834 : p. 650. — In this connection it is well worthy of note that in the Japanese cosmogony the predecessor or "father," of our present sun and moon is represented as beginning his activities in the new-created world by repeatedly performing *in a horizontal plane* a circumambulation of the "Island of the Congealed Drop;" also that in Chinese tradition the first man *held the primeval sun and moon one in each hand.* Our latest Chinese writer upon the subject speaks of this as particularly noticeable. *Revue des Deux Mondes,* May 14, June 1, and June 14, 1884. A few passages are cited in *The Catholic World,* December, 1884, pp. 320–323.

nith, and that the revolutions of the stars were round a perpendicular axis.[1] What could have led an astronomer to *invent* such a doctrine it is impossible to say. On the other hand, if it was one of the interesting and seemingly paradoxical traditions of the early postdiluvian world, it is perfectly easy to see how imperishable a story it would be, particularly among the star-loving Chaldæans and Babylonians, from whom the earliest Greek astronomers and scientists received no small share of their doctrines.[2] And that the Chaldæans and probably the Egyptians had precisely this idea is not a notion here advanced for the first time.[3]

Another interesting question now suggests itself. When and under what circumstances was this alleged " declination " of the Pole imagined to have taken place ? Was it gradual, or sudden ? Did the ancients suppose it to have resulted from a movement in the regular order of nature, or from one in

---

[1] Since writing the above I have read Richard A. Proctor's " New Theory of Achilles' Shield," and have been particularly struck with his argument, from the position of the aquatic constellations in the most ancient astronomy, that the celestial equator at the time of the invention of the constellations must have been " *in a horizontal position.*" *Light Science for Leisure Hours.* London, 1870 : pp. 309–312.

[2] The instructor of Thales was a Chaldæan, a fact which writers on the early cosmological speculations of the Greeks have almost uniformly overlooked. See also L. von Schroeder, *Pythagoras und die Inder.* Leipsic, 1884.

[3] " Il est de même vraisemblable que les Chaldéens ont eu l'idée d'une destruction et d'un renouvellement du monde, c'est-à-dire, de la surface de notre globe, et conjointement avec cette destruction, *d'un déplacement des corps célestes du firmament.* . . . Diverses inscriptions dans les temples Égyptiens et des hiéroglyphes . . . me paraissent aussi être des essais de représenter distinctement la catastrophe du déluge et le *changement qui alors s'est opéré dans l'ancien ciel.*" — Klee, *Le Déluge.* Paris, 1847 : p. 307.

13

violation thereof? Was it to them a normal and
ever on-going change, or was it the record of a natural catastrophe?

Our hypothesis would lead us to expect the latter
of these suppositions.[1] The only rational and credible explanation of the declination is to be found in
a transfer of the theatre of human history from the
circumpolar home to some land of lower latitude.
Now if, during the prevalence of the Deluge, or
later, in consequence of the on-coming of the Ice
age, the survivors of the Flood were translocated
from their antediluvian home at the Pole to the
great Central Asian "plateau of Pamir," the probable starting-point of historic postdiluvian humanity, the new aspect presented by the heavens in this
new latitude would have been precisely as if in the
grand world-convulsion the sky itself had become
displaced, its polar dome tilted over about one third
of the distance from the zenith to the horizon.
The astronomical knowledge of those survivors very
likely enabled them to understand the true reason
of the changed appearance, but their rude descendants, unfavored with the treasures of antediluvian
science, and born only to a savage or nomadic life
in their new and inhospitable home, might easily
have forgotten the explanation. In time such children's children might easily have come to embody
the strange story handed down from their fathers
in strange myths, in which nothing of the original
facts remained beyond an obscure account of some
mysterious displacement of the sky, supposed to have

[1] Bailly in his *Histoire de l'Astronomie des Anciens* inclines to the
opinion that the ancient Egyptians thought the declination a gradual
one, but Klee expresses decided doubt. *Le Déluge*, p. 301.

occurred in a far-off age in connection with some appalling natural cataclysm or world-disaster.[1]

Now it is difficult to believe it a mere accident that in various ancient authors we find allusion both to an extremely ancient displacement of the sky and to its supposed original state. None of these allusions have ever been explained by writers on the subject. One of them occurs in Plato's Timæus, where, in language ascribed to an Egyptian priest of Solon's time, "a declination of the bodies revolving round the earth" is spoken of, and this declination is offered as the true explanation of the partial destruction of the world commemorated in the myth of Phaëthon. As this destruction was by fire there would at first sight seem to be no connection between it and the destruction at the time of the Deluge; nor is there in the context anything to suggest such a connection. Fortunately, however, we have in Hyginus a fuller version of the myth, from which it appears that the Greeks supposed Deukalion's universal flood to have been providentially sent to extinguish the fearful conflagration which Phaëthon's unskillful driving of the steeds of the sun had

[1] The only other plausible explanation of the facts now under consideration would be that furnished by the long ago proposed but emphatically rejected theory, that in some distant geological age in consequence of some cataclysm the axis of the earth's rotation was changed, bringing the new or present Pole into a region before temperate or torrid. C. F. Winslow, M. D., in his pamphlet on *The Cooling Globe*, Boston, 1865, was one of the most recent theorists to favor this view. But see Maedler, *Populäre Astronomie*, p. 370 ss., who states that, according to the calculations of Bessel, the bodily plucking up of one hundred and fourteen cubic miles of the Himalaya mountains and the transfer of them to North America would change the position of the earth's axis less than one hundred feet. Still stronger statements are made in the paper read before the London Geological Society, Feb. 21, 1877, by Professor J. F. Twisden.

occasioned. This makes the connection clear and direct. The Flood and the "declination of the heavenly bodies revolving round the earth" are at once brought into a true historic relation.[1]

In like manner, in the Bundahish, in the first five chapters, and in Zäd Sparam's paraphrase of the same, it is stated that during the first three thousand years, before the incoming of the Evil One, "the sun, moon, and stars stood still," but as soon as the Destroyer of the good creation came he assaulted and deranged the sky, as well as the earth and sea.[2] And remarkably enough, it is stated that as a result of this assault the Evil One mastered as much as "*one third* of the sky" and overspread it with darkness.[3] Moreover, in the thirtieth chapter, in giving a prophetic account of the final restoration of the material world to its primeval state, there seems to be an allusion in verse thirty-two to a necessary resetting or readjustment of the celestial vault by the hand of its Creator.[4]

To all such facts, wherever found, we have in the hypothesis of an Arctic Eden and a transfer of the human horizon at the time of the Deluge to lower latitudes a perfect key.

[1] Compare Milton, *Paradise Lost*, x. 648–690.

[2] "The Aztecs said that when the sun had risen for the first time, at the beginning, it *lay on the horizon, and moved not.*" Dorman, *Primitive Superstitions.* Phila., 1881 : p. 330. Both of these reports look as if they had sprung from misapprehension of the original tradition given by Anaxagoras.

[3] West, *Pahlavi Texts.* London, 1880: Pt. i., p. 17. West translates uncertainly. Justi renders the passage, "Er nahm vom Inneren des Himmels ein Drittheil ein." *Der Bundahish.* Leipsic, 1868 : p. 5.

[4] West, *Pahlavi Texts*, Pt. i., p. 129. This last remark is based upon West's version ; it is not supported by Windischmann's.

CHAPTER II.

THE EDEN DAY.

*Such day
As heaven's great year brings forth.*
MILTON.

To the first men, if the Garden of Eden was located at the Pole, there could have been but one day and one night in a year. Moreover, at the break of that strange day the sun must have risen, not in the East, as in postdiluvian times, but in the South. Do the traditions or sacred books of the ancient world afford any hint of such a sunrise and of such an Eden day?

A partial answer to this question is found in the beliefs of the ancient Northmen. A learned Danish writer pronounces it "remarkable" that the Scandinavian mythology informs us that, before the establishment of the present order of the world, the sun, which now rises in the East, "*rose in the South.*" [1]

Equally striking confirmations appear in other mythologies. Turning to the second Fargard of the Avesta, we find the most ancient Iranian account of Yima, the first man and "the King of the Golden Age." A detailed account is also given of a certain

---

[1] " Ce qu'il y a de plus remarquable dans la mythologie du Nord, c'est qu'elle nous reconte qu'avant l'ordre actuel des choses (avant que les fils de Bor, c'est-à-dire les dieux, eussent créé Midgard), le soleil se levait au Sud, tandis qu'à présent il se lève à l'Est." — Frédérik Klee, *Le Déluge,* Fr. ed. Paris, 1847 : p. 224.

Vara, or inclosure, which as a safe habitation — a kind of Garden of Eden — he was divinely commanded to make. Then comes this singular question and answer : "O Maker of the material world, thou Holy One! What lights are there in the Vara which Yima made ?"

"Ahura Mazda answered : There are uncreated lights and created lights. There the stars, the moon, and the sun are only *once a year* seen to rise and set, and *a year seems only as a day.*" [1] Haug's version of the last clause is, " And they think that a day which is a year." [2] Spiegel's is the same,[3] although in his Commentary he confesses himself perplexed as to the meaning of so remarkable a declaration. "The really genuine words," he observes, "are very difficult." They are not so when once the key is found.

That the East Aryans had the same idea is also evident from the Laws of Manu. Among this people Yama — the same as the Iranian Yima — was the first man. His first abode, as we have seen, was at the North Pole, and at death he became a god, the guardian of the South Pole, at which was the region of the dead. But though the Hindus no longer associated him with the North at the time of the writing of this ancient book, they well understood that Yama's primitive Eden in Ilâvrita, around the north polar Meru, where the gods reside, has only one day and one night in the year. This is the language of the Code : " A year of mortals is a day

[1] Darmesteter's Translation, vol. i., p. 20.

[2] Haug's *Essays on the Religion of the Parsis*, 2d ed., p. 235.

[3] " Diese (die Bewohner) halten für einen Tag was ein Jahr ist." Spiegel, *Avesta.* Leipsic, 1852 : vol. i., p. 77. See also his *Commentar über das Avesta.* Wien, 1864 : vol. i., pp. 78, 79.

and a night of the gods, or regents of the universe seated around the North Pole ; and again their division is this : their day is the northern and their night the southern course of the sun." [1]

In like manner, in the Sûrya Siddhânta we read, "The gods behold the sun, after it is once arisen, for half a year." [2]

Equally unmistakable is the language of the probably more ancient work, lately translated under the title of " The Institutes of Vishnu : " —

"The northern progress of the sun is a day with the gods.

"The southern progress of the sun is (with them) a night.

"A year is (with them) a day and a night." [3]

---

[1] *Code of Manu,* i. 67.

[2] Chapter xii., 74.

[3] *The Institutes of Vishnu,* translated by Julius Jolly. Ch. **xx., 1, 2, 3.** *Sacred Books of the East,* vol. vii., p. 77. I cannot help thinking that in these alternate approaches and recessions of the sun we have the true explanation of the origin of the old Rabbinical idea of half-yearly cold and heat in hell, this latter being located, as we have shown, at the South Pole : " The great Jalkut Rubeni gives us the following account of hell : Sheol is *half fire* and *half hail,* and therein are many rivers of fire. The seven abodes (or divisions) of hell are very spacious ; and in each there are seven rivers of fire and seven rivers of hail. The uppermost abode is sixty times less than the second, and thus the second is sixty times larger than the first, and every abode is sixty times larger than that which precedes it. In each abode are seven thousand caverns, and in each cavern seven thousand clefts, and in each cleft seven thousand scorpions ; and each scorpion hath seven limbs, and on each limb are one thousand barrels of gall. There are likewise seven rivers of rankest poison, which when a man toucheth he bursteth ; and the destroying angels judge him and scourge him every moment, *half a year* in the fire and *half a year* in the hail and snow. And the cold is more intolerable than the fire." Eisenmenger, *Entdecktes Judenthum,* vol. ii., p. 345 (English translation, vol. ii., p. 52). According to the *Sûrya Siddânta,* the demons as well as the gods behold the sun for six months at a time.

This strange notion is perfectly clear and comprehensible the moment we assume that the long-lived fathers and first regents of the human race originally dwelt at the North Pole, and that these, apotheosized and glorified in the imagination of later generations, in time became the gods which ancient nations worshiped.

Both in the Iliad and Odyssey the learned Anton Krichenbauer finds two kinds of days continually referred to. In what he considers the more ancient portions of the poems, the day is a period of one year's duration, especially when used in describing the life and exploits of the gods ; in what he considers the more modern portions, the term has its modern meaning as a period of twenty-four hours. He quotes Lepsius as recognizing a similar " one-day year " in the Egyptian and other ancient chronologies ; also the mention made of it by Palaifatos and Suidas.[1]

In all such hitherto unnoticed testimonies — and we have not exhausted the list of them [2] — we have new and singularly unimpeachable evidences that in the thought of these ancient peoples the land in which the generated gods and men alike originated was a land in which, as in our Polar Eden, a day and a night filled out the year. And if such was their

---

[1] *Beiträge zur homerischen Uranographie.* Wien, 1874 : pp. 1-34. Comp. p. 68.

[2] Even the Bushmen of South Africa have the strange idea that the sun did not shine on their country in the beginning. Only after the children of the first Bushmen had been sent up to the [Northern ?] top of the world and had launched the sun was light procured for this [subterranean] South African region. *Bushman Folk-lore.* By W. II. J. Bleek, Ph. D., Parliament Report. Capetown and London, 1875 : p. 9. A similar myth was found among the Australian aborigines.

idea, whence, save from actual tradition, could they have derived it? As cautious a scientific authority as Sir Charles Lyell, speaking of these cosmological and chronological traditions of the Hindus, says: "We can by no means look upon them as a pure effort of the unassisted imagination, or believe them to have been composed without regard to opinions and theories *founded on the observation of Nature.*" [1]

Even where the tradition has become distorted or inverted among barbarians, the parallelism of the year and the day is not always lost. A curious instance of this has come under the notice of the writer since the present chapter was begun: "In those days (in the world before the present) the seasons were much shorter than they are now. A year then was but as a day of our time." [2]

---

[1] *Elements of Geology,* 11th ed., vol. i., p. 8.

[2] W. Matthews, "The Navajo Mythology," in *The American Antiquarian and Oriental Journal.* Chicago, July, 1883: p. 209. Compare the expression given by Garcia as from the Mixteque cosmogony, in P. Dabry de Thiersant, *Origine des Indiens du Nouveau Monde.* Paris, 1883: p. 140 n. 2.

CHAPTER III.

THE EDEN ZENITH.

. . . The shrine where motion first began,[1]
And light and life in mingling torrent ran,
From whence each bright rotundity was hurled,
The Throne of God,—the Centre of the World.

CAMPBELL's Pleasures of Hope.

EL *walketh in the* CHUG *of heaven.* — Book of Job.

To the first men, on the hypothesis of an Arctic Eden, the zenith and the north pole of the heavens were identical. Such an aspect of the starry vault the humanity of our late historic ages has never seen. Under such an adjustment of the rotating firmament, how regular and orderly would nature appear! What profound significance would of necessity attach to that mysterious unmoving centre-point of cosmic revolution directly overhead! As intimated on page 50, that polar centre must naturally have seemed to be the top of the world, the true heaven, the changeless seat of the supreme God or gods. "And if, through all the long life-time of the antediluvian world, this circumpolar sky was thus to human thought the true abode of God, the

[1] The poet is speaking of the North Pole. The first three lines are illustrated by the closing chapters of Part third, above; the last sums up the facts to be set forth in the present chapter. A word from Menzel is here in place: " Nysa wird in vielen griechischen Mythen als im Centralpunkt bezeichnet von wo das Weltleben ausging und wohin es zurückkehrt. . . . Das ideale Nysa können wir nirgend anders als im Ausgangspunkte des Welt, im Nordpol suchen." *Die vorchristliche Unsterblichkeitslehre,* i. 65; also p. 42.

oldest postdiluvian peoples, though scattered down the sides of the globe half or two thirds the distance to the equator, could not easily forget that at the centre and true top of the firmament was the throne and the palace of its great Creator."

The religions of all ancient nations signally confirm and satisfy this antecedent expectation. With a marvelous unanimity *they associate the abode of the supreme God with the North Pole, "the centre of heaven," or with the celestial space immediately surrounding it.* No writer on Comparative Theology has ever brought out the facts which establish this assertion, but the following outline of them will suffice for our present purpose : —

First. *The Hebrew Conception.* — In so pure and lofty a monotheism as that of the ancient Hebrews, we must not expect to find any such strict localization of the supreme God in the circumpolar sky as we shall find among polytheistic peoples. "Do I not fill heaven and earth ?" is the language of Jehovah. Nevertheless, as the Hebrews must be supposed to have shared, in some measure, the geographical and cosmological ideas of their age, it would not be strange if in their sacred writings traces of these ideas were here and there discernible. Some of these traces are quite curious, and they have attracted the attention of not a few Biblical scholars, to whom their origin and *rationale* are entirely unsuspected. Thus a learned writer on Hebrew geography, after blindly repeating the common assumption that "the Hebrews conceived the surface of the earth to be an immense disk, supported, like the flat roof of an Eastern house, by pillars," yet uses such language as this : "The North appears to have been regarded as the highest part of the earth's surface, in consequence, perhaps, of the mountain ranges which existed there." [1]

Another, touching upon the same subject, says, "The Hebrews regarded what lay to the North as *higher,* and what lay to the South as *lower:* hence they who traveled from South to North were said to 'go up,' while they who went from North to South were said to 'go down.'" [2]

In Psalm seventy-fifth, verse sixth, we read, "Promotion cometh not from the East, nor from the West, nor from the South." Why this singular enumeration of three of the points of the compass, and this omission of the fourth? Simply because heaven, the proper abode of the supreme God, being conceived of by all the surrounding nations, if not by the Hebrews themselves, as in the North, in the circumpolar sky, that was the sacred quarter, and it could not reverently be said that promotion cometh not from the North.[3] It would have been as offensive as among us to say that promotion cometh not from above. Therefore, having completed his negative statements, the Psalmist immediately adds, "But God is the judge; He putteth down one, and setteth up another."

A curious trace of the same conception appears in the book of Job, in the eighth and ninth verses

[1] Rev. William Latham Bevan, A. M., in *Smith's Dictionary of the Bible,* Art. "Earth," vol. i., p. 633, 634 (Hackett's ed.). McClintock and Strong's *Cyclopædia,* Art. "Geography," vol. iii., p. 792.

[2] McClintock and Strong, *Cyclopædia,* Art. "North," vol. vii., p. 185. The Akkadians had the same idiom. Lenormant, *Beginnings of History,* p. 313.

[3] "A peculiar sanctity is attached to the North in the Old Testament records." T. K. Cheyne, *The Book of Isaiah.* London, 1870: pp. 140, 141. [See our cut: "The Earth of the Hindus," p. 152.]

of the twenty-third chapter. In Old Testament times, the Hebrews and the Arabians designated the cardinal points by the personal terms, " before " for East, "behind" for West, "left hand " for North, and " right hand " for South. Thus Job, in the passage indicated, is complaining that he can nowhere, East or West, North or South, find his divine judge.[1] But, in speaking of one of these points, he adds this singular qualification, "*where God doth work.*" This is said of the left hand, or North. It seems to be inserted to render peculiarly emphatic the declaration, "I go . . . [even] to the left hand where He doth work, but I cannot behold Him." If at first blush such an apparent localizing of the divine agency seems inconsistent with Job's splendid descriptions of God's omnipresence in other passages, it should be remembered that we, too, speak of the omnipresent deity as dwelling " on high," and address Him as " Our Father which art *in Heaven.*"

A natural counterpart to this idea of a northern heaven would be a belief or impression that spiritual perils and evils were in a peculiar degree or manner to be apprehended from the right hand, or South, as the proper abode of demons, — the quarter to which Asmodeus fled when exorcised by the angel.[2] We cannot positively affirm that such a belief con-

---

[1] Adam Clarke, *Commentary, in loc.* The best explanation the oldest commentators know how to give is this: There were more human beings and more intelligent ones North of Job's country than in either of the three other cardinal directions ; especially was the North the seat of the great Assyrian empire ; but God desires to reside and to work preëminently among men, hence the language of the text ! Matthew Poole, in *Dietelmair and Baumgarten's Bibelwerk*, vol. v., p. 634.

[2] Tobit, viii. 3. Compare *The Book of Enoch*, xviii. 6–16; xxi. 3–10.

sciously prevailed among the ancient Hebrews, but, holding the possibility in mind, we find passages of Scripture which seem to stand out in a new and striking light. Thus, in case there was such a belief, how great the force and beauty of the expression, " Because [the Lord] is at my right hand [the side exposed to danger] I shall not be moved." [1] With this may be compared the confident expressions of the one hundred and twenty-first Psalm : " The Lord is thy keeper : the Lord is thy shade upon thy right hand." So also in the ninety-first it is on the right hand that destruction is anticipated : " A thousand shall fall at thy side, and [or even] ten thousand at thy right hand ; but it shall not come nigh thee." Again, in the one hundred and forty-second it is said, " I looked on my right hand, but there was no man that would know me : refuge failed me ; no man cared for my soul." Notice also the imprecation, " Let Satan stand at his right hand" (Ps. cix. 6), and the vision of Zechariah, where the great adversary makes his appearance on the right of the one whom he came to resist (Zech. iii. 1).

But as Satan here reveals himself from beneath and from the South, so to Ezekiel the true God reveals himself from above and from the North (Eze. i. 4). In that quarter was God's holy mountain (Is. xiv. 13), the city of the Great King (Ps. xlviii. 2), the land of gold (Job xxxvii. 22, marg.), the place where divine power had hung the earth upon nothing (Job xxvi. 7).[2] Hence the priest officiating at

---

[1] Ps. xvi. 8. The reference seems all the more unmistakable since the next two verses speak of Sheol, or Hades.

[2] " Im Norden sind die höchsten Berge, vor allen der heilige Götterberg Is. 14, 13. . . . Vom Norden her kommt in der Regel Jeho-

the altar, both in the tabernacle and later in the temple, faced the North. According to the Talmud, King David had an Æolian harp in the North window of his royal bed-chamber, by means of which the North wind woke him every night at midnight for prayer and pious meditations.[1] Probably it is not without significance that in Ezekiel's vision of the ideal temple of the future the chamber prepared for the priests in charge of the altar was one "whose prospect was toward the North."[2] (Eze. xl. 46.)

vah." Herzog's *Real-Encyklopädie,* Art. "Welt," Bd. xvii., S. 678. "Like the Hindus, Persians, Greeks, and Teutons, . . . the She-mitic tribes spoke of a mountain of their gods in the far North (Is. xiv. 13; Eze. xxviii. 14); and even with the Jews, notwithstanding the counteracting influence of the Mosaic creed, traces of such a pop-ular belief continued to be visible (Ps. xlviii.), the North being, *e. g.,* regarded as the sacred quarter (Lev. i. 11; Eze. i. 4)." Dillmann, in *Schenkel's Bibel Lexicon.* Leipsic, 1879: vol. ii., p. 49.

[1] "Daily from the four quarters of the world blow the four Winds, of which three are continually attended by the North wind; otherwise the world would cease to be. The most pernicious of all is the South wind, which would destroy the world were it not held back by the angel Bennetz." Quoted from the Talmud by Bergel, *Studien über die naturwissenschaftlichen Kenntnisse der Talmudisten.* Leipsic, 1880: p. 84. Compare Dillmann, *Das Buch Henoch,* Kap. lxxvi.; lxxvii.; xxv. 5; xxxiv.; xxxvi. W. Menzel, *Die vorchrist-liche Unsterblichkeitslehre,* Bd. ii., p. 35, 101, 168, 345. See also p. 177 of this volume.

[2] At first view it seems strange that in the Middle Ages, in Chris-tian Europe, the North should have come to be regarded as the special abode of Satan and his subjects, and that on the north side of some churches, near the baptismal font, there should have been a "Devil's Door," which was opened to let the evil spirit pass to his own place at the time of the renunciation of him by the person baptized. The simple explanation of this is found in the fact that the people were taught that their old gods, whom they had worshiped when pagans, were devils. Compare Grimm, *Deutsche Mythologie,* p. 30, 31. Con-way, in his *Demonology and Devil Lore* (London, 1879: vol. ii., 115; i., 87), entirely misconceives the philosophy of the fact. A similar change seems to have occurred among the Iranians after Mazdeism

Second. *The Egyptian Conception.* — The correspondence of the ancient Egyptian conception of the world and of heaven with the foregoing would be remarkable did we not know that Egypt was the cradle of the Hebrew people. The ancient inhabitants of the Nile valley had the same idea as to the direction of the true summit of the earth. To them, as to the Hebrews, it was in the North. This was the more remarkable since it was exactly contrary to all the natural indications of their own country, which continually ascended toward the South. As stated in a previous chapter, Brugsch says, " The Egyptians conceived of the earth as rising toward the North, so that *in its northernmost point it at last joined the sky.*" [1] In correspondence herewith the Egyptians located their *Ta-nuter,* or "land of the gods," in the extreme North.[2] On this account it is on the *northern* exterior wall of the great temple of Ammon at Karnac that the divinity promises to King Rameses II. the products of that heavenly country, " silver, gold, lapis-lazuli, and all the varieties of precious stones of the land of the gods." Hence, also, contrary to all natural indications, the northern hemisphere was considered the realm of light, the southern the realm of darkness.[3]

had transformed their ancient Daêvas from gods to demons. Hence, while in portions of the Avestan literature (generally the older) the heaven of Ahura Mazda is in the North, in other portions the North is the world of death and demons. See Bleek's *Avesta,* i., pp. 3, 137, 143 ; ii. 30, 31 ; iii. 137, 138, *et passim.* Darmesteter, Introduction, p. lxvii., lxxx. Haug, *Religion of the Parsis,* pp. 267 ff.

[1] *Geographische Inschriften altægyptischer Denkmäler.* Leipsic, 1858 : vol. ii., p. 37.

[2] In one place Brugsch translates *ta-nutar-t mahti* " das nördliche Gottesland." *Astronomische und astrologische Inschriften,* p. 176.

[3] " To the twelve great gods of heaven are immediately subjected

The passage out of the secret chambers of the Great Pyramid was pointed precisely at the North Pole of the heavens. All the other pyramids had their openings only on the northern side. That this arrangement had some religious significance few students of the subject have ever doubted. If our interpretation is correct, such passages from the burial chamber toward the polar heaven intimated a vital faith that from the chamber of death to the highest abode of life, imperishable and divine, the road is straight and ever open.[1]

Third. *The Conception of the Akkadians, Assyrians, Babylonians, Indians, and Iranians.* — After what has been said in former chapters respecting the location of Kharsak Kurra, Sad Matâti, Har-Moed, Su-Meru, and Harâ-berezaiti, no further proof is needed that all the peoples above named associated the true heaven, the abode of the highest gods,

the stars dispersed in infinite number through all the ethereal space, and divided into four principal groups according to the four quarters of the world. They were then divided into two orders more elevated, the one filling the northern hemisphere and belonging to light, to the good principle, the other to the southern hemisphere, dark, cold, *funeste*, and to the sombre abodes of Amenti." Guigniaut's Creuzer, *Religions de l'Antiquité*, vol. ii., p. 836. A very curious survival of the above conception is found in the Talmudic *Emek Hammeleck*. See Eisenmenger, *Entdecktes Judenthum*, Stehelin's version, vol. i., p. 181 ; comp. p. 255 ff.

[1] The association of Set with the constellation of the Great Bear, reported by Plutarch and lately confirmed by original astronomical texts (Brugsch, *Astronomische Inschriften altægyptischer Denkmäler*, Leipsic, 1883, pp. 82-84, 121-123), seems at first view inconsistent with the south polar location of demons and destructive divinities. But the apparent difficulty is transformed into an all the stronger proof of the correctness of our theory when it is remembered that in the most ancient times Set " was not a god of evil," but the supreme world-sovereign from whom the Egyptian kings derived their authority over the two hemispheres. " *It was not till the decline of the Em-*

with the northern celestial pole.[1] In each case the apex of their respective mounts of the gods pierced the sky precisely at that point. To this day the Haranite Sabæans — the most direct heirs of the religious traditions of the Tigro-Euphratean world —construct their temples with careful reference to the ancient faith.[2] Their priests also, in the act of sacrifice, like all ancient priesthoods, face the North.[3]

In the Rig Veda, ii., 40, 1, we read of the *amŕtasya nắbhim*, " the Navel of the Heavens." The same or similar expressions occur again and again in the Vedic literature. They refer to the northern celestial Pole, just as the expression *nắbhir pṛthivyắs,* " Navel of the Earth," R. V. iii., 29, 4, and elsewhere, signifies the northern terrestrial Pole. To each is ascribed preëminent sanctity. The one is the holi-

---

pire that this deity came to be regarded as an evil demon, that his name was effaced from the monuments, and other names substituted for his in the Ritual." Renouf, *Religion of Ancient Egypt*, pp. 119, 120. The expression *navel* or *centre of heaven*, as a designation for the northern celestial Pole, so common among ancient nations, would seem to have been current among the Egyptians also. Brugsch, Ibid., p. 122, 123. In the text as translated, however, there is some obscurity. Compare p. 154.

[1] " There can be no doubt that ' the Heaven of Anu ' was the particular limited celestial region, centring in the Pole star and penetrated by the summit of the Paradisaical Mount." — Rev. O. D. Miller, *The Oriental and Biblical Journal.* Chicago, 1880 : p. 173.

[2] " L'église n'a que deux fenêtres et une porte qui est toujours ouverte du côté du sud, afin que celui qui y entre ait l'étoile polaire devant lui." — N. Siouffi, *Études sur la Religion des Soubbas ou Sabéens, les Dogmes, leur Mœurs.* Paris, 1880 : p. 118.

[3] " Cette position de la victime permet au sacrificateur, qui a le morgno appuyé sur l'épaule gauche, de se placer, pour remplir son rôle, de façon qu'il ait la figure tournée vers l'étoile polaire qui couvre Avather, tout en ayant en même temps la tête de l'animal à sa droite." — Ibid., p. 112.

est shrine in heaven, the other the holiest shrine on earth. That no translator has hitherto caught the true meaning of the terms seems unaccountable.[1]

In Buddhism, the heir and conservator of so many of the ancient ideas of India, the same notion of a world ruler with his throne at the celestial Pole lived on.[2] Very curiously, if we follow the authority of the Lalitavistara, the first actions and words ascribed to the infant Buddha on his arrival in our world unmistakably identify the North with the abode of the gods, and *its nadir* with the abode of the demons.[3] Even the modern relics of the non-Aryan aboriginal tribes of India, as for example the Gonds, have retained this ancient ecumenical ethnic belief.[4]

---

[1] In his heading to Hymn I., 185, 5. Grassman parenthetically conjectures that the Navel of the World therein spoken of may be "*im Osten,*" but suggests no reason for its location in that or any other quarter. Not by accident, however, did the ancient bard elsewhere (X., 82, 2) place the abode of God "beyond the Seven Rishis," in the highest North.

[2] "The omnipotence of Amitâbha is dwelt on in some fine *gâthâs.* In *the centre of heaven* he sits on the lotus throne and guides the destinies of mortals." Arthur Lillie, *Buddha and Early Buddhism.* London, 1882: p. 128. Compare also p. 7 : "This Pole-star (*Alpha Draconis*) was believed to be the pivot round which the cosmos revolved. . . . The symbol of God and the situation of Paradise got to be associated with this star."

[3] "Le Lalitavistara, 97, rapporte ces paroles d'une manière un peu différente : 'Je suis le plus glorieux dans ce monde, etc.' Ensuite, après avoir fait sept pas dans la direction du septentrion : 'Je serai le plus grand de tous les êtres,' puis après sept pas dans la direction du nadir : 'Je détruirai le Malin et les mauvais esprits, je publierai la loi suprême qui doit éteindre le feu de l'Enfer au profit de tous les habitants du monde souterrain.'" Note to Professor Kern's *Histoire du Bouddhisme dans l'Inde. Revue de l'Histoire des Religi ns.* Paris : tom. v., nro. 1, p. 54. Compare the less explicit account in Beal's *Romantic History of Buddha,* p. 44.

[4] "In burying they lay the head to the South and the feet to the

Fourth. *The Phœnician, Greek, Etruscan, and Roman Conception.* — That the Phœnicians shared the general Asiatic view of a mountain of the gods in the extreme North appears from Movers' learned work upon that people.[1]

The evidence that in ancient Hellenic thought, also, the heaven of the gods was in the northern sky is incidental, but cumulative and satisfactory. For example, heaven is upheld by Atlas, but the terrestrial station of Atlas, as we have elsewhere shown, is at the North Pole. Again, Olympos was the abode of the gods ; but if the now generally current etymology of this term is correct, Olympos was simply the Atlantean pillar, pictured as a lofty mountain, and supporting the sky at its northern Pole.[2] In fact, many writers now affirm that the Olympos of Greek mythology was originally simply the north polar " World-mountain " of the Asiatic nations.[3]

North, *as the home of their gods is supposed to be in the latter direction.* They call the North Deoguhr sometimes, and the South, Muraho, is looked upon as a region of terror ; so the feet are laid towards Deoguhr in order that they may carry the dead man in the right direction." — *Report of Ethnological Committee,* quoted in Spencer's *Descriptive Sociology,* Div. I., Pt. 3, A., p. 36.

[1] *Die Phönizier.* Bonn, 1841–56, vol. i., pp. 261, 414.

[2] " Here the idea is that the gods reside above this mountain [Su-Meru], which is, as it were, the support of their dwellings. This brings to our mind the fable of Atlas supporting the heavens ; the same idea may probably be traced in the Greek Olympos (Sanskrit, *âlamba,* a ' support ')." Samuel Beal, *Four Lectures on Buddhist Literature in China.* London, 1882 : p. 147. Compare Grill.

[3] Compare A. H. Sayce, *Transactions of Society Bib. Archeology,* vol. iii., 152. — Even in the mathematical cosmos of Philolaos, though the *sedes deorum* seems to be placed in Hestia, at the centre of the system, there is yet a steep way leading perpendicularly to the polar summit of the heavens, by means of which the gods and holy souls attain the diviner realm of all perfection : " Dii vero, quando ad convivium pergunt, tum quidem acclivi via proficiscuntur sub summum

In prayer the Greeks turned towards the North, and from Homer we know that when they addressed the "Olympian" gods they stretched out their hands "toward the starry heavens;" Greek prayers, therefore, must have been addressed toward the northern heavens.   Entirely confirmatory of this is the account Plato gives of "the holy habitation of Zeus," in which the solemn convocations of the gods were held, and which, he explains, "was placed in the Centre of the World." [1]

That this Centre is the northern celestial Pole is placed beyond question by a well-known passage from Servius Maurus,[2] where it is called the "*domicilium Jovis,*" and where we are informed that the Etruscan and Roman augurs considered thunder and lightning in the northern sky more significant than in any other quarter, being "higher and *nearer to the abode of Jove.*" [3]   Countries in high northern latitudes shared in this peculiar sanctity.   "Toward

qui sub cœlo est fornicem (ἀψῖδα), et immortales quæ dicuntur animæ, quando ad summum pervenerunt, extra progressæ in cœli dorso consistunt, circumlatæque cum iis animabus, quæ comitari eas potuerunt, loca supra cœlum spectant, ubi pura et absoluta veritas, cognitio virtus, pulchritudo, atque omnis omnino perfectio patet." Aug. Bœckh, "De vera indole astronomiæ Philolaicæ." *Gesammelte Kleine Schriften.* Leipsic, 1866: vol. iii., p. 288. Compare pp. 290–292.

[1] *Critias,* 120.   [2] *Æneid,* ii. 693.

[3] "*E' ideo ex ipsa parte significantiora esse fulmina, quoniam altiora et viciniora domicilio Jovis.*" Compare Regell, "*Das Schautempel der Augurn*" in the *Neue Jahrbücher der Philologie,* Bd. cxxiii., pp. 593–637. "The Hawaiian soothsayer, or *kilo-kilo,* turned always to the North when observing the heavens for signs or omens, or when regarding the flight of birds for similar purposes. The ancient Hindus turned also to the North for divining purposes, and so did the Iranians before the schism, after which they placed the devs in the North; so did the Greek, and so did the Scandinavians before their conversion to Christianity." A. Fornander, *The Polynesian Race.* London, 1878: vol. i., p. 240.

the end of the official or state paganism," says M.
Beauvois, "the Romans regarded Great Britain as
nearer heaven and more sacred than the Mediterranean countries."[1] Varro and other Latin writers
confirm this general representation, so that all modern expounders of the old Etruscan religion unite
in locating the abode of the gods of Etruria in the
Centre of Heaven, the northern circumpolar sky.[2]
Niebuhr and other authorities of the highest rank
assure us that the Romans shared the same faith.[3]

[1] "*Sacratiora sunt profecto Mediterraneis loca vicina cœlo.*" Beauvois, in *Revue de l'Histoire des Religions.* Paris, 1883 : p. 283. The
statement is based upon expressions in the official panegyric of the
Emperor Constantine Augustus. Compare the following : " Diodorus Siculus speaks of a nation whom he calls the Hyperboreans, who
had a tradition that their country is nearest to the moon, on which
they discovered mountains like those on the earth, and that Apollo
comes there once every nineteen years. This period, being that of the
metonic cycle of the moon, shows that if this could have been really
discovered by them they must have had a long acquaintance with
astronomy." Flammarion, *Astronomical Myths.* London : p. 88.

[2] " Im Nordpunkte der Welt." K. O. Müller, *Die Etrusker.* Breslau, 1828 : Bd. ii., pp. 126, 129. " Suivant eux, ceux-ci devaient habi-
ter dans la partie septentrionale du ciel, à raison de son immobilité.
C'est de la région polaire qu'ils veillaient sur toute la terre." A.
Maury, in *Religions de l'Antiquité,* Creuzer et Guigniaut, tom. ii., p.
1217. " La théologie étrusque, accueillant une doctrine que nous
avons déjà recontrée à l'état de rêve confus dans la théologie grecque,
plaçait à l'extrême nord le séjour des Æsars ou dieux. Mais, tandis
que l'Hellène se tourne vers les dieux pour les interroger, le Toscan
imite leur attitude supposée, afin de voir l'espace comme ils le voient
eux-mêmes. Ayant donc le visage tourné vers le midi, il appelle
antica la moitié méridionale du ciel," etc. A. Bouche-Leclercq, La
Divination chez les Étrusques. *Revue de l'Histoire des Religions.*
Paris, 1881 : tom. iii., p. 326.

[3] " Der Wohnsitz der Götter ward im Norden der Erde geglaubt."
Niebuhr, *Römische Geschichte,* vol. ii., Anhang, p. 702. " It is well
known that the Romans placed the seat of the gods in the extreme
North." *The Oriental Journal.* Chicago, 1880 : vol. i., p. 143. Niebuhr's remark, " Der Augur dachte sich schauend wie die Götter auf
die Erde schauen," explains the somewhat unqualified and mislead-

Fifth. *The Japanese Conception.* — We have already seen that in the Japanese cosmogony the down-thrust spear of Izanagi becomes the upright axis of heaven and earth. Izanagi's place, therefore, at the upper end of this axis can be nowhere else than at the North Pole of the sky.[1]

But we are not left to inference. So inseparably was the Creator associated with the Pole in ancient Japanese thought that one of his loftiest and divinest titles was derived from this association. Writing of the primitive ideas of this people, one of our best authorities uses the following language : " I shall do the *Ko-ji-ki*, and the Shinto religion, and the Japanese philosophy, strict justice by saying that, according to them, there existed in the beginning one god, and nobody and nothing besides.

> " ' Far in the deep infinitudes of space,
> Upon a throne of silence,'

sat the god Ame-no-mi-naka-nushi-no-kami, whose name signifies THE LORD OF THE CENTRE OF HEAVEN." [2]

What this Centre of Heaven is cannot well be doubtful to any careful reader of the present chapter.

Sixth. *The Chinese Conception.* — The oldest traceable worship among the Chinese is that of Shang-te, the highest of all gods. It is believed to have existed more than two thousand years before Christ. Shang-te is usually and correctly described

ing statement of Professor Kuntze touching the rotary posture of the Roman in prayer. *Prolegomena zur Geschichte Roms. Oraculum, Auspicium Templum, Regnum.* Leipsic, 1882 : p. 15.

[1] See above, pt. iv., ch. 2.

[2] Sir Edward J. Reed, *Japan*, vol. i., p. 27. Compare Léon de Rosny, in *Revue de l'Histoire des Religions.* Paris 1884 : p. 208 ; also p. 211.

as the god of heaven. But his proper place of
abode, his palace, is called Tsze-wei. And if we inquire as to the meaning and location of Tsze-wei,
the native commentators upon the sacred books in-
form us that it is "a celestial space about the North
Pole." [1]

Here, as in Japan, and in Egypt, and in India, and
in Iran, and in Greece, the Pole is "*the centre*" of
the sky. A writer in the "Chinese Repository"
quotes from authoritative religious books these declarations: "The Polar star is the Centre of Heaven."
"Shang-te's throne is in Tsze-wei, *i. e.*, the Polar
star." "Immediately over the central peak of
Kwen-lun appears the Polar star, which is Shang-
te's heavenly abode." "In the central place the
Polar star of Heaven, the one Bright One, the
Great Monad, always dwells." [2]

In accordance with this conception, the Emperor
and his assistants, when officiating before the Altar
of Heaven, always face the North.[3] The Pole-star
itself is a prominent object of worship.[4] And how
prevalent this localization of the abode of God at

---

[1] Legge, *The Chinese Classics*, vol. iii., Pt. i., p. 34 n. See further,
Legge, *Spring Lectures on the Religions of China*, London, 1880, p.
175, and the not well understood prayer in Douglas, *Confucianism
and Tauism*, London, 1879, p. 278. From these and other references
it is plain that Confucians and Tauists alike identified the northern
sky with the abode of God.

[2] Vol. iv., p. 194. So, likewise in West Mongolian thought the
celestial pole and the "apex of the Golden Mountain" are identical :
"*Altan kadasu niken nara Tagri-dschin urkilka.* Apex montis
aurei, nomine Cardo Cœli, stella polaris." *Uranographia Mongolica.
Fundgruben des Orients*, Bd. iii., p. 181.

[3] See *English Translation of the Chinese Ritual for the Sacrifice to
Heaven.* Shanghai, 1877 : pp. 25, 26, 27, 28, 31, 48.

[4] Joseph Edkins, *Religion in China*, p. 115. Compare G. Schlegel,
Uranographie Chinoise, pp. 506, 507.

the Pole remains after four thousand years may be illustrated by the following incident narrated by Rev. Dr. Edkins : " I met on one occasion a schoolmaster from the neighborhood of Chapoo. He asked if I had any books to give away on astronomy and geography. Such books are eagerly desired by all members of the literary class. . . . The inquiry was put to him 'Who is the Lord of heaven and earth?' He replied that he knew none but the Polestar, called in the Chinese language *Teen-hwang-ta-te,* — the Great Imperial Ruler of Heaven." [1]

Seventh. *The Ancient German and the Finnic Conception.* — Like the ancients, when praying and sacrificing to the gods, the pagan Germans turned their faces toward the North.[2] There, in the northern heaven, at the top of Yggdrasil, the world-axis, stood the fair city of Asgard, the home of the Asen. The Eddas expressly say of it that it was built " in the Centre of the World." [3] At that point, whence alone

---

[1] *Religion in China,* p. 109. This title irresistibly suggests the Assyrian one, *Dayan-Same,* " Judge of Heaven." *Transactions Society Bib. Archæology,* iii. 206.

[2] Jakob Grimm, " Betende und opferende Heiden schauten gen Norden." *Deutsche Mythologie,* Bd. i., p. 30.

[3] Grimm, " Im Mittelpunkte der Welt." *Deutsche Mythologie,* p. 778. The following is from the Prose Edda : " Then the sons of Bör built in the middle of the universe the city called Asgard, where dwell the gods and their kindred, and from that abode work out so many wondrous things both on the earth and in the heavens above it. There is in that city a place called Hlidskjálf, and when Odin is seated there upon his lofty throne he sees over the whole world, discerns all the actions of men, and comprehends whatever he contemplates. His wife is Frigga, the daughter of Fjörgyn, and they and their offspring form the race that we call the Æsir, — a race that dwells in Asgard the old, and in the regions around it, and that we know to be entirely divine." Mallet, *Northern Antiquities,* p. 406. The expression, " from that abode work out so many wondrous things," recalls to mind Job's description of the North as the place " where God doth work."

the whole world of men is ever visible by night and
by day, stood Hlidskjálf, the watch-tower of Odin.
From this "*partie septentrionale du ciel*" he and
Frigga, like the great gods of the Etruscans, "*veillaient sur toute la terre.*" [1]

Among the ancient Finns the name of the supreme god was Ukko. In their mythology he is
sometimes represented as upbearing the firmament,
like Atlas, and sometimes he is called *Taivahan Na-
panen*, "the Navel of Heaven." As Castrén shows,
this curious title is given him simply because he resides in the centre or Pole of heaven.[2] In the great
epic of this people, the Kalevala, the abode of the
supreme God is called Tähtela,[8] which word simply
means " Place of *Tähti :* Esthonian, *Täht*, the Polar
star."

We have not exhausted our materials in hand for
the illustration of this point,[4] but surely we have
presented enough. Reviewing this singular unanimity of the ancient nations, no thoughtful reader
can fail to be impressed with its significance. No
other explanation of it can be so simple and obvious
as the supposition that the heaven which overarched the cradle of humanity was a heaven whose
zenith was the northern Pole.

Before concluding the present chapter, another
point of considerable interest should be noticed. In
reading the Edenic traditions of the ancient nations

---

[1] *Vide supra*, p. 214 n. 2.

[2] Castrén, *Finnische Mythologie* (Tr. Schiefner), pp. 32, 33.

[8] Rune 11, 32, 36, 40.

[4] See, for example, Gill, *Myths and Songs of the South Pacific.* London, 1876 : p. 17.

as given in Part fourth, the question may well have suggested itself to the reader, "How is it that, with such perfect unanimity on the part of contemporary nations in respect to the north-polar position of the cradle of mankind, the traditions of the Hebrews alone should have placed it in the East?" In the facts just now reviewed we have a key to this puzzle. The only word in Genesis which connects Eden with the East is Kedem (*Qedem*). This term "properly means that which is *before* or *in front of* a person, and was applied to the East from *the custom* of turning in that direction when describing the points of the compass."[1] From Gen. xiii. 14, it would seem to have acquired this association with the East as early as the days of Abraham, but according to "the custom" of a particular time or people it could mean one point of the compass as well as another. It was simply the "front-country." In late historic times among the Hebrews it was the East, and accordingly the West was the country "behind," the North the "left hand," the South the "right," as before noticed. In Egypt, however, the usage was different, — the "front-country" being either the North or the South, — which we cannot certainly tell, as Egyptologists are divided on the question. Pierret thinks that it was South, and that accordingly the right hand was West and the left East.[2] Chabas and others, however, exactly reverse the meaning of the hieroglyphics translated "right" and "left," and hold that in designating the points of the compass the ancient Egyptian faced the North.

---

[1] Smith's *Bible Dictionary*, Art. "East."

[2] *Dictionnaire d'Archéologie Égyptienne.* Paris, 1875 : p. 191. Comp. pp. 116, 118, 187, 344, 351, 364, 371, 392, 399.

Among the Akkadians and Assyrians, if we may rely upon a questionable statement of Lenormant, still another adjustment prevailed : the right hand was the North, the left the South, and the "front" direction, of course, the West.[1]

In view of these facts it is plain that, anterior to the fixation of Hebrew usage, that is in pre-Abrahamic times, *Qedem*, or the "front-country," may as well have meant the North as any other quarter. And there is much reason to suppose that it did have this meaning. We have seen that this was peculiarly the sacred quarter of the whole Asiatic and Egyptian world. Toward it faced all earliest priesthoods and worshipers of whom we have any knowledge.[2] What so natural as that they should contemplate and designate the different quarters of the world from the standpoint of their normal posture in worship ? And if once we assume that such was the usage of all the Noachidæ anterior to their dispersion, and that accordingly "the front-country" meant the North, all at once becomes plain. Genesis then unites with universal ethnic tradition in locating the cradle of mankind in the North. The record then reads, "And the Lord God planted a garden in the North country, in Eden." And, in precise agreement herewith, it is down from the mountainous heights of this North country — "from

---

[1] *Fragments de Bérose*, p. 367 ; also, 380, 419. But compare *Chaldæan Magic*, pp. 168, 169, where, by identifying the West with the point " behind the observer," he directly contradicts the account given in his Commentary on Berosus. The paragraph does not appear in the original French edition of the work.

[2] Even among the aborigines of America and Africa we are told that "the West is the left hand and the East the right." Massey, *The Natural Genesis*, vol. ii., p. 231.

Qedem " — that the descendants of Noah in after
time come into " the plain in the land of Shinar "
(Gen. xi. 2). So is cleared up simultaneously another mystery, for how to bring the first colonizers
of Shinar into the Tigro-Euphrates valley, from any
probable Ararat by any probable " journeying *from
the East*," or, as the margin gives it, " *eastwards*,"
has always perplexed the commentator.[1]

This interpretation harmonizes for the first time
Gen. ii. 8 with Eze. xxviii. 13, both now referring to
one and the same point of the compass, the sacred
North. Again, the well-known difficulty of harmonizing the references to " the children of Qedem,"
found in the oldest of the Hebrew Scriptures, such
as Gen. xxix. 1, and Job i. 3, is solved at once by
this interpretation. At the same time it gives us a
location for "the land of Uz" exactly corresponding with the explicit declaration of Josephus : " Uz
founded Trachonitis and Damascus ; this country
lies between Palestine and Cœlosyria." [2]

To most readers, this solution of the problem of
the exceptional character of the Hebrew tradition
will probably at once commend itself as eminently
satisfactory. To some, however, it may seem a little
difficult of belief that one and the same term could
in successive ages have found application to different points of the compass.[3] To such the following,

---

[1] Of course, this interpretation proceeds upon the common assumption that *Miqqedem* is translocative in signification, and that the land
of Shinar was in the Tigro-Euphrates basin. In another note I have
indicated the possibility that the land of Shinar was in primeval Qedem, in which case *Miqqedem* in Gen. xi. 2 should be translated precisely as in Gen. ii. 8, " *in* the North country."

[2] *Antiquities of the Jews*, Bk. i., 6, 4.

[3] See diagram illustrative of the discrepancy between Euphratean
and Egyptian orientations in Brown, *Myth of Kirké*. London, 1883 :

written, of course, with no reference to our problem,
will be of special interest: "The names of the four
cardinal points, and, what is very remarkable, the
hieroglyphic signs by which they are expressed, are
in a certain measure the same in the Akkadian and
Chinese cultures. This I intend to show in a special monograph upon the subject; but that which is
here of importance to note is the displacement of
the geographical horizon produced in the establishing of the 'hundred families.' The South, which
was so termed on the cuneiform tablets, corresponds
in Chinese to the East, the North to the West, the
East to the South, making thus a displacement of
quarter of a circle. It would be interesting if, on
examination of the Akkadian and Assyrian names,
we could find that they in their turn denoted an
early displacement of which only these traces remain to us." [1]

p. 99. Comp. p. 101, bot. Mr. G. Massey, in his vast astrotypolog-
ical medley, refers to the horizon-displacement, but affords no intelligible explanation. He says, "In making the change to a circle of
twelve signs, the point of commencement in the North was 'slewed'
round eastward. Hence the Akkadian Mountain of the World became the Mountain of the East. Mount Meru, the primordial birth-
place in the North, likewise became the Mountain eastward. This
may be followed in the Adamah of the Genesis; and in the Book of
Enoch it says, 'The fourth wind, which is named the North, is divided
into three parts, and the third part contains Paradise.' Thus Eden,
which began at the summit of the Mount, and descended into the
Circle of Four Quarters prepared by Yima, in the Avesta, against
the coming Deluge, was finally planted in the twelfth division of the
zodiac of twelve signs, as the garden eastward." *The Natural Genesis.* London, 1883: vol. ii., p. 263.

[1] Terrien de Lacouperie, *Early History of the Chinese Civilization.*
London, 1880: p. 29. On this curious matter Mr. T. G. Pinches
threw some new light at a meeting of the Society of Biblical Archeology, Feb. 6, 1883. In May Mr. Terrien de Lacouperie read a paper
before the Royal Asiatic Society, entitled "The Shifting of the Car-

Possibly the usage of ancient Egypt may enable us to put our solution in yet simpler form. If we may accept the teachings of the learned Maspéro, the Egyptians often reduced the four quarters or directions to two, using the term East in a sense sufficiently broad to include both East and North, and the term West in a sense sufficiently broad to include both West and South.[1] If, then, Moses, who in his education was an Egyptian, wrote in accord-

dinal Points in Chaldæa and China," which will appear in his forthcoming work on *The Origin of Chinese Civilization.* Similar interchanges and identifications of the North and West are referred to by Menzel, *Die vorchristliche Unsterblichkeitslehre,* i., p. 101. See also *Asiatic Researches,* vol. viii., pp. 275–284.

[1] "J'ai exposé depuis longtemps dans mes cours au Collége de France une théorie d'après laquelle les Egyptiens auraient divisé les quatre points en deux séries groupées : Nord-Est, Sud-Ouest. . . . Ce n'est que par suite de la classification dont je viens de parler qu'on met souvent à l'Ouest les régions proprement situées au Sud, ou reciproquement au Sud les régions situées à l'Ouest. L'application de cette idée à l'Est nous mène aussi à croire que l'on a pu dire du *Tanoutri* qu'il était au Nord." (M. Maspéro, in a letter to the author, under date of December 20, 1882.) This usage could hardly have arisen among any people not acquainted with the spherical figure of the earth. How easily it could arise among us is illustrated by Sir John de Maundeville, who, writing in A. D. 1356, located Paradise so far to the East of England that *he could no longer correctly describe the place by this term.* Thus, after speaking of the Terrestrial Paradise as situate far " to the East, at the *beginning* of the earth," he says, " But this is not that East which we call our East, on this half, where the sun rises to us ; for when the sun rises is East in those parts towards Terrestrial Paradise, it is then midnight in our parts on this half, on account of the roundness of the earth, of which I have told you before ; for our Lord God made the earth all round in the middle of the firmament." Wright, *Early Travels in Palestine.* London, 1848 : p. 276. The nearest way to an Eden thus located would, of course, be northward. Its location could therefore be described with equal correctness either by the term " eastward " or " northward." Still another interesting theory of its origin will suggest itself to the thoughtful student of such facts as those alluded to by Mr. Scribner in *Where did Life Begin?* pp. 32, 33.

ance with such a usage, it would be quite possible to use Qedem for a "front-country" in the North, and again, without embarrassment, to use the same term in speaking of the East.[1]

[1] Compare the arrangement of the winds on the ceiling of the Pronaos of the temple at Dendera. Brugsch, *Astronomische Inschriften altägyptischer Denkmäler.* Leipsic, 1883 : pp. 26 bot., and 27 top.

CHAPTER IV.

THE NAVEL OF THE EARTH.[1]

He is the god who sits in the centre, on the Navel of the Earth; and he is the interpreter of religion to all mankind. — PLATO.

But at the Navel of the Earth stands Agni, clothed in richest apparel. — Rig Veda.

To whom then will ye liken God? It is HE *that sitteth upon the* CHUG *of the Earth, and the inhabitants thereof are as grasshoppers.* — ISAIAH.

After proceeding some distance we paused to take breath where the crowd was more dense and obstinate than usual: and I was seriously informed that this was the exact Navel of the Earth, and that these obstinate pilgrims were bowing and kissing it. — The Land and the Book.

Jedes Volk hat einen Nabel der Erde. — KLEUKER.

STUDENTS of antiquity must often have marveled that in nearly every ancient literature they should encounter the strange expression " the Navel of the Earth." Still more unaccountable would it have seemed to them had they noticed how many ancient mythologies *connect the cradle of the human race with this earth-navel.* The advocates of the different sites which have been assigned to Eden have seldom, if ever, recognized the fact that no hypothesis on this subject can be considered acceptable which cannot account for this peculiar association of man's first home with some sort of natural centre of the earth. Assuming, however, that the human race began its history at the Pole, and that

[1] Printed in advance in the *Boston University Year Book*, vol. xi., 1884.

15

all traditional recollections of man's unfallen state were connected with a *polar* Eden, the mystery which otherwise envelops the subject immediately vanishes.

We have already seen that the term "navel" was anciently used in many languages for "centre," and that the Pole, or central point of the revolving constellations, was the "Navel of Heaven." But as to the celestial Pole there corresponds a terrestrial one, so it is only natural that to the term the "Navel of Heaven" there should be the corresponding expression the "Navel of the Earth."

Beginning with Christian traditions, let us make a pilgrimage to the Church of the Holy Sepulchre at Jerusalem. There, in the portion belonging to the Greek Christians, we shall discover a round pillar, some two feet high, projecting from the marble pavement, but supporting nothing. If we inquire as to its purpose, we shall be informed that it is designed to mark the exact centre or "Navel" of the Earth.[1] Early pilgrims and chroniclers refer to this

---

[1] As my own inspection of this monument was nearly thirty years ago, I have thought it well to make inquiry as to its present state. The following, written under date of Oct. 28, 1884, by my obliging friend, Dr. Selah Merrill, the United States Consul at Jerusalem, and well known as an Oriental archæologist, will be read with much interest: "The stone to which you refer still stands in the middle of the Church (Greek) of the Holy Sepulchre, and is called the Centre or Navel of the Earth. It is called a 'pillar,' although it is not a pillar, but a vase, conforming in its general shape to a large, tall fruit dish. The top is in the form of a basin, with a raised portion in its centre; that is, in the bottom of the basin. I was told that at every feast bread was laid on this pillar. I am assured that it is called the Centre of the Earth only by the Arab or native Christians of Syria, and not by the Greeks proper; also, that every Greek church in Syria that is built after the form of this one has such a 'pillar' in the centre. Within two or three years past, an old church has been

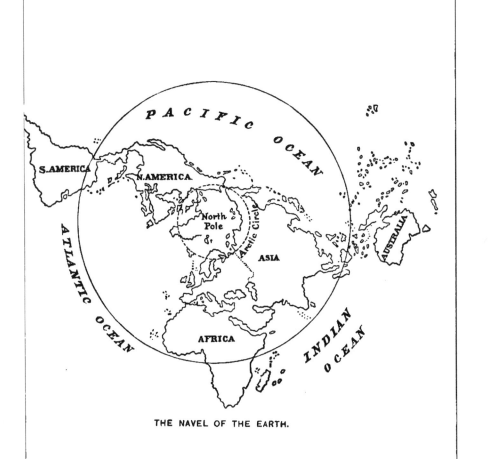

THE NAVEL OF THE EARTH.

curious monument, but its antiquity no one knows.[1] As usually described, it is a monument of the geographical ignorance of those who placed it there, a proof that they supposed the edge of the "flat disk" of the earth to be everywhere equidistant from this stone. In reality, it is a monument of primeval astronomic and geographic science.

excavated a little distance north of the Damascus gate. In the *Palestine Fund Report* for October, 1883, I wrote some account of this to supplement what had been written before by others. In the centre of that church there is a similar stone, but that is a real pillar. This church is no doubt very old, and is popularly spoken of as the 'Church of St. Stephen.' In my judgment it stands on the site of an older church.

"It seemed to me a little singular that this object should be called a 'pillar' (*Amûd*), when it is only a vase, or vase-shaped; but as the tradition connected with it is very old, the name may have come down from the time when the object used for this purpose was actually a pillar or column."

It is interesting to compare with the foregoing the description given by Bernard Surius, of Brussels, in the year 1646, particularly as at that time the "Oriental Greeks" seem to have had no scruple in calling the pillar the Centre of the Earth: "Omtrent het midden steckt eenen witten marmer-steen uyt, van twee voeten in syn vierkant, daer een rondt putteken in is, 't welck soo de Oostsche Griecken seggen, het midden van den aerdt-bodem is." *Reyse van Jerusalem.* Antwerp, 1649: p. 664.

[1] Bishop Argulf, in his pilgrimage, A. D. 700, "saw some other relics, and he observed a lofty column in the holy places to the north of the Church of Golgotha, in the middle of the city, which at midday at the summer solstice casts no shadow; which shows that this is the centre of the earth." Wright, *Early Travels in Palestine*, p. 4. As late as A. D. 1102, it still seems to have been outside the then existing Church. Bishop Sæwulf says, "At the head of the Church of the Holy Sepulchre, *in the wall outside*, not far from the place of Calvary, is the place called *Compas*, which our Lord Jesus Christ himself signified and measured with his own hand as the middle of the world according to the words of the Psalmist, 'God is my king of old, working salvation in the midst of the earth.'" Ibid., p. 38. In 1322, however, it is described by Sir John de Maundeville as "in the midst of the Church." Ibid., p. 167. At one time in the Middle Ages, the spot seems to have been marked by a letter or inscription.

To find the true symbolical and commemorative character of this pillar, we need to remind ourselves of a tendency ever present and active among men. We have already alluded to the scores of " Calvaries " which have been set apart in Roman Catholic lands, and hallowed as memorial mounts. Up the side of each leads a *Via dolorosa*, with its different "stations," each recalling to the mind, by sculptured reliefs or otherwise, one of the immortal incidents of the Passion. On the summit is the full crucifixion tableau, — the Saviour hanging aloft upon the cross, between two crucified malefactors. The spear, the reed with the sponge, the hammer, — all are there, sometimes the ladder also ; and near by, the tomb wherein never man was laid. In the minds of the worshipers it is a holy place.

Even in our Protestant republic, on the shore of Lake Chautauqua, we have seen successfully carried out, in our own day, a complete reproduction of Palestine. Thousands have visited it to take object-lessons in Sacred Geography. From it these thousands have gained clearer ideas of the relative positions and bearings of Hermon and Tabor and Olivet, of Kedron and Cherith and the Jordan, of Nazareth and Hebron and the Holy City, than else they ever would have had. What here has been done for purposes of instruction has elsewhere and often upon a greater or smaller scale, been done for purposes of direct religious edification, and for the gratification of religious sentiment.

Now, just as Christians love to localize in their

Barclay, *City of the Great King.* Philadelphia, 1858 : p. 370. See Michelant et Reynaud, *Itinéraires à Jerusalem.* Genève, 1882 : pp. 36, 104[4], 182, 230, etc.

own midst their " Holy Places," so the early nations of the world loved to create miniature reproductions of Eden, the fair and sacred country in which man dwelt in the holy morning hours of his existence.[1] The traditional temple architecture of many early religions was determined by this symbolical and commemorative motive. This was eminently true of the sacred architecture of the Babylonians, Egyptians, Hebrews, and Chinese.[2] Koeppen assures us that "every orthodoxly constructed Buddhist temple either is, or contains, a symbolical representation of the divine regions of Meru, and of the heaven of the gods, saints, and Buddhas, rising above it." [3] Lillie says, "The thirteen pyramidal layers at the top of every temple in Nepâl represent the thirteen unchangeable heavens of Amitâbha." [4] With what

---

[1] "The Hindus generally represent Mount Meru of a conical figure, and kings were formerly fond of raising mounds of earth in that shape, which they venerated like the divine Meru, and the gods were called down by spells to come and dally upon them. They are called *Meru-sringas*, or the peaks of Meru. There are four of them either in or near Benares ; the more modern, and of course the more perfect, is at a place called Sár-náth. It was raised in the year of Christ 1027. . . . This conical hill is about sixty feet high, with a small but handsome octagonal temple on the summit. It is said in the inscription that this artificial hill was intended as a representation of the worldly Meru, the hill of God, and the tower of Babel, with its seven steps or zones, was probably raised with a similar view and for the same purpose."— Wilford in *Asiatic Researches*, vol. viii., p. 291.

[2] Miller, "The Pyramidal Temple," in the *Oriental and Bib. Journal.* Chicago, 1880 : vol. i., pp. 169–178. Also, Boscawen, in the same, 1884, p. 118. Perrot and Chipiez, *History of Art in Chaldæa and Assyria.* London and New York, 1884 : vol. i., pp. 364–398.

[3] *Die Religion des Buddha*, vol. ii., 262.

[4] *Buddha and Early Buddhism*, p. 51. We find the same symbolism even among the civilized aborigines of America. Thus " the temple at Tezcuco was of nine stories, *symbolizing the nine heavens.*" Bancroft, *Native Races*, vol. iii., p. 184. Compare pp. 186, 195, 197; also 532–537.

astonishing elaboration this idea has sometimes been carried out may be seen in the Senbyoo temple in Mengoon, near the capital of Burmah.[1] That the natural features of the landscape were often utilized in producing these symbolic shrines and holy places is only what we should expect. "The Buddhists of Ceylon," as Obry states, " have endeavored to transform their central mountain, *Dêva-Kuta* (Peak of the Gods), into Meru, and to find four streams descending from its sides to correspond with the rivers of their Paradise."[2]

Again, in the "rock-cut" temples of Ellora, we have, in like manner, a complete representation of the Paradise of Siva. Faber develops the evidence of this practice among the ancients with great fullness, and with respect to the Hindus and Buddhists says, "Each pagoda, each pyramid, each montiform 'high-place,' is invariably esteemed to be a copy of the holy hill Meru," the Hindu's Paradise.[3]

From "Records of the Past," vol. x., p. 50, we see that the Egyptians had the same custom of building temples in such a manner that they should be symbolical of the abode of the gods. So in Greece and

[1] See *Journal of the Royal Asiatic Society.* London, 1870: pp. 406–429.

[2] *Le Berceau de l'Espèce Humaine*, p. 118.

[3] *Origin of Pagan Idolatry.* London, 1816: vol. i., p. 345. So an American writer says, "Akkad, Aram, and all the other 'highlands' of antiquity were but reproductions, traditionary inheritances from this primitive highland, this Olympus of all Asia. . . . Similar notions were associated at a later period with Mount Zion in Jerusalem, and with the Mohammedan Mecca and other sacred localities. Such ideas [as that they were respectively in the centre of the world] are no indication of the ignorance of the ancients : they were symbolical and traditionary conceptions inherited from the sacred mount of Paradise." *The American Antiquarian and Oriental Journal.* Chicago, 1881 : p. 312. Compare 1884, p. 118.

Rome the citadel mounts in their cities had quite as great religious as military significance. Lenormant, speaking of Rome and Olympia, remarks, " It is impossible not to note that the Capitoline was first of all the *Mount of Saturn,* and that the Roman archæologists established a complete affinity between the Capitoline and Mount Cronios in Olympia, from the standpoint of their traditions and religious origin (Dionysius Halicarn., i., 34). This Mount Cronios is, as it were, the *Omphalos* of the sacred city of Elis, the primitive centre of its worship. It sometimes receives the name Olympos." [1] Here is not only symbolism in general, but also a symbolism pointing to the Arctic Eden, already shown to be the primeval mount of Kronos, the *Omphalos* of the whole earth.[2]

Now, as Jerusalem is one of the most ancient of the sacred cities of the world, and, at the same time, the one where the tradition of the primeval Paradise was preserved in its clearest and most historic form, it would be strange if, in all its long history, no king or priesthood had ever tried to enhance its attractiveness and sanctity by making it, or some part of it, symbolize Earth's earliest Holy Land, and commemorate man's earliest Theocracy. That the at-

---

[1] *Beginnings of History,* pp. 151, 153.

[2] Among the Romans no city, or even camp, was *rite* established and founded without a sacred *Umbilicus.* It "fiel in den Schnittpunkt des *Decumanus* und *Cardo Maximus,* d. h., wohin die *Via decumana,* sich mit der *Via principalis* kreuzt ; dieser Schnittpunkt befand sich vor dem *introitus Praetorii ;* da stand auch die *Ara castrorum,* da war der *Umbilicus* des Systems. Diesen Umbilicus nun finden wir in Rom noch in Mauerresten vorhanden am nordöstlichen Anfang des Forum wieder, welche Stelle als Umbilicus bezeichnet wurde." J. H. Kuntze, *Prolegomena zur Geschichte Roms.* Leipsic, 1882: p. 154. See notes below, on the cities of Cuzco and Mexico.

tempt was made is beyond a doubt. To this day the visitor is shown the spot where, according to one tradition, Adam was created.[1] Not many feet away, under the custody of another religion, he finds the sacred rock-hewn grave in which at least the head of the first of men was buried.[2] In the little Gihon, the name of one of the Paradise rivers still lives. The miraculous virtue of the Pool of Bethsaida was ascribed in early Christian legend to its being in subterranean contact with the Tree of Life, which grew in the midst of Paradise.[3] Christ's cross was said to have been made of the wood of the same tree. The very name, Mount Sion, is a memorial one. The Talmudic account of " The Strength of the Hill of Sion" shows that the Palestinian mount was named after the heavenly one, and not *vice versa,* as commonly supposed. The true sacred name of the Holy City is, therefore, not Sion (though it is often called by the heavenly appellation also), but " Daughter of Sion." She is simply

---

[1] Murray's *Handbook for Syria and Palestine.* London, 1858: Pt. i., p. 164. Another account reads, " E de Iherusalem à Seint Habraham sunt. viii. liwes, e là fust Adam fourmé." *Itinéraires à Jerusalem, et Descriptions de la Terre Sainte.* Rédigés en français aux XI*, XII*, XIII* siècles. Publiés par Michelant et Reynaud. Genève, 1882: p. 233.

[2] See F. Piper, *Adams Grab auf Golgotha. Evangelischer Kalender,* 1861: p. 17 ff. (illustrated). Philippe Mousket (A. D. 1241), in his descriptive poem on the Holy Places, makes it the tomb of both Adam and Eve: —

> " Et là tout droit à li Iudeu
> Crucifiiérent le fil Deu,
> Fu Adam, li premiers om. mis
> Et entierés et soupouiis,
> Et Eve, sa feme, avoec lui." etc.
>
> (Michelant et Reynaud, *ut supra,* p. 115.)

[3] W. Henderson, *Identity of the Scene of Man's Creation, Fall, and Redemption.* London, 1864: p. 10.

a copy, a miniature likeness, of the true mount and
city of God "in the sides of the North."[1]

So confident is Lenormant that Solomon and
Hezekiah intentionally conformed their capital to
the Paradisaic mount, and intentionally introduced
in their public works features which should symbolize and commemorate peculiarities of Eden, that
he uses the fact as an unanswerable argument
against those imaginative critics who would place
the composition of the second chapter of Genesis
subsequent to the Babylonian exile. He says, —

"Another proof, and a very decisive one in my
opinion, of the high antiquity of the narrative of
Genesis concerning Eden, and of the knowledge of
it possessed by the Hebrews long before the Captiv-
ity, is the intention — so clearly proved by Ewald —
to imitate 'the four rivers' which predominated in
the works of Solomon and Hezekiah for the distribution of the waters of Jerusalem, which, in its turn,
was considered as the *Umbilicus* of the Earth (Ezek.
v. 5), in the double sense of centre of the inhabited
regions and source of the rivers. The four streams
which watered the town and the foot of its ram-
parts — one of which was named Gihon (1 Kings
i. 33, 38; 2 Chron. xxxii. 30, xxxiii. 14), like one of
the Paradisaic rivers — were, as Ewald has shown,
reputed to issue through subterranean communications from the spring of fresh water situated beneath the Temple, the sacred source of life and
purity to which the prophets (Joel iii. 18; Ezek.
xlvii. 1–12; Zech. xiii. 1, xiv. 8; *cf.* Apoc. xxii. 1) attach a high symbolic value."[2]

---

[1] See chapter iii. of the present Part.

[2] "Ararat and Eden." *The Contemporary Review*, vol. iii., No. 27
(Am. ed., p. 46).

In this citation, in addition to a strong assertion of the symbolical character of the topography and waterworks of Jerusalem, we have the location itself included in this symbolism. The city is said to have been the *Umbilicus* or Navel of the Earth, for two reasons : first, because of its relation to surrounding countries ;[1] and, second, because of its containing the source of the rivers. In our next chapter, this last reason will become more significant than even the writer intended. At present we will only add that the true philosophy of this symbolical centrality of Jerusalem is found in two facts : first, the Hebrews had a tradition that *primeval Eden was the Centre of the Earth :*[2] and, second, by styling Jerusalem the Navel of the Earth, as they did, it was symbolically all the more assimilated to the primitive Paradise which in so many other ways it sacredly commemorated.

Passing to the field of Hellenic tradition, we are told by all modern interpreters that the Greeks shared the "narrow conceit and ignorance of all ancient nations," and supposed their own land to occupy the middle of the "flat earth-disk." And because of certain expressions in Pindar and a passage in Pausanias, it is affirmed as a first principle in the geography of the ancient Greeks that Delphi was believed to be the exact topographical centre-point of the whole earth.

[1] That this traditionally-given first reason for the appellation is not well founded is evident from the fact that the Hebrews had a "Navel of the Earth," farther to the North, before ever they had possessed themselves of the site of Jerusalem (Judg. ix. 37).

[2] In Origen, *Selectis ad Genesin,* we read, "Tradunt Hebræi locum, in quo Paradisum plantavit Deus, Eden vocari, et ajunt *ipsum mundi medium esse, ut pupillam oculi.*" Compare Hershon, *Talmudic Miscellany,* p. 300.

Such a representation is far from satisfactory. For while the term " *Omphalos* of the Earth " was undoubtedly applied in a sense to Delphi, it belonged to it only as the name Athens belongs to many a town thus designated in America. It had other and older topographical connections and associations. We find traces of the same title in connection with Olympos, with Ida, with Parnassos, with Ogygia, with Nyssa, with Mount Meros, with Delos, with Athens, with Crete, and even with Meroë. In the multiplicity of these localizations, the people seem to have lost the clue to the original significance of the conception, and to have contrived crude etymological myths of their own for the explanation of what seemed to them a remarkable designation.[1]

The moment we make the true original *Omphalos* of the Earth the North Pole, and invest it with sacred traditionary recollections of Eden life, all this confusion becomes clear. The "centre-stone" of Delphi, like the Omphalium of the Cretans, becomes merely a memorial shrine, an attempted copy of the great original. And if all the Olymps and Idas and Parnassos mounts were alike convenient reproductions and localizations of the one celestial mountain of the gods at the North Pole, what wonder if we find each of them in some way designated as the Centre of the Earth.

Homer's " *Omphalos* of the sea," Calypso's isle,

---

[1] " À peine l'enfant [Zeus] venoit de naître, que les Curètes le portèrent sur l'Ida. Dans le trajet, le cordon ombilical se detacha et tomba au milieu d'une plaine qui prit de là le nom de ὀμφαλὸς, *nombril* (nom qu'elle devoit avoir auparavant)." — T. B. Eméric-David, *Jupiter ; Recherches sur ce Dieu, sur son Culte,* etc., Paris, 1833, t. i., p. 248, referring to Callimachus, *Hymnus in Jovem,* v. 44 ; Diodorus Sic., v. 70.

has in like manner all the marks of a mythico-tradi-
tional north polar Eden. Its name, Ogygia, connects
it with a far-off antediluvian antiquity.[1] It is situated in the far North, and Odysseus needs the blast
of Boreas to bring him away from its shores on
the homeward journey. Its queen, Calypso, is the
daughter of Atlas ; and Atlas' proper station in
Greek mythology, as elsewhere shown, is at the terrestrial Pole. Its beauty is Paradisaic, it being
adorned with groves and " soft meadows of violets,"
— so beautiful, in fact, that " on beholding it even an
Immortal would be seized with wonder and delight."[2]
Finally, identifying the place beyond all question,
we have the Eden "fountain," whose waters part
into "four streams, flowing each in opposite directions." [3]

In Mount Meros we have only the Greek form
of Meru, as long ago shown by Creuzer.[4] The one
is the Navel of the Earth for the same reason that
the other is. Egyptian Meroë (in some Egyptian
texts *Mer*, in Assyrian *Mirukh*, or *Mirukha*), the
seat of the famous oracle of Jupiter Ammon, was
possibly named from the same "World-mountain."
This would explain the passage in Quintus Curtius, which has so troubled commentators, wherein
the object which represented the divine being is
described as resembling a "navel set in gems." [5]

---

[1] See Welcker, *Griechische Götterlehre*, i., 775 *et seq.*

[2] *Odyssey*, v. 63–75.

[3] Ibid.

[4] *Symbolik*, vol. i., p. 537.

[5] " Id quod pro deo colitur, non eandem effigiam habet, quam
vulgo diis accommodaverunt : umbilico maxime similis est habitus,
smaragdo et gemmis coagmentatus." Quintus Curtius, *De Reb. Ges.*,
iv. 7, 23. See notes in Lemaire's ed., Paris, 1822; also Diodorus
Siculus, iii. 3. Capt. Wilford notices another coincidence : " The

When the two doves of Zeus, flying from the two opposite ends of the world, determine the cosmic centralness of "Parnassos," it is of an antediluvian Parnassos that the myth is speaking.[1] It is that mount on whose polar top we have already found the "*domicilium*" of Zeus.

Nonnos, in describing the symbolical *peplos* which Harmonia wove on the loom of Athene, says, "First she represented the earth with its *omphalos* in the centre ; around the earth she spread out the sphere of heaven varied with the figures of the stars. . . . Lastly, along the exterior edge of the well-woven vestment she represented the Ocean in a circle."[2] That Delphi or the Phocian Parnassos is the *omphalos* here mentioned is far enough from credible. It is the Pole, and the manner in which the term is introduced shows that it was perfectly understood by every reader, and needed no explanation. The true shrine of Apollo was not at Delphi, but in that older earth-centre of which Plato speaks in the motto prefixed to this section. His real home is among "the Hyperboreans," in a land of almost perpetual light ; and it is only upon annual visits that he comes to Delphi.[3] The remembrance of this fact would have

Pauranics say that . . . the first climate is that of Meru ; among the Greeks and Romans the first climate was that of Meroë." — Wilford in *Asiatic Researches*, vol. viii., p. 289.

[1] "Before this time" — the time of the deluge of Deucalion — "Zeus had once wanted to know where the middle of the earth was, and had let fly two doves at the same moment from the two ends of the world, to see where they would meet ; they met on Mount Parnassos, and thus it was proved beyond a doubt that this mountain must be the centre of the earth." — C. Witt, *Myths of Hellas.* London, 1883 : p. 140.

[2] Lenormant, *Beginnings of History*, p. 549.

[3] "Au début de l'hiver Apollon quitte Delphes pour le pays mystérieux des Hyperboréens, où règne une lumière constante, et qui

helped the interpreters of Pindar out of more than one perplexity.[1] According to Hecatæus, Lêtô, the mother of Apollo and his sister Artemis, was born on an island in the Arctic Ocean, "beyond the North wind." Moreover, on this island inhabited by the Hyperboreans, Apollo is unceasingly worshiped in a huge round temple, in a city whose inhabitants are perpetually playing upon lyres and chanting to his praise.[2] So reports Diodorus (ii., 47); and herewith agrees the imaginary journey of Apollonius of Tyana, — a namesake of Apollo, — who tells of his journey far to the North of the Caucasus into the regions of the pious Hyperboreans, among whom he found a lofty sacred mountain, the *Omphalos* of the Earth.[3]

In the Phædo we have a charming description of Plato's terrestrial Paradise. "In this fair region,"

échappe aux rigueurs de l'hiver." Maxime Collignon, *Mythologie Figurée de la Grèce.* Paris, 1883: p. 96. See Alcæus' Hymn, referred to by Menzel, *Unsterblichkeitslehre,* i., p. 87. The present writer is not the first to be reminded here of polar Meru: "Bei ihnen (den Hyperboreern), wohnen beständig der Sonnengott Apollo und seine Schwester Artemis, wie auf dem indischen Meru ebenfalls Indra, der Lichtgeist und Sonnengott, wohnt." Dr. Heinrich Lüken, *Die Traditionen des Menschengeschlechts, oder die Uroffenbarung unter den Heiden.* Münster, 2d ed., 1869: p. 73.

[1] See *Olympian Odes,* iv., 74; vi., 3; viii., 62; xi., 10. *Nemean,* vii., 33. *Frag.,* i., 3, and *passim ;* comp. *Olymp.,* ii., iii.; *Pyth.,* iv., etc.

[2] "The Dorian worship of Apollo was *primitively* Boreal." Humboldt, *Cosmos* (Bohn's ed.), ii., 511. Compare Pindar's expression in second *Olympian Ode :* "the Hyperborean folk who serve Apollo."

[3] "Cette montagne est sacrée; c'est l'ombilic du monde." Moreau de Jonnès, *L'Océan des Anciens,* p. 162. As to the Ægean Delos, the best explanation Keary can give is this : "Delos was afterward deemed to be the navel of the earth, because, being in special favor with Apollo, *it might be thought to stand under the eye of the midday sun.*" (!) *Primitive Belief,* p. 183. Compare, on the other hand, Pindar's *Fragment* in honor of Delos, the Homeric *Hymn to Apollo,* and the Japanese myth of Onogorojima before described.

Socrates is made to say, "all things that grow — trees and flowers and fruit — are fairer than any here; and there are hills and stones in them smoother and more transparent and fairer in color than our highly-valued emeralds and sardonyxes and jaspers and other gems, which are but minute fragments of them : for there all the stones are like our precious stones, and fairer still. The temperament of their seasons is such that the inhabitants have no disease, and live much longer than we do, and have sight and hearing and smell and all the other senses in much greater perfection. And they have temples and sacred places in which the gods really dwell, and they hear their voices, and receive their answers, and are conscious of them, and hold converse with them, and they see the sun, the moon, and the stars as they really are." [1]

If we ask as to the location of this divinely beautiful abode, every indication of the text agrees with our hypothesis. It is right under the eye when the world is looked at from its summit, the Northern celestial pole.[2] Viewed from the standpoint of Greece and its neighbor lands it is *"above,"* — it is *" the upper Earth,"* the dazzling top of the *" round"* world. In it, moreover, is the Navel of the Earth, μεσογαία, inhabited by happy men.

If anything is needed to disprove the common notion that geographical ignorance and national self-esteem first governed the ancient peoples in locating in their own countries "navels" of the earth, it is furnished by what is, in all probability, the oldest epic in the world, that of Izdhubar, fragments of

---

[1] *Phædo*, 110, 111.
[2] Εἴ τις ἄνωθεν θεῷτο.

which have survived in the oldest literature of Babylonia. These fragments show that the earliest inhabitants of the Tigro-Euphrates basin located "the Centre of the Earth," *not in their own midst*, but in a far-off land, of sacred associations, where "the holy house of the gods" is situated, — a land "into the heart whereof man hath not penetrated;" a place underneath the "overshadowing world-tree," and beside the "full waters."[1] No description could more perfectly identify the spot with the Arctic Pole of ancient Asiatic mythology. Yet this testimony stands not alone; for in the fragment of another ancient text, translated by Sayce in "Records of the Past," we are told of a "dwelling" which "the gods created for" the first human beings, — a dwelling in which they "became great" and "increased in numbers," and the location of which is described in words exactly corresponding to those of Iranian, Indian, Chinese, Eddaic, and Aztec literature; namely, "in the Centre of the Earth."[2]

In the Hindu Puranas we are told over and over that the earth is a sphere, and that Mount Meru is its Navel or Pole.[3] But the expression *nâbhi*, or "Navel" of the earth, is older than the Puranas, though the very meaning of Purana is "ancient." Like the term "Navel of Heaven," it occurs in the

---

[1] A. H. Sayce, *Babylonian Literature.* London, 1878: p. 39. The Sunis of Northwestern Africa, in our own day, fix the centre of the world outside their own territory, "between themselves and the Soudan." R. G. Haliburton, *Notes on Mount Atlas and its Traditions.* Salem, Mass., 1883: p. 8.

[2] *Records of the Past*, xi., pp. 109 *seq.* George Smith, *Chaldæan Account of Genesis*, 2d ed., p. 92. Lenormant, *Beginnings of History*, app., pp. 508–510.

[3] "The convexity in the centre is the navel of Vishnu." — *Asiatic Researches*, vol. viii., p. 273.

hymns of the earliest Veda. But where was the
sacred shrine to which it was applied? It was no
holy place in Bactria, or in the Punjâb. Nothing
tends to locate it in India. On the other hand, the
fifth verse of the one hundred and eighty-fifth hymn,
mandala first, of the Rig Veda, seems most plainly
to fix it at the North Pole. In this verse Night and
Day are represented as twin sisters in the bosom
of their parents Heaven and Earth; each bounding
or limiting the other, but both kissing simultaneously the *Nâbhi* of the Earth. Now, everywhere
upon earth, except in the polar regions, Night and
Day seem ever to be pursuing and supplanting
each other. They have no common ground. At
the Pole — and only there — they may be said, with
locked arms, to spin round and round a common
point, and unitedly to kiss it from the opposite sides.[1]
This plainly is the meaning of the poet; and remembering all the legendary splendors of the polar
mountain around which sun and moon are ever moving, we must pronounce the figure as beautiful as
it is instructive.[2]

[1] The following versions may be compared: " Zusammenkommend,
die beiden Jungen, deren Enden zusammenstossen, die verbündeteten
Schwestern in der beiden Aeltern Schosse, küssend den Nabel der
Welt, schützt uns, Himmel und Erde, vor Gewalt." — Ludwig, i. 182.

"Going always together, equally young and of like termination,
sisters and kindred, and scenting [*sic*] the navel of the world, placed
on their lap as its parents; defend us, Heaven and Earth, from great
danger." — Wilson, ii., 188.

> " Die Beiden Jungfraun an einander grenzend,
> " Die Zwillingsschwestern in dem Schoss der Eltern,
> " Die im Verein der Welten Nabel küssen, —
> " Beschirmt vor grauser Noth uns Erd' und Himmel."
>
> (Grassmann, ii., 177.)

Compare *R. V.*, i., 144, 3; ii., 3, 6, and 7; *et passim.*

[2] A later poet has borrowed the same idea: —

In perfect accord herewith, we find the bard asking, in another hymn, where the Navel of the Earth
is ; and in doing it he associates it as closely as possible, not with some central home-shrine in his own
land, but with the extreme *"End of the Earth,"* — an
expression used again and again, in ancient languages, for the Pole and its vicinity.[1]

Again, in another Vedic passage, the Navel of the
Earth is located upon " the mountains," and this association points us to the North.[2]   Still stronger evidence of its polar location is found in other hymns,
where the supporting column of heaven — the Atlas
pillar of Vedic cosmology — is described as standing in or upon the Navel of the Earth.[3]

Finally, so unmistakable is the Vedic teaching on
this subject that a recent writer, after asserting with
all his teachers that the cosmography of the Vedic
bards was " embryonic," and their earth a " flat
disk" overarched by a solid firmament, which was
"soldered on to the edge of the disk at the horizon,"
nevertheless, later, in studying one of the cosmo-
gonical hymns of Dīrghatamas, the son of Mamata,
reaches the conclusion that the singer had knowledge both of the celestial and of the terrestrial Pole,
and that, in seeking to answer the question as to *the*

" Around the fire in solemn rite they trod,
    The lovely lady and the glorious god ;
    Like Day and starry Midnight when they meet
    In the broad plains at lofty Meru's feet."
(Griffiths' Translation of *Kumâra Sambhava,* or *The Birth of the War-God.*
London, 1879.)

[1] The following is Grassmann's translation : " Ich frage nach dem
äussersten Ende der Erde, ich frage wo der Welt Nabel ist," etc.
Rig Veda, i., 164, 34 ; comp. 35.

[2] *Rig Veda,* ix., 82, 3.

[3] Ibid., ix., 86, 8 ; ix., 79, 4; ix., 72, 7, etc.

birth-place of humanity, he locates it precisely at the point of contact between the polar mountain and the Pole of the northern sky.[1]

We have seen that, according to Old-Iranian tradition also, man was created in the *"central"* division of the earth. The primordial tree, which "kept the strength of all kinds of trees," was "in the vicinity of the *Middle* of the Earth."[2] The primeval ox, which stood by the Paradise river when the destroyer came, was "in the *Middle* of the Earth."[3] Mount Taéra (Pahl.: Térak), the celestial Pole, and Kakâd-i-Dâîtîk, the mountain of the terrestrial Pole, are each described in similar terms: the one as "Centre of the World," the other as "Centre of the Earth."[4] The expression *Apâm Nepât*, the "Navel of the Waters," occurs in the Avestan writings again and again, and is always applied either to the world-fountain from which all waters proceed, or to the spirit presiding over it.[5] But as this world-foun-

[1] The reader will no doubt be glad to see the exact language: "Le contact de la terre et du ciel, serait-il l'hymen mystérieux d'où l'humanité naquit? Le ciel, ce serait le père qui engendre; la mère, ce serait la grande terre, ayant sa matrice dans la partie la plus haute de sa surface, sur les hauts monts; et ce serait là que le père 'féconderait le sein de celle qui est en même temps, son épouse et sa fille.' On a cru voir ce point de contact dont parle Dîrghatamas, — *Outtânâyah tchamwâh*, 'endroit septentrional où les deux surfaces se touchent,' — au pôle nord, connu de l'auteur; l'étoile polaire se nommant *outtanapada*. Il est certain que la somme des connaissances positives collectionées par ce philosophe était relativement important." — Marius Fontane, *Inde Védique.* Paris, 1881: pp. 94, 200.

[2] West, *Pahlavi Texts*, pt. i., p. 161.

[3] West, *Pahlavi Texts*, pt. i., p. 162.

[4] Ibid., pp. 22, 36. So, in consequence of the duality and opposite polarity alluded to in the context, "Hell is in the middle of the earth," at the South Pole, p. 19.

[5] See Index to Darmesteter's *Zend-Avesta*. Compare the Vedic hymn (ii., 35), "*An den Sohn der Wasser*," *Apâm napât*, whose loca-

tain, Ardvî Sûra, is located in the north polar sky
(see next chapter), we have here also a recognition
of a world-*omphalos*, inseparable from the ancient
and sacred Paradise-mountain at the Pole.[1]

The Chinese terrestrial Paradise is described not
only as "at the Centre of the Earth," but also as
directly under Shang-te's heavenly palace, which is
declared to be in the North star, and which is sometimes styled "Palace of the Centre."[2] Very probably the historic designation, "The Middle Kingdom," was originally a sacred name,[3] commemorative of that primeval middle country which the
Akkadian called Akkad, the Indian Ilâvrita, the Iranian Kvanîras, and the Northman Idavollr. In the
funeral rites of China, this supposition finds a cogent confirmation.[4]

tion is "*an dem höchsten Orte*" (v., 13, Grassmann). Compare quotation from Ritter, in part iv., chapter first, *supra*.

[1] "Dieser Albordj, der Lichtberg, der Nabel der Erde, wird von
Sonne Mond und Sternen umgeben." — Carl Ritter, *Erdkunde*, Bd.
viii., p. 46.

[2] "In Kwen-lun is Shang-te's lower recreation-palace. . . . Shang-
te's wife dwells in this region, immediately over which is Shang-te's
heavenly palace, which is situated in the centre of the heavens, as his
earthly one is in the centre of the earth. . . . The Queen mother
dwells alone in its midst, in the place where the genii sport. At the
summit there is a resplendent azure hall, with lakes inclosed by precious gems, and many temples. Above rules the clear ether of the
ever-fixed, the polar, star." — Condensed from the *Chinese Recorder*,
vol. iv., p. 95.

[3] Frédérik Klee, *Le Déluge*. Paris, 1847 : p. 188, note.

[4] "Quand je vous ai parlé des libations en usage à la Chine, je
vous ai dit, Monsieur, qu'on se tournait vers le pôle septentrional
pour faire les libations en l'honneur des morts. En considérant la
vénération de ce peuple pour ses ancêtres, on n'aperçoit qu'une explication naturelle de cet usage ; c'est de dire que les Chinois se tour-
nent vers le pays du monde, où ils ont pris naissance, et où leur ancêtres reposent." — Bailly, *Lettres sur l'Origine des Sciences et sur
celle des Peuples de l'Asie*. Paris, 1777 : p. 236.

Passing to Japan, it is curiously interesting to note that the Ainos, who are supposed to have been the first inhabitants, are believed to have come into the archipelago " from the North ; " [1] that their heaven is on inaccessible mountain-tops in the same quarter ; [2] and that their name, according to some authorities, etymologically signifies " *Offspring of the Centre.*" [3] In burial, their dead are always so placed that when resurrected their faces will be set toward the lofty northern country from which their ancestors are believed to have come, and to which their spirits are believed to have returned.[4]

[1] Griffis, *The Mikado's Empire*, p. 27.

[2] " These [a mythological pair] were the ancestors of the Ainos. Their offspring, in turn, married ; some among each other, others with the bears of the mountains [the Bear Tribe ?]. The fruits of this latter union were men of extraordinary valor and nimble hunters, who, after a long life spent in the vicinity of their birth, departed to the far North, where they still live on the high and inaccessible table-lands above the mountains ; and, being immortal, they direct, by their magical influences, the actions and the destiny of men ; that is, the Ainos." — Ibid., p. 28.

[3] Ai-no-ko. Ibid., p. 29.

[4] " It may not be devoid of interest to mention here that the Ainos bury their dead with the head to the South. . . . The Aino, to-day, as he did in ancient times, buries his dead by covering the body with matting, and placing it with the head to the South in a grave which is about three feet deep." *Notes on Japanese Archæology with especial reference to the Stone Age*, by Henry von Siebold, Yokohama, 1879, p. 6. Let no reader imagine this a meaningless rite of undeveloped savages. " From all these observations, as well as from the traditions of the Ainos, in which are ever-recurring laments for a better past ; and from many peculiarities in their customs, we must conclude that the Ainos are to be classed with those peoples that have earlier been more richly supplied with the implements of civilization, but have become degraded through isolation. Prehistoric discoveries . . . favor this view. The pits found there for dwellings indicate that the Ainos came from the North to Yezo." Professor Brauns, of Halle. Translated from Memoirs of the Berlin Anthropological Society, in *Science*. Cambridge, 1884 ; p. 72.

Taking these facts in connection with those presented in chapter second of the preceding part, one ·can hardly evade the conclusion that, when Griffis informs us that the Japanese considered their country as lying at "the top of the world," and when others say that the Japanese once regarded their country as the "Centre of the World," [1] it is most probable that these writers have applied to the Japan of to-day ideas which originally belonged to a far-distant prehistoric polar Japan, the primitive seat of the race, as it has lived on in these most ancient traditions of the Ainos.

In Scandinavian mythology we meet with a similar idea. In the Eddas, both Asgard and Idavollr are represented as in "the Centre of the World;" and at least one author, in explaining the reason of it, has come within a hair's-breadth of the truth, though missing it. [2]

The ancient Mexicans conceived of the cradle of the human race as situated in the farthest North, upon the highest of mountains, cloud-surrounded,

[1] "The Japanese *in their earlier separation* regarded their country as the centre and most important part of the world." — J. J. Rein, *Japan, Travels and Researches,* English translation. London, 1884: p. 6.

[2] " Nos ancêtres scandinaves plaçaient la demeure de leurs dieux, Asgard, au milieu du monde, c'est-à-dire au centre de la surface de la terre d'alors. Il est assez remarquable qu'une telle idée n'est pas sans fondement, puisqu'il faut admettre, comme je crois l'avoir démontré, que l'Europe, l'Asie, et l'Amérique, unis vers le pôle nord, formaient avant le déluge un seul continent." Frédérik Klee, *Le Déluge,* Fr. ed. Paris, 1847: p. 188 n. But, by clinging to " the highest mountains of Asia," as the centre originally meant, M. Klee loses the chief advantage of his supposed union of the continents at the Pole. — The Teutonic *omphalos* of the world is preserved at Finzingen, near Altstädt, in Saxe-Weimar. See Kuhn and Schwartz, *Norddeutsche Sagen.* Leipsic, 1848 : p. 215.

the residence of the god Tlaloc. Thence come the rains and all streams, for Tlaloc is the god of waters. The first man, Quetzalcoalt, after having ruled as king of the Golden Age in Mexico, returned by divine direction to the primeval Paradise in the North (*Tlapallan*), and partook of the draught of immortality. The stupendous terraced pyramid-temple in Cholula was a copy and symbol of the sacred Paradise-mountain of Aztec tradition, which was described as standing "in the *Centre* of the *Middle-country.*" [1] Some of the Mexican myths represent the mountain as now "crooked," or turned partly over. For the true explanation of this see above, pp. 192–196.

Among the ancient Inca-subjects of Peru [2] was

---

[1] *Im Centrum des Mittellands.* Lüken, *Traditionen*, p. 75; citing Clavigero, *Storia del Messico*, tom. ii., 13, 14. "Die Mexicaner op- ferten auf den höchsten Bergen weil sie glaubten, dass auf ihnen Tlaloc, der Herr des Paradieses wohne. Sie wurden einerseits als der *Mittelpunkt der Erde* betrachtet, andererseits aber als die Stätte, welche *dem Himmel am nächsten* ist, und ihm in näherer Berührung als die Erde selbst steht." Keerl, *Die Schöpfungsgeschichte*, p. 799. In like manner the national temple of Tlaloc and Vizilputzli, his brother, stood in the centre of the city of Mexico, whence four cause- way roads conducted East, West, North, and South. In the centre of the temple was a richly ornamented Pillar of peculiar sanctity. Bancroft, *Native Races*, vol. iii., p. 292. The Quiché prayer to the "Heart of Heaven, Heart of Earth," would seem to rest upon similar conceptions of the true abode of God. Popol Vuh. Max Müller, *Chips from a German Workshop*. New York, 1872: vol. i., p. 335.

[2] "The centre and capital of this great territory was Cuzco (i. e., 'navel'), whence to the borders of the kingdom branched off four great highways, North and South and East and West, each traversing one of the four provinces or vice-royalties into which Peru was di- vided." *The Land of the Incas*, by W. H. Davenport Adams. Lon- don, 1883: p. 20. In the central temple here, too, there was a Pillar, *placée dans le centre d'un cercle dans l'axe du grand temple et tra- versée par un diamètre de l'est à l'ouest.* P. Dabry de Thiersant,

found the same idea of a Navel of the Earth, and even among the Chickasaws of Mississippi.[1]

Thus is all ancient thought full of this legendary idea of a mysterious, primeval, holy, Paradisaic Earth-centre, — a spot connected as is no other with the "Centre of Heaven," the Paradise of God. Why it should be so no one has ever told us; but the hypothesis which places the Biblical Eden at the Pole, and makes all later earth navels commemorative of that primal one, affords a perfect explanation. In the light of it, there is no difficulty in understanding that Earth-centre in Jerusalem with which we began. The inconspicuous pillar in the Church of the Holy Sepulchre symbolizes and commemorates far more than the geographical ignorance of mediæval ages. It stands for the Japanese pillar by which the first soul born upon earth mounted to the sky. It stands for the World-column of the East-Aryans and the Chinvat Bridge of Iran. It stands for the law-proclaiming pillar of orichalcum in Atlantis, placed in the centre of the most central land. It stands for that Talmudic pillar by means of which the tenants of the terrestrial Paradise mount to the celestial, and, having spent the Sab-

De l'Origine des Indiens du Nouveau-Monde et de leur Civilisation. Paris, 1883 : p. 125. Still more interesting is it to note that the predecessors of the Peruvians are reported to have had an idea of the work of the creation of the world as proceeding from the North to the South. Dorman, *Origin of Primitive Superstitions.* Philadelphia, 1881, p. 334.

[1] "Some of the large mounds left in Mississippi were called '*navels*' by the Chickasaws, although the Indians are said not to have had any idea whether these were natural mounds or artificial structures. They thought Mississippi was at *the centre of the earth*, and the mounds were as the navel in the middle of the human body." — Gerald Massey, referring to Schoolcraft, i. 311.

bath, return to pass the week below. It symbolizes Cardo, Atlas, Meru, Harâ-berezaiti, Kharsak-
Kurra, — every fabulous mountain on whose top
the sky pivots itself, and around which all the heavenly bodies ceaselessly revolve. It perpetuates a
religious symbolism which existed in its region before ever Jerusalem had been made the Hebrew
capital, — recalling to our modern world the *tabbur
ha-arets* of a period anterior to the days of Samuel.[1]
In tradition it is said to mark the precise spot
"whence the clay was taken, out of which the body
of Adam was modeled." It does so, but it does it
in a language and method which were common to
all the most ancient nations of the earth. It points
not to the soil in which it stands, but to the holier
soil of a far-away primitive Eden.[2]

[1] Judg. ix. 37 (margin).
[2] The genuinely scientific basis of this ancient symbolism is vividly
shown in our above given sketch-map of the actual relations of all
the continents to the North Pole.

CHAPTER V.

THE QUADRIFURCATE RIVER.

Als ich erfunden han,
Us dem paradise ran
Zu führten baum und gras,
Und alles das darynne was,
Zu guter moss ein wasser gross,
Das in vier teil darnachefloss.

LUTWIN.

Wir haben hier ein merkwürdiges Stromsystem. — GRILL.

"AND a river went out of Eden to water the garden, and from thence it was parted and became into four heads."

In chapter second of Part Second we presented the simple and natural interpretation suggested by the hypothesis of a primitive circumpolar continent. If the reader will kindly turn back to the statement there made (p. 51), he will see in how natural a manner the water system of that lost "land of delights" might have become, in after tradition, the one disparted river which waters the whole earth.

The insuperable difficulties of all hitherto attempted identifications of the four rivers are too numerous to present here in detail.[1] In our interpreta-

---

[1] "We entirely agree with Delitzsch [the elder] that ʻ Paradise is lost,' and the four streams are on this account a riddle which cries, ʻ Where is Paradise ?ʼ the question remaining without an answer." Ebers, *Ægypten und die Bücher Mose*, p. 30. See McClintock and Strong's *Cyclopædia*, Arts. "Gihon," "Pison," "Eden," etc. "Wherever there is a river-head that can be made to run on all-fours, even by assuming the existence of water-channels no longer extant,

tion the original river is from the sky ; the division takes place on the heights at the Pole, and the four resulting rivers are the chief streams of the circumpolar continent as they descend in different directions to the surrounding sea. Does such a view find any support in the traditions of the ancient world ?

That it does will be clear to any one who has carefully read thus far. Let us take the rivers of the Persian cradle of the race. Where do they rise? If the investigator of this question have made no previous studies in Comparative Sacred Hydrography, he will be surprised to find that in Persian thought, not only the Paradise rivers, but also all the rivers of the whole earth, *have but one head-spring and but one place of discharge.*

This head-spring is the Ardvî-Sûra, situated in heaven, — the heaven of the Pole. " This heavenly fountain," says Haug, summarizing the contents of the Abân Yasht, — " this heavenly fountain has a thousand springs and a thousand canals, each of them forty days' journey long. Thence a channel goes through all the seven *keshvares*, or regions of the earth, conveying everywhere pure celestial waters." [1]

the Biblical Eden has been discovered, — whether in Asia, Africa, Europe, or America." Gerald Massey, *The Natural Genesis*, vol. ii., p. 162. We may add that Mr. Samuel Johnson's suggestion (*Oriental Religions ; Persia.* Boston, 1885 : p 253), to the effect that the " four rivers " of the Hebrew story consisted of two real rivers, the Tigris and the Euphrates, *plus* two imaginary " words, that simply mean ' flowing waters,' and that were used as generic terms for the purpose of making up the number *four*, the conventional sign of completeness in all Eastern mythologies," is a characteristic specimen of the unscholarly and dogmatic caprice of pantheistic exegesis in the field of ancient religious ideas and their history.

[1] *Essays*, 2d ed., p. 198. See Darmesteter's translation : " From this river of mine alone flow all the waters that spread all over the

The following is an ancient invocation to Anâhita, the spirit of these heavenly waters : " Come before me, Ardvî-Sûra Anâhita ! — come down from yonder stars on to the earth created by Ahura-Mazda ! Thee shall worship the handy lords, the rulers of countries, sons of the rulers of countries." [1]

From its elevation the heavenly height is called Hûgar, i. e., "the lofty :" " Hûgar, the lofty, is the mount from which the water of Ardvî-Sûra leaps down the height of a thousand men." [2] Again it is written, "Hûgar, the lofty, on which the water of Ardvî-Sûra flows and leaps, is the chief of summits, since it is that above which is the revolution of Satavês, the chief of reservoirs." [3]

As all the rivers of the earth's seven regions, so all lakes and seas and the ocean itself, are from this one celestial fountain. "Through the warmth and clearness of the water, purifying more than other seven keshvares ; this river of mine alone goes on bringing waters both in summer and in winter." *The Zend-Avesta*, Pt. ii., pp. 52-84.

[1] Haug, Ibid., p. 198. Darmesteter, Ibid., p. 73.

[2] *Bundahish* (West), xii. 5. *The Zend-Avesta* (Darmesteter), ii. p. 54.

[3] *Bundahish*, xxiv. 17. When West (*Pahlavi Texts*, Pt. i., p. 35, note 6) uses the last clause of this quotation to show that the location of Hûgar is "probably" in the western quarter, his argument rests upon two mistakes, both of which seem to be shared by all modern Avestan students. The first mistake is to suppose Satavês a different star from Tishtar (Tistrya) ; and the second is the notion that Tishtar was the star now called Sirius. The fact is that originally Satavaêsa and Tistrya were simply two designations for one and the same object, and that object was not our Sirius, but the Pole star. I say *our* Sirius, because there is evidence that this name also once belonged to a very different heavenly body, and to one situated in " *die Mitte des Himmels*," i. e., at the Pole. (Ideler, *Sternennamen*, p. 216.) Hûgar (Hukairya) is the heavenly height of the polar sky, high above Harâ-berezaiti, whenever this term is applied, as originally, to the *terrestrial* polar mount. *Abân Yasht*, 88. See Windischmann, *Zoroastrische Studien*, p. 171.

waters, everything continually flows from the source Ardvî-Sûra." [1] However named, all waters are simply portions of the same heaven-descending stream. "The other innumerable waters and rivers, springs and channels, are one in origin with those, so in various districts and various places they call them by various names." [2] Even plant-sap, and blood, and milk, and all the seventeen kinds of liquid enumerated in the Yashts, are parts of the one cosmic current. "All these, through growth, or the body which is formed, mingle again with the rivers, for the body which is formed and the growth are both one." [3]

Everything of a liquid nature, therefore, in the whole world is conceived of as proceeding from one source high in the north-polar sky. Whither is it tending? What becomes of it all in the end? Where do its myriad rills and rivers at last discharge? As according to the cosmological conception so often illustrated in these pages, all start from the zenith, we should naturally expect all to reunite at last in the nadir. This is found to be the fact. But in this nether gathering place the waters, now polluted from their contact with all the filth and vileness of the world, are not allowed to rest and ac-

[1] *Bundahish*, ch. xiii., 3. The chapter on Seas.
[2] Ibid., xx. 33. *Ranha*, the original Avestan name of the world-river, became corrupted into *Arañhâm — Arang — Aring* — and finally into *Arg*. Windischmann, *Zoroastrische Studien*, pp. 187, 189.
[3] Ibid., xxi. 2. Henry Bowman, in his *Eighteen Hundred and Eighty-one; or the End of the Æon* (St. Louis, Mo., 1884, p. 36), gives the following remarkable interpretation to the heaven-descending river: "The throne of God is the apex, culmination, directly over the pole's axis, and so in the centre of the city, — corresponding to the tree of life, which in the old creation was situated in the centre of the garden, — from which proceeds the ELECTRICAL CURRENT, the 'pure river of the water of life, clear as crystal.'"

cumulate.[1] This cesspool of the universe has a *pervious* bottom. By the various processes of straining, vaporizing, aeration, etc., the polluted waters are by Tishtar brought back distilled and purified, and are re-discharged into the zenith-reservoir which perpetually supplies the gushing streams of Ardvî-Sûra.[2] Into such a marvelously complete cosmical circulatory water system did the Iranic imagination develop the primitive head-stream of Eden. But never, even in the most extravagant mythological adornments of the idea, was it for a moment forgotten that the original undivided stream originates in the north polar sky; and that its division into earthly streams and rivers is on the holy mount which stands in the centre of Kvanîras, the central and circumpolar *keshvare* of the whole habitable earth.[3]

The various fragmentary allusions of the oldest Greek poets to Okeanos and the rivers would seem to imply the early existence, and perhaps early loss, of a similar Hellenic conception of the water circulation of the entire earth. Thus, according to Homer's familiar couplet, it is from Okeanos, in

---

[1] This underworld is the long-misunderstood " cave," in which, in the Vedic myth, the demons try to imprison the stolen rain-cows, so that the earth may be cursed with drought.

[2] Ibid., xx. 4. *Vendidâd*, v. 16–19. More fully and graphically described in *Dâdistân-î Dînîk*, ch. xciii. The ancient idea seems yet to survive in modern folk-lore : " In der Geschichte von Ikirma und Chuseima (in den Erzählungen der 1001 Nächte) sitzen zwei Engel der eine in Gestalt eines Löwen, der andere in der eines Stieres vor einer Pforte, Wache haltend und Gott preisend. Die Pforte, welche nur der Engel Gabriel öffnen kann, führt zu einem von Rubingebirgen umflossenen Meere, der Quelle aller Wasser auf Erden ; aus ihm schöpfen Engel die Gewässer der Welt bis zum Auferstehungstage." Justi, *Geschichte des alten Persiens*, 1879, p. 80.

[3] Compare Spiegel, *Erânische Alterthumskunde.* Leipsic, 1871 : vol. i., pp. 198–202.

some application of the term, that "all rivers and
every sea and all fountains flow." [1] Euripides presents the same idea.[2] There is, therefore, *one fountain* of all the world's waters. The same conception
is expressed by Hesiod in his Theogony, where all
rivers, as sons, and all fountains and brooks, as
daughters, are traced back to Okeanos. Then we
have a constant descending movement of all waters
until they reach the world-surrounding Ocean-river
at the equator, beyond which is the Underworld.
From this equatorial ocean, parting off from the
southern or under shore, new branches diverge and
form the river system of the Hadean kingdom.
Other Underworld rivers were perhaps conceived of
as percolating through the earth and emerging to
the surface in the lower hemisphere. There is at
least some evidence that the Greeks, like the Persians, had this idea of interterranean water-courses,
and even rivers, resembling the circulation of the
blood in the human body.[3] Sometimes these Underworld rivers are represented as four in number, thus
making the circumpolar water system of the Underworld a perfect counterpart of the Eden rivers at
the summit of the upper hemisphere.[4] All, moreover, like those of the Persian Underworld, seem to
be plunging forward and ever downward, until in
the last glimpse which the imagination can catch
they are seen streaming from the roof of the grot
of the goddess Styx, and, as Preller expresses it,

---

[1] *Iliad,* xxi. 195.

[2] Hippolytus, 119.

[3] *Bundahish,* viii. 4.

[4] "In der Unterwelt gab es ausser dem Styx noch drei Flüsse.
Die Vierzahl entspricht derjenigen der vier Paradiesflüsse." — Wolfgang Menzel, *Die vorchristliche Unsterblichkeitslehre,* vol. ii., p. 6.

" falling thence, beneath the Earth, downward into the deep, deep Night." [1]

Here, then, we have a unitary water system, embracing the whole earth, and the remarkable Homeric and Hesiodic term ἀψόῤῥοος, " refluent," may well imply that the Underworld προχοή, or "outflow," [2] *returns* in nature's perfect order to feed its original fountain, thus conforming the whole, in every part, to the sacred hydrography of the Persians. [3]

Granting this, one should locate the Okeanosfountain, not where Preller and Welcker and Völcker and the other mythographers have hitherto placed it, but in the farthest North, and in the sky. That this location was the original one is plain from all the local implications of the mythological accounts of the proper home of Okeanos and Tèthys, and is further confirmed by many incidental evidences connected with such myths as those of the Eridanus, [4] the Acheloös, the birth of Zeus, and particularly those of Atlas and his children. [5]

---

[1] Preller, *Griechische Mythologie,* i. 29. Plato, in his cosmical sketch in Phædo, makes the Hadean rivers pour into Tartaros.

[2] *Odyssey,* xx. 65.

[3] " Fountful Ida " corresponds almost perfectly to the Iranian Hûgar, down whose sides leap and flow the waters of Ardvî-Sûra. Moreover, in its very name Lenormant and others see a root connecting it with Ilâvrita, the circumpolar paradisaic *varsha* of Puranic geography. It should be added that to Ilâvrita corresponds significantly the Norse Idavöllr, or " plain of Ida," which is " *in the middle* of the divine abode." Mallet, *Northern Antiquities,* p. 409.

[4] " Der Eridanus ist *ursprünglich* ein mythischer Fluss." Ideler, *Ursprung der Sternennamen,* p. 229. See especially Robert Brown, Jr., *Eridanus.* London, 1883.

[5] Compare the like conclusion of Grill, *Die Erzväter der Menschheit.* Leipsic, 1875 : i., pp. 222, 223. Grill also claims that the ancient Germans had a similar world-river, p. 223. I cannot help thinking that in the descending Ukko's stream and in the ascending Ämmä's stream of Finnish mythology we have traces of a like cosmic

In the most ancient Akkadian, Assyrian, and Babylonian literature there are expressions which seem clearly to indicate the presence among these peoples of a precisely similar conception with respect to the waters of the world.[1] The same is true of Egyptian literature, but in both these cases the data are as yet too meagre to make them entirely conclusive in argument.[2] We therefore pass them by, and close with a glance at the Eden river of the ancient Aryans of India.

This, as already seen, is the heaven-born Gangâ. The Vedas call it "the river of the three worlds," for the reason that it flows through Heaven and Earth and the Underworld. In Vedic times "the original source and home of the waters was thought to be the highest heaven (*paramam vyoman*), the region peculiarly sacred to Varuna." [3] This is clearly

water circulation. See Castrèn, *Mythologie*, p. 45. After reading the long note in Buxtorfii, *Lexicon Chaldaicum, Talmudicum et Rabbinicum*, Lipsiae, 1865, pp. 341, 342, one could also readily believe that we have here the true origin of the two movements or paths set forth in the omnifluent philosophy of Heraclitus: τὴν ὁδὸν κάτω, and τὴν ὁδὸν ἄνω. Again, "In the Edda all rivers derive their origin from that called *Iver gelmer.*" *Asiatic Researches*, vol. viii., p. 321.

[1] Attention is only called to the ancient Akkadian hymn given by George Smith, *Assyrian Discoveries*, pp. 392, 393; to the exceedingly interesting article by Professor Sayce on "The Encircling River of the Snake-God of the Tree of Life," in *The Academy*, London, Oct. 7, 1882, p. 263; and finally to the instructive account of the Akkadian "mother of rivers" given in Lenormant's *Origines*, ii. 1, p. 133, a citation from which has already been made on p. 171. See also Robert Brown, *The Myth of Kirkê*, p. 110.

[2] "Die Ægypter wussten schon frühe von einem die Erde umfliessenden Strom." — Grill, *Die Erzväter der Menschheit*, i., p. 277.

[3] E. D. Perry, *Journal of the American Oriental Society*, 1882, p. 134. He adds in a foot-note, "In the Veda, 'water' and all corresponding terms, such as stream, river, torrent, ocean, etc., are used indiscriminately of the water upon the earth and of the aqueous vapor in the sky or of the rain in the air." Compare M. Bergaigne: "L'eau

17

illustrated in scores of passages : for example, in the beautiful prayer for immortality, where the fourfold [1] head-spring of all waters is located in the sacred Centre of Heaven.[2] Sometimes the heaven-sprung stream is called the Sindhu,[3] sometimes the Sarasvatî.[4] In the later Mahâbhârata its head-spring is placed in the heaven of Vishnu, high above the lofty Pole-star (Druva). On their descent the ethereal waters wash the Pole-star, and the Seven Rishis (the Great Bear), and the polar pivot of "the lunar orb,"[5] thence falling upon the top of beautiful

des rivières terrestres est reconnue identique par sa nature et son origine à celle des rivières célestes," etc., etc. *La Religion Védique,* tom. i., p. 256. See pp. 251–261.

[1] *Rig Veda,* ix. 74, 6.

[2] *Rig Veda,* ix. 113, 8. Grassmann translates it :—

> "Wo König ist Vivasvats Sohn,
> Und wo des Himmels Heiligthum
> Wo ewig strömt des Wassers Born,
> Da mache du unsterblich mich."

See the "Hymns to the Waters" generally, and particularly that addressed to *Apâm Napât,* the "Navel of the Waters," *R. V.,* ii. 35, comparing therewith the invocations to the "Navel of the Waters" in the Yashts. Darmesteter, *Zend-Avesta,* ii. 6 n., 12, 14, 20, 36, 38, 39, 71, 94, 102, 202. Windischmann, *Zoroastrische Studien,* pp. 177–186.

[3] "Der vedische Inder redet von dem Sindhu κατ' ἐξοχήν, dem Einen himmlischen Strom oder Weltstrom, in dem er die Gesammtheit der atmosphärischen Dünste und Wasser als in Bewegung begriffener und die Erde rings umfliessender sich zur Anschauung bringt."—Grill, *Die Erzväter der Menschheit,* Th. i., p. 197.

[4] See the Vedic passages in Bergaigne, *La Religion Védique,* tom. i., pp. 325–328.

[5] Wilkins, *Hindu Mythology.* London, 1882 : p. 102. In Indian cosmology the lunar sphere is concentric with and includes the earth-sphere ; hence water falling perpendicularly from the celestial to the terrestrial pole can yet on its way "wash the lunar sphere." So too a mountain at the North Pole, if only high enough, will reach to the "lunar sphere." Such, in fact, was the case with the Paradise mountain of Indian cosmology, and traces of the idea live on in the Tal-

Meru. "On the summit of Meru," says the Vishnu Purana, "is the vast city of Brahma, . . . inclosed by the river Gangâ, which, issuing from the foot of Vishnu and washing the lunar orb, falls here [on the top of Meru] from the skies, and, after encircling the city,[1] divides into four mighty rivers, flowing in opposite directions. These rivers are Sítá, the Alakanandá, the Chakshu, and the Bhadrá. The first, falling on the tops of the inferior mountains on the east side of Meru, flows over their crests, and passes through the country of Bhadráswa to the ocean. The Alakanandá flows south to the country of Bhárata, and, dividing into seven rivers on the way, falls into the sea. The Chakshu falls into the sea after traversing all the western mountains and passing through Ketumála. And the Bhadrá washes the country of the Uttarakurus and empties itself into the northern ocean."[2]

mud and in Patristic theology too plain for even Massey to render valueless : "Meru is shown to be the mount which reached to the moon and became a figure of the four lunar quarters. . . . Hence the tradition that Paradise was preserved during, or was exempt from, the Deluge because it was on the summit of a mountain that reached to the moon (Bereshith Rabba, xxxiii.) ; which shows the continuation of the typical mount of the seven stars into the lunar phase of time-keeping, where the mount of the four quarters carried Eden with it." *The Natural Genesis*, vol. ii., p. 244.

[1] Here is probably the origin of the curious notion of the Sabæans touching the Euphrates. Or was the borrowing on the other side ? "Les Soubbas ont la certitude que l'Euphrate, qui, d'après eux, prend sa source sous le trône d'Avather (personnage qui préside au jugement des âmes et dont le trône est placé sous *l'étoile polaire*), passait autrefois à Jérusalem." M. N. Siouffi, *La Religion des Soub-bas ou Sabéens.* Paris, 1880: p. 7, note. Jehovah's city here takes the place of Brahma's.

[2] *The Vishnu Purana,* Wilson's version, vol. vii., p. 120. Compare herewith the notions of the Chinese Buddhists : " With reference to this land of Jambu-dwîpa [the earth], the Buddhists say that in the

Here, again, as our interpretation of Genesis requires, the four rivers traced back to their origin bring us to the summit of the earth at the Pole, — to the one river which descends from the north polar sky. Curious confirmations of this primitive conception come even from the most distant continents.[1] Late Christian legend shows evident traces of it, for in Maundeville's description of the Paradise-fountain he says, "All the sweet waters of the world *above and beneath* take their beginning from that well of Paradise;" and again, "Out of that well all waters *come and go*," — giving thus clear expression to the idea of a unitary cosmic water circula-

midst of it is a centre (heart), called the lake A-nieou-to (Anavataptu); it lies to the south of the Fragrant Mountains, and to the north of the great Snowy Mountains (Himavat). It is 800 li in circuit. In the midst of this lake is the abode of a Naga, who is in fact the transformed appearance of Dasabhumi Bodhisatwa (or of the Bodhisatwas of the ten earths). From his abode proceed four refreshing rivers, which compass Jambu-dwipa. At the east side of the lake, from the mouth of a silver ox, flows out the Ganges River. After compassing the lake once it enters the sea towards the southeast. From the south side of the lake, from the mouth of a golden elephant, flows the Sindhu [Indus] River. After compassing the lake once it enters the sea on the southwest. On the west side of the lake, flowing from the mouth of a horse of lapis-lazuli, flows the river Foh-tzu (Vakshu, *i. e.*, Oxus), which, after compassing the lake once, enters the sea on the northwest. On the north side of the lake, flowing from a crystal lion, flows the river Sida [Hoang-ho], which after making one circuit flows into the sea on the northeast." Beal, *Buddhist Literature in China.* 1882 : p. 149.

[1] Thus in Africa, among the Damaras, "the highest deity is Omakuru, the Rain-giver, who dwells in the far North." E. B. Tylor, *Primitive Culture,* Am. ed., vol. ii., p. 259. So also in America: "Die alten Mexikaner glaubten, das Paradies liege auf dem höchsten Berge, wo die Wolken sich versammeln, von wo sie Regen bringen, und von wo auch die Flüsse herabkommen." Lüken, *Traditionen,* i., p. 115. And this Paradise-mountain was in the farthest North. See the pathetic prayer to Tlaloc in Bancroft, *Native Races,* vol. iii., pp. 325–330.

tion.[1] So, again, in the apocryphal " Revelation of
the Holy Apostle Paul," the angel who was showing
the apostle the wonders of the heavenly city brought
him to just such a World-river, whose spring was
in heaven, but whose main body surrounded the
earth.

"And he set me upon the river whose source
springs up in the circle of heaven, and it is this river
which encircleth the whole earth. And he says unto
me : This river is Ocean." [2]

---

[1] Compare verses 482–487 of the Old German legend of Brandan
in Carl Schroeder, *Sanct Brandan.* Erlangen, 1871 : p. 61 : —

> "Vor dem sale stûnt ein brunne,
> "ûz dem vlôz milch und wîn,
> "waz mohte wunderlicher sin.
> "ouch olei und honicseim darûz vlôz
> "daz *an vier enden* sich ergôz."

The editor (p. 105) connects this last line with the quadripartite
river of Paradise, and the lines immediately following give it an unequivocally cosmical significance : —

> "Von dem selben brunnen
> "haben die wurze saf gewunnen
> "die got liez gewerden ie."

[2] *The Apocryphal Gospels, Acts and Revelations. Ante - Nicene
Christian Library,* vol. xvi., p. 483.

CHAPTER VI.

THE CENTRAL TREE.

The Tree of Life,
The middle tree, and highest there that grew.
MILTON.

Sowohl der Apfelbaum und die Quelle, als auch der Drache des Hesperidengartens, werden in den Mythen und Märchen der meisten Völker in das Centrum der Natur, an den Gipfel des Weltberges, an den Nordpol verlegt. — WOLFGANG MENZEL.

IN the centre of the Garden of Eden, according to Genesis iii. 3, there was a tree exceptional in position, in character, and in its relations to men. Its fruit was "good for food," it was "pleasant to the eyes," "a tree to be desired."[1] At first sight it would not perhaps appear how a study of this tree in the different mythologies of the ancient world could assist us in locating primitive Paradise. In the discussions of such sites as have usually been

[1] Was this "tree of knowledge" identical with the "tree of life"? Possibly. "The tradition of Genesis," says Lenormant, *Beginnings*, p. 84, "at times appears to admit two trees, one of Life and one of Knowledge, and again seems to speak of one only, uniting in itself both attributes (Gen. ii. 17 ; iii. 1–7)." Compare Ernst von Bunsen, *Das Symbol des Kreuzes bei allen Nationen.* Berlin, 1876 : p. 5. To make the whole account relate to one tree it would only be necessary first to translate the last clause of ch. ii. 9 " the tree of life also in the midst of the garden, *even* the tree of knowledge of good and evil ; " and then the last clause of ch. iii. 22 "and now lest he continue to put forth his hand and to take of the tree of life," etc., — for both of which constructions there are abundant precedents, if only the *gam* be rendered with the freedom used in some other passages. As to the first, see 1 Sam. xvii. 40 ; xxviii. 3 ; Dan. iv. 10 ; as to the second, the Hebrew grammars on the use of the future. Compare also Prov. iii. 13, 18, where *wisdom* is a tree of *life.*

proposed it could not ; but if the Garden of Eden was precisely at the North Pole, it is plain that a goodly tree standing in the centre of that Garden would have had a visible and obvious cosmical significance which could by no possibility belong to any other. Its fair stem shooting up as arrow-straight as the body of one of the "giant trees of California," far overtopping, it may be, even such gigantic growths as these, would to any one beneath have seemed the living pillar of the very heavens. Around it would have turned the "stars of God," as if in homage ; through its topmost branches the human worshiper would have looked up to that unmoving centre-point where stood the changeless throne of the Creator. How conceivable that that Creator should have reserved for sacred uses this one natural altar-height of the Earth, and that by special command He should have guarded its one particular adornment from desecration ! (Gen. ii. 16, 17.) If anywhere in the temple of nature there was to be an altar, it could only be here. That it was here finds a fresh and unexpected confirmation in the singular agreement of many ancient religions and mythologies *in associating their Paradise-Tree with the axis of the world, or otherwise, with equal unmistakableness, locating it at the Arctic Pole of the Earth.*[1]

That the Northmen conceived of the universe as

---

[1] "The Mythical Tree, like the Pillar and the Mount, is a type of the celestial Pole." Massey, *The Natural Genesis*, vol. i., p. 354. The arguments of Professor Karl Budde in favor of eliminating the Paradise-tree from the original Genesis account of the Garden of Eden betray a strange lack of insight. *Die biblische Urgeschichte.* Giessen, 1883: pp. 45-88. Even Kuenen refuses to entertain so arbitrary a notion, and M. Réville well exclaims, What would a Paradise be without *l'Arbre de Vie !*

a tree (the Yggdrasil) is well known to ordinary
readers. Its roots are in the lowest hell, its mid-
branches inclose or overarch the abode of men, its
top reaches the highest heaven of the gods. It was
their poetical way of saying that the whole world
is an organic unity pervaded by one life. As the
abode of the gods was in the north polar sky, the
summit of the tree was at that point, its base in
the south polar abyss, its trunk coincident with the
axis of heaven and earth.[1] It was, therefore, in position and in nature precisely what an idealizing
imagination magnifying the primitive tree of Paradise to a real World-tree would have produced.[2]

But while most readers are familiar with this
Norse myth, few are aware how ancient and universal an idea it represents. This same tree appears
in the earliest Akkadian mythology.[3] And what is
precisely to our purpose, it stood, as we have before
seen, at "the Centre" or Pole of the earth, where
is "the holy house of the gods."[4] It is the same

---

[1] Menzel, "Dieses Sinnbild entsteht ursprünglich aus der Vorstellung der Weltachse." *Die vorchristliche Unsterblichkeitslehre*, i. 70.

[2] See "Les Cosmogonies Aryennes," par J. Darmesteter, *Revue
Critique.* Paris, 1881 : pp. 470–476.

[3] "By the full waters grew the giant 'overshadowing tree,' the
Yggdrasil of Norse mythology, whose branches were of 'lustrous
crystal,' extending downwards even to the deep." Sayce, *Babylonian
Literature*, p. 39. Compare Lenormant, *Beginnings of History*, pp. 83–
107. Had Professor Finzi duly considered the Tree of Life in Akkadian tradition, he could hardly have felt "constrained" to ascribe
the origin of the sacred tree of the Assyrian monuments to "Aryan,
more particularly Iranian influences." *Ricerche per lo Studio dell'
Antichità Assira*, p. 553, note.

[4] "In Eridu a dark pine grew. It was planted in a holy place.
Its crown was crystal white, which spread towards the deep vault
above. The abyss of Hea was its pasturage in Eridu, a canal full of
waters. Its station was the centre of this earth. Its shrine was the
couch of Mother Zikum. The (roof) of its holy house like a forest

tree which in ancient Egyptian mythology inclosed the sarcophagus of Osiris, and out of which the king of Byblos caused the roof-pillar of his palace to be taken. But this was only another form of the Tat-pillar, which is the axis of the world.[1] In the light of comparative cosmology it is quite impossible to agree with Mr. Renouf in his treatment of the Tree in Egyptian mythology. It is neither "the rain cloud," nor "the light morning cloud," nor "the transparent mist on the horizon." His own citations of texts clearly show that under all its names the Egyptian Tree of Life is a true World-tree, whose trunk is coincident in position and direc-

---

spread its shade. There were none who entered not within it. It was the seat of the mighty Mother." —*Records of the Past*, vol. ix., p. 146.

[1] "It was most likely at Memphis, too, that he [Ptah] was imaged as a pillar *beginning in the lowest and ending in the highest heaven*, a conception which is undoubtedly referred to in that feature of the myth, as related by Plutarch, where the king of Byblos causes a pillar to be made in his palace out of the tree which had grown around the sarcophagus of Osiris. In fact, we possess delineations of Osiris as well as of Ptah answering to this description. On a post, on which is graven a human countenance, and which is covered with gay clothing, stands the so-called Tat-pillar, entirely made up of a kind of superimposed capitals, one of which has a rude face scratched upon it, intended, no doubt, to represent the shining sun. On the top of the pillar is placed the complete head-dress of Osiris, the ram's horns, the sun, the ureus-adders, the double feather, all emblems of light and of sovereignty, and which, in my judgment, must have been intended to represent the highest heaven. [See the plate in Wilkinson, M. and C., 2d series, suppt. plate 25 and 33, No. 5. Mariette, *Abydos*, I., pl. 16.] The Tat-pillar is the symbol of durability, immutability. This representation of Osiris, which its rude and simple character, without trace of art, proves to have been one of the most ancient, must apparently be held to be symbolical of him as 'Lord of the length of time and of eternity.'" Ticle, *History of the Egyptian Religion*, pp. 46, 47. See also G. Massey, *The Natural Genesis*, vol. i., pp. 417, 418, 422 ; and Brugsch, *Astronomische und Astrologische Inschriften*, p. 72.

tion with the axis of the world ; a tree in whose
sky-filling branches Bennu, the sun-bird, is seated ;
a tree from whose north polar top the "*North-
wind*" proceeds ; a tree which, like the Yggdrasil,
yields a celestial rain that is as life-giving as Ardvî-
Sûra's, and that descends, not merely upon the fields
of Lower Egypt, but, like Ardvî-Sûra's, to the Underworld itself, refreshing "those who are in *Amenti.*"[1]
The super-terrestrial portion of the Egyptian's Yggdrasil, therefore, — like that of the Northman's, —
stands at the Arctic Pole.

The Phœnicians, Syrians, and Assyrians had each
their sacred tree in which the universe was symbolized.[2] In the lost work of Pherecydes the former
is represented as a "winged oak."[3] Over it was
thrown the magnificent veil, or *peplos*, of Harmonia, on which were represented the all-surrounding
Ocean with his rivers, the Earth with its *omphalos*
in the centre, the sphere of Heaven varied by the
figures of the stars.[4] But as this self-interpreting

---

[1] See Renouf, "Egyptian Mythology, particularly with Reference to
Mist and Cloud." *Transactions of the Society for Biblical Archæology.*
London, 1884 : pp. 217-220. A beautiful confirmation of our view
is found in the important text in which "the abyss under the earth"
(*die Tiefe unter der Erde*) is poetically expressed by the term "the
cavity of the Persea (*die Höhle der Persea*). Brugsch's version, from
which the above German expressions are taken, may be seen in the
Zeitschrift für Aegyptische Sprache und Alterthumskunde. Leipsic,
1881 : pp. 77 ff. Surely no opening in an ordinary cloud could be
called the subterranean deep.

[2] " W. Baudissin is wrong in supposing it unknown to the Phœnicians." — Lenormant, *Beginnings of History*, vol. i., p. 104 n.

[3] But δρῦς was originally a generic term for tree. See Curtius,
Etymologie, s. v.

[4] " This veil is identical with the starry peplos of Harmonia."
Robert Brown, Jr., *The Unicorn.* London, 1881 : p. 89. *The Myth
of Kirkê.* London, 1883 : p. 71.

symbol was furnished with wings to facilitate its constant rotation, it is plain that we have in it, not only a World-tree, but also one the central line of whose trunk is one with the axis of heaven and earth.[1] In the language of Maury, "It is a conception identical with the Yggdrasil of Scandinavian mythology."[2] That section of the tree, therefore, which reaches from the abode of men into the holy heavens rises pillar-like from the Pole of the earth to the Pole of the sky.

Among the Persians the legendary tree of Paradise took on two forms, according as it was viewed with predominant reference to the universe as an organic whole, or to the vegetable world as proceeding from it. In the first aspect it was the Gaokerena (Gôkard) tree, or "the white Hôm" (Haoma = Soma); in the second, the "tree of all seeds," the "tree opposed to harm." Of the former it is written, "Every one who eats of it becomes immortal; . . . also in the renovation of the universe they prepare its immortality therefrom; it is the chief of plants."[3] Of the second we read, "In like manner

---

[1] "Thus the universe definitively organized by Zeus, with the assistance of Harmonia, was depicted by Pherecydes as an immense tree, furnished with wings to promote its rotary motion, — a tree whose roots were plunged into the abyss, and whose extended branches sustained the unfolded veil of the firmament decorated with the types of all terrestrial and celestial forms." Lenormant, *Beginnings of History*, p. 549. Compare Louis de Ronchaud, "Le Péplos d'Athéné Parthénos," *Revue Archéologique.* Année, xxiii. (1872) pp. 245 *seq.*, 309 *seq.*, 390 *seq.*; xxiv. 80 *seq.* Also W. Swartz, "Das Halsband der Harmonia und die Krone der Ariadne." *Neue Jahrbücher der Philologie,* 1883: pp. 115–127. This writer's view of the connection of the *Halsband* with the *foot* of the Yggdrasil is very curious and not wholly clear.

[2] *Religions de la Grèce Antique,* iii. 253.

[3] *Bundahish,* xxvii. 4. Compare the *Vendîdâd,* Farg. xx.

as the animals, with grain of fifty and five species and twelve species of medicinal plants, have arisen from the primeval ox, so ten thousand species among the species of principal plants, and a hundred thousand species among ordinary plants, have grown from all these seeds of the tree opposed to harm, the many-seeded. . . . When the seeds of all these plants, with those from the primeval ox, have arisen upon it, every year the bird (Kamros) strips that tree and mingles all the seeds in the water; Tîshtar seizes them with the rain-water and rains them on to all regions." [1]

Where stood this tree which, in its dual form, was at once the source of all other trees and the giver of immortality? Every indication points us to the northern Pole. It was in Aîrân-Vej,[2] the Persian Eden, and this we have already found. It was at the source of all waters, the north polar fountain of Ardvî-Sûra.[3] It was begirt with the starry girdle of the zodiacal constellations, which identifies it with the axis of the world.[4] It grew on "the highest height of Harâ-berezaiti," [5] and this is the celestial mountain at the Pole. Finally, although Grill mis-

---

[1] Ibid., xxvii. 2, 3.

[2] *Bundahish*, xxix. 5.

[3] Ibid., xxvii. 4. Compare Windischmann : " Also der Baum des Lebens wächst in dem Wasser des Lebens, in der Quelle Ardviçûra Anâhita." *Zoroastrische Studien.* Berlin, 1863 : p. 171.

[4] *Homa Yasht*, 26. Haug, *Essays*, 2d ed., p. 182.

[5] *Yasht*, IX. (*Gosh.*), 17. Compare *Bundahish*, xviii., as translated by Justi and Windischmann. See Grill, *Die Erzväter*, i., pp. 186–191. Windischmann, *Zoroastrische Studien*, p. 165 *seq.* Spiegel, *Erânische Alterthumskunde*, i. 463 *seq.* It is by no means inconsistent herewith that, according to the Minokhired, the tree grows in the sea *Var-Kash* "am verborgensten Orte," since this statement has reference to the subterranean rooting of the tree in the lowest part of the Underworld. Kuhn, *Herabkunft*, p. 124.

takenly makes the Chinvat bridge "correspond with
the Milky Way and the rainbow," he nevertheless
correctly discerns some relationship between Chinvat and the Persian Tree of Life.[1] By this identification we are again brought to the one unmistakable location toward which all lines of evidence
perpetually converge.

The Aryans of India, as early as in the far-off
Vedic age, had also their World-tree, which yielded
the gods their soma, the drink which maintains immortality. As we should anticipate, its roots are in
the Underworld of Yama at the hidden pole, its top
in the north polar heaven of the gods, its body is the
sustaining axis of the universe.[2] Weber long ago
expressly identified it with the World-ash of the
Edda;[3] and Kuhn,[4] Senart,[5] and all the more recent
writers accept without question the identification.
Grill's interesting sketch of the historic developments of the myth may be seen in the Appendix to
this volume.[6] Some of the late traces of it in Hindu

---

[1] Grill, *Ibid.*, p. 191. Compare the original Zend invocation in the
Homa Yasht: "*Amereza gayêhê stûna,*" "*O imperishable Pillar of
Life.*" Haug, *Essays*, p. 177 n.

[2] *Rig Veda*, x. 135, 1; *Atharvan Veda*, vi. 95, 1. See Kuhn, *Herabkunft des Feuers und des Göttertranks.* Berlin, 1859: p. 126 *seq.* J.
Grill, *Erzväter*, i., pp. 169-175. Obry, *Le Berceau de l'Espèce Humaine*, pp. 146-160. Windischmann, *Zoroastrische Studien*, pp. 176,
177. It is true that the roots of this divine *Asvattha* are sometimes
represented as in the heaven of the gods, its growth being downwards;
but this is only to symbolize the emanation of Nature and of Nature's
life from the divine source, as clearly expressed in the opening verses
of the fifteenth reading of the *Bhagavad Gîtâ.* See John Davies'
translation, London, 1882, p. 150; and for a parallel, M. Wolff, *Mu-
hammedanische Eschatologie*, Leipsic, 1872, p. 197.

[3] *Indische Studien*, Bd. i., p. 397.

[4] *Herabkunft*, etc., p. 128.

[5] *La Légende du Bouddha*, p. 240.

[6] See APPENDIX, Sect. V.

art betray the ancient conception of the Pole as a means of ascent to heaven, a bridge of souls and of the gods, a stair substituted for the slippery pillar up which the Tauist emperor vainly sought to climb.[1]

Among the Greeks [2] it is more than probable that the "holy palm" in Delos, on which Lêtô laid hold at the birth of Apollo, represents the same mythical World-tree. If so, and if we follow Hecatæus in locating the scene, we shall be brought to the Arctic Pole.[3] The eternally flourishing olive of Athênê (Euripides, Ion 1433) seems also but another form of the holy palm, and this in some of its descriptions brings us again to the land of the Hyperbo-

---

[1] "In the Naga sculptures (Fergusson, *Tree and Serpent Worship*, pl. 27), the Tree of the Mount or Pole is identified at the bottom by one tree, and at the top by another, and between the two there is a kind of ladder, with a series of steps or stairs which ascend the tree, in the place of a stem. These denote the Tree of the Ascent, Mount, or Height, now to be considered as representing the Pole."—G. Massey, *The Natural Genesis*, vol. i., p. 354.

[2] Kuhn, *Herabkunft*, etc., pp. 133-137.

[3] Menzel, *Unsterblichkeitslehre*, i. 89. Its "central" position with respect to the world of men is recognized by old Robert Burton in his *Anatomy of Melancholy*, New York, 1849, p. 292. Compare Massey: "The Tree of the Pole is extant in Celebes, where the natives believe that the world is supported by the Hog, and that earthquakes are caused when the Hog rubs itself against the Tree. . . . At Ephesus they showed the Olive and Cypress Grove of Lêtô, and in it the Tree of Life to which the Great Mother clung in bringing forth her twin progeny. There also was the Mount on which Hermes announced the birth of her twins Diana and Apollo [sun and moon]. The imagery is at root the same as the Hog rubbing against the Tree of the Pole." *The Natural Genesis*, vol. i., p. 354. And again, the cosmical imagery of Hesiod: "Das leitende Bild eines Baumes, dessen Stamm sich von den Wurzeln erhebt und oben ausbreitet, tritt in den Worten der Theogonie v. 727: vom Tartarus aufwärts seien die Wurzeln der Erde und des Meeres, deutlich hervor." W. F. Rinck, *Die Religion der Hellenen*. Zurich, 1853: Bd. i., p. 60.

reans.[1] In the Garden of the Hesperides, the tree
which bore the golden apples was unquestionably
the Tree of Paradise ; but following Æschylus, Pherecydes, and Apollodorus, we must place it in the
farthest North, beyond the Rhipæan mountains.[2]
Traces of the same mythical conception among the
Romans are presented by Kuhn.[3]

The sacred tree of the Buddhists figures largely
in their sculpture. An elaborate specimen representation may be seen on the well-known Sanchi
Tope. One inconspicuous feature in the representation has often puzzled observers. Almost invariably,
at the very top of the tree we find a little umbrella.
So universal is this that its absence occasions remark.[4] This little piece of symbolism has a curious
value. In Buddhist mythological art the umbrella
symbolizes the north polar heaven of the gods,[5] and
by attaching it to the tip of the sacred tree the ancient sculptors of this faith unmistakably showed
the cosmical character and axial position of that to
which it was attached.

But this cosmic tree was the mythical Bôdhi tree,
the Tree of Wisdom, —

> " Beneath whose leaves
> It was ordained that Truth should come to Buddh." [6]

---

[1] Nonnus, *Dionysiac*, xl. 443 *seq.*   Lüken, *Traditionen*, p. 74.

[2] Preller, *Gr. Mythologie*, i. 149.   Völcker, *Mythische Geographie*.
Leipsic, 1832 : p. 134.

[3] *Herabkunft*, etc., pp. 179, 180.

[4] James Fergusson, *Tree and Serpent Worship*. London, 2d ed.,
1873 : pp. 134, 135.

[5] Lillie, *Buddha and Early Buddhism*. London, 1881 : pp. 2, 19.
A different study of the cosmical nature of this tree may be found in
Senart, *Légende du Bouddha*. Paris, 1875 : pp. 239–244.

[6] Arnold, *Light of Asia*, Book vi.

Its location is in " the Middle of the Earth." [1] Notwithstanding his doctrine of an African origin of mankind, Gerald Massey says, " In the legendary life of Gautama, Buddha is described as having to pass over the celestial water to reach Nirvana, which is the land of the Bôdhi Tree of Life and Knowledge. He was unable to cross from one bank to the other, but the spirit of the Bôdhi tree stretched out its arms to him and helped him over in safety. By aid of this tree he attained the summit of wisdom and immortal life. It is the same Tree of the Pole and of Paradise all mythology through. The Tree of the Guarani garden, the Hebrew Eden, the Hindu Jambu-dwîpa, is likewise the Tree of Nirvana. This final application of the imagery proves its origin. The realm of rest was first seen at the polar centre of the revolving stars." [2]

The ancient Germans called their World-tree the *Irmensul, i. e.,* " Heaven-pillar." Grimm speaks of its close relationship with the Norse Yggdrasil, and

---

[1] " The Buddhists assert that this tree marks *the middle of the earth.*"—E. C. Brewer, *Dictionary of Miracles.* Philadelphia, 1884: p. 314.

[2] *The Natural Genesis,* vol. ii., 90. On the independence of the Buddhist cosmogony and cosmology Beal remarks, " But whilst we may regard Buddhism in the light of a reformation of the popular belief in India, we must bear in mind that the stream of tradition which reappears in its teaching, and may be traced in its books, is independent and probably distinct from the Brahmanical traditions embodied in the Puranas and elsewhere. At any rate, this is the case so far as the primitive question of creation and of the cosmic system generally is concerned. Mr. Rhys Davids has already remarked that ' the Buddhist archangel or god Brahma is different from anything known to the Brahmans, and is part of an altogether different system of thought' (*Buddhist Suttas,* p. 168 n.). I am inclined to go further than this, and say that the traditions of the Buddhists are different from those of the Brahmans in almost every respect." Samuel Beal, *Buddhist Literature in China.* London, 1882 : p. 146.

lends his high authority to the view that it was simply a mythical expression of the idea of the world's axis.[1] The same view was advanced still earlier by the distinguished Icelandic mythographer, Finn Magnusen.[2] How profoundly the myth affected mediæval Christian art is illustrated in many places, among the rest in the sculptures on the south portal of the Baptistery at Parma.[3] It is also not without a deep significance that "in the mediæval legend of Seth's visit to the Garden of Eden, to obtain for his dying father the Oil of Compassion, the Tree of Life which he saw lifted its *top to heaven* and sent *its root to hell;*"[4] and that on the crucifixion of Christ, himself the

"*Arbor, quæ ab initio posita est,*"

this cosmical Tree of the Garden died, and became the "*Arbre Sec*" of mediæval story.[5]

---

[1] "Mir scheint auch die im deutschen Alterthum tief gegründete Vorstellung von der *Irmensäule,* jener altissima, universalis columna quasi sustinens omnia, dem Weltbaum Yggdrasil nah verwandt." — J. Grimm, *Deutsche Mythologie,* p. 759. Compare pp. 104-107.

[2] *Den aeltre Edda.* Kjöbenhavn, 1822 : Bd. ii., 61. Compare the following : " Yggdrasil has never been satisfactorily explained. But at all events the sacred tree of the North is, no doubt, identical with the '*robur Jovis,*' or sacred oak of Geismar, destroyed by Boniface, and the Irminsul of the Saxons, the *columna universalis,* the terrestrial tree of offerings, an emblem of the whole world as far as it is under divine influence." Thorpe, *Northern Mythology,* vol. i., p. 155.

[3] See F. Piper, *Evangelischer Kalender* für 1866, pp. 35-80 (illustrated). Also Piper's " Baum des Lebens," in the same *Kalender* for 1863, pp. 17-94.

[4] Gubernatis, *Zoölogical Mythology.* London, 1872 : vol. ii., p. 411, note.

[5] *The Book of Marco Polo.* Edition of Col. H. Yule. London, 1871 : pp. 120-131. Notice particularly the picture on p. 127, which corrects Polo's blunder in confounding the *Arbre Sol* with the *Arbre Sec.* The bird at the top of the central and highest of the trees depicted conclusively identifies it with the World-tree of universal Aryan tradition. On this bird see Kuhn.

The Paradise-tree of the Chinese Tauists is also a World-tree. It is found in the centre of the enchanting Garden of the Gods on the summit of the polar Kwen-lun. Its name is Tong, and its location is further defined by the expression that it grows "hard by the closed Gate of Heaven." [1] As in many of the ancient religions, the mount on which, after the Flood, the ark rested was considered the same as that from which in the beginning the first man came forth, it is not strange to find the tree on the top of the mountain of Paradise remembered in some of the legends of the Deluge. In the Tauist legend it seems to take the place of the ark. Thus we are told that "one extraordinary antediluvian saved his life by climbing up a mountain, and there and then, in the manner of birds plaiting a nest, he passed his days on a tree, whilst all the country below him was one sheet of water. He afterwards lived to a very old age, and could testify to his late posterity that a whole race of human beings had been swept from the face of the earth." [2]

It is at least suggestive to find this same idea of salvation from a universal deluge by means of a miraculous tree growing on the top of the divine Mountain of the North among the Navajo Indians of our own country. Speaking of the men of the world before our own, and of the warning they had received of the approaching flood, their legends go on : "Then they took soil from all the *four corner mountains of the world*, and placed it on top of the mountain that stood *in the North;* and thither they all went, including the people of the mountains,

---

[1] Lüken, *Traditionen*, p. 72.
[2] *The Chinese Repository*, vol. viii., p. 517.

the salt-woman, and such animals as then lived in the third world. When the soil was laid on the mountain, the latter began to grow higher and higher, but the waters continued to rise, and the people climbed upwards to escape the flood. At length the mountain ceased to grow, and they planted on the summit a great reed, into the hollow of which they all entered. The reed grew every night, but did not grow in the daytime; and this is the reason why the reed grows in joints to this day: the hollow internodes show where it grew by night, and the solid nodes show where it rested by day. Thus the waters gained on them in the day-time. The turkey was the last to take refuge in the reed, and he was therefore at the bottom. When the waters rose high enough to wet the turkey, they all knew that danger was near. Often did the waves wash the end of his tail, and it is for this reason that the tips of the turkey's tail-feathers are to this day lighter than the rest of his plumage. At the end of the fourth night from the time it was planted the reed had grown up to the floor of the fourth world, and here they found a hole through which they passed to the surface." [1]

The opening sentence of the above citation gives us a topography exactly corresponding to Mount Meru, the Hindu "mountain of the North," with its "four corner mountains of the world," in the four opposite points of the horizon. Moreover, in the Deluge myths of the Hindus, as in this of the Nava-

[1] W. Matthews, "The Navajo Mythology." *The Am. Antiquarian,* July, 1883, p. 208. The difficulty of any interpretation of this cosmology other than the true is illustrated by the efforts of M. Réville. *Les Religions des Peuples Non-civilisés.* Paris, 1883: vol. i., pp. 271–274.

jos, it was over this central mountain that the survivors of that world-destruction found deliverance.
However explained, the coincidences are remarkable.

In Keltic tradition the Tree of Paradise is represented by the tree which bore golden apples in
Avalon. But Avalon is always represented as an
island in the far North, and its "loadstone castle"
self-evidently connects it with the region of the magnetic Pole.[1]

In the ancient epic of the Finns, the Kalevala, we
see the World-tree of another people. If any doubt
could rise as to its position in the universe, the constellation of *the Great Bear in its top* would suffice
to remove it.[2]

---

[1] Menzel, *Unsterblichkeitslehre,* i. 87, 95 ; ii. 10. Keary, *Outlines
of Primitive Belief,* p. 453. Especially see Humboldt's references to
"*Monte Calamitico,*" the mediæval magnetic mountain in the sea to
the north of Greenland. *Cosmos* (Bohn's ed.), ii. 659 ; v. 55. Also,
Le Cycle mythologique irlandais et la Mythologie celtique. Par H. d'Ar-
bois de Jubainville. Paris, 1884. Dr. Carl Schroeder, *Sanct Brandan.* Erlangen, 1871 : pp. 57, 111, 167, etc.

[2] The German translation by Anton Schiefner. Helsinfors, 1852 :
Rune x., 31-42. Compare Schiefner, *Heldensagen der minussinischen
Tataren,* p. 62 *seq.* Traces of the same myth are found among the
Samoans (*Samoa a Hundred Years Ago and Long Before.* By George
Turner, LL. D. London, 1884 : pp. 199, 201). Also, among the
Ugrian tribes (Peschel, *Races of Man,* p. 406) ; and among many of
the tribes of the American aborigines, and in Polynesia. See M.
Husson, *La Chaine Traditionnelle, Contes et Légendes au point de vue
mythique.* Paris, 1874 : especially pp. 140-160. Massey, *The Natural
Genesis.* "It was at the top of the Tree of Heaven — the Pole —
that the Guaranis were to meet once more with their Adam, Atum,
Tum, or Tamoi, who was to help them from thence in their ascent to
the higher life. Here the Tree of Life becomes a tree of the dead to
raise them into heaven. So in the Algonkin myth the tree of the dead
was a sort of oscillating log for the deceased to cross the river by, as
a bridge of the abyss, beyond which the Dog, as in the Persian mythos,
stands waiting for the souls of the dead, just as the Dog stands at

Thus the sacred trees, like the sacred waters, of every ancient people invariably conduct the investigator to lands outside the historic *habitats* of the peoples in question, and ever to one and the same primeval home-country, the land of light and glory at the Arctic Pole.[1]

the Northern Pole of the Egyptian, and is depicted in the tree of the Southern Solstice, — the Tree of the Pole which was extended to the four quarters." Vol. i., p. 404.

[1] Since completing the foregoing chapter I have seen the work entitled *Plant Lore, Legends, and Lyrics ; embracing the Myths, Traditions, Superstitions, and Folk-lore of the Plant Kingdom*. By Richard Folkard, Jun. London, 1884. In the first three chapters the reader will find valuable supplementary reading on " The World-Trees of the Ancients," "The Trees of Paradise," "The Tree of Adam," " Sacred Trees of all Nations," etc. Other chapters treat of " Plant Symbolism," " Plant Language," and of the fabulous trees and miracle plants which play so important a part in the history of religious and scientific credulity. Should any reader thereof be inclined to claim that "the progress of science " has forever done away with such ignorant mediæval mystagogy, he will do well to turn to *The Weekly Inter-Ocean*, Chicago, Dec. 11, 1884, in which, in an illustrated article entitled "The Tree of Life," we are informed that "science has now discovered in a most unexpected manner both the Tree and the River of Life." The former is the brain and spinal cord of man. " We do not mean that the brain merely looks like a tree or resembles one externally. We are not dealing with analogies. But we do mean that the brain and spinal cord are an actual tree. By the most rigid scientific examination it is shown to fill the ideal type and plan of a tree more completely than any tree of the vegetable kingdom. The spinal cord is the trunk of this great tree. Its roots are the nerves of feeling and motion branching out over the body. . . . The Tree of Life is planted in the midst of many others, for the heart is a tree, the lungs are a tree, and the pancreas, stomach, liver, and all those vital organs. The brain is its radiant and graceful foliage. The mental faculties are classified in twelve groups by the most recent scientific analysis. This Tree bears twelve kinds of fruit. . . . On each side of the Tree of Life is the great River of Life. Let us lay a man down with his head to the north, and his arms stretched to the west and to the east. The River of Life has its four heads in the four chambers of the heart, the two auricles and the two ventricles. The branches of this river pass upward to the head, 'the land of gold,'

eastward to the left and westward to the right arm and lung. But greatest of all the branches, 'The River, or Phrath,' are the aorta and vena cava, reaching southward to the trunk and lower limbs. In branching over the body this river divides into four parts at seventeen different points. Two branches of the river form a network around the very trunk of the tree, and spread upward among its expanding branches. The blood is the ' Water of Life,' and it looks 'as clear as crystal' when seen through the microscope, the eye of science. It is three fourths water, and through this are diffused the red cells and the living materials which are to construct and to maintain the bodily organs." Had this article and its antique-looking illustration been found in one of the Church fathers, it would have afforded to a certain class of " scientists " great edification.

CHAPTER VII.

THE EXUBERANCE OF LIFE.

And the Lord God planted a garden. And out of the ground made the Lord God to grow every tree that is pleasant to the sight and good for food. — The Book of Genesis.

Moreover, there were a great number of elephants in the island; and there was provision for animals of every kind. Also whatever fragrant things there are in the earth, whether roots, or herbage, or woods, or distilling drops of flowers or fruits, grew and thrived in that land. — The Critias of Plato.

Wie verkehrt man überhaupt geht, wenn man lediglich aus dem Kreise unsrer jetzigen Erfahrung die Urwelt construiren will, haben uns die paläontologischen Entdeckungen der neuern Zeit gelehrt, die eben in der Urwelt uns die riesenhaftesten und wunderbarsten Thiergestalten vorführen. — Dr. H. Lüken.

According to all ancient traditions and beliefs, the cradle of the human race was in a portion of the world characterized by an altogether extraordinary exuberance of life. Of all lands the sun shone upon it was the fairest and best. Even down to the Deluge, and later, something of the divine goodness of that primeval home-land remained. In the eyes of Plato, the steady deterioration has been going on from the beginning, the good soil washing down from the heavenly mountains of the earth's summit and disappearing in the abyss, until, "in comparison with what then was, there are remaining only the bones of the wasted body, as they may be called, — all the richer and softer parts of the soil having fallen away, and the mere skeleton of the land being left." [1]

[1] *Critias*, III.

The deterioration of the climate of the mother-region of the race is particularly described in the first Fargard of the Avesta : " The first of the good lands and countries which I, Ahura Mazda, created was the Airyana Vaêjô [Aîran Vêj, " Iran the Ancient "] by the good river Dâitya. Thereupon came Angra Mainyu [Ahriman], who is all death, and he counter-created by his witchcraft the serpent in the river, and winter, a work of the daêvas. There are [now] ten winter months there, two summer months, and these are cold for the waters, cold for the earth, and cold for the trees." [1] So in Fargard second we have a legendary account of the successive migrations of the earliest remembered men out of the original North country " *southwards,* to meet the sun," and nearly all commentators ascribe these repeated "southward" movements to the gradual refrigeration and glaciation of the primitive home in " Iran the Ancient." [2]

The same idea of a perfect primeval climate is found among all ancient peoples. Ovid represents

[1] Darmesteter, i., p. 8. Haug, p. 227. It will be observed that the winter and summer here described are the exact counterpart or "counter-creation" of the original polar day (the growing season) of ten months, and the original polar night (or winter of rest from growth) of two months. This is another incidental evidence that " Iran the Ancient " was situate at the Pole.

[2] " Or l'avènement de la période glaciaire pourrait seule expliquer un tel fait, car on ne connaît aucune autre cause capable de rendre inhabitable, à cause de froid, une contrée qui est representée comme ayant été à l'origine un pays d'excellente nature. On serait donc obligée d'en inférer que les Éraniens avestiques avaient conservé, non seulement le souvenir de la période glaciaire, mais aussi celui des beaux jours qui l'ont précédée, et c'est ce qu'en général on n'admittra pas facilement. L'âge d'or primitif n'est pas un souvenir traditionnel des temps préglaciaires," etc. Piétrement, *Les Aryas et leur Première Patrie.* Paris, 1879 : p. 15. How near the truth !

the spring, in Saturn's reign, to have been perennial. The spring of our world-age is only an ab-
breviated reminder of that great original.[1] So Lac-
tantius has preserved a fragment of the old ethnic
creed when he tells us that only upon the loss of
Paradise, darkness and winter came over the earth.[2]

With this supposed deterioration of soil and climate the deterioration of man kept pace. Hence
ancient writers, with hardly an exception, represent
the men of their own day as far inferior in stature,
in strength, and in longevity to the first progenitors
of the race. Hesiod, Aratus, Ovid, Vergil, and Clau-
dian vary somewhat in their accounts of the Golden,
Silver, and later ages of human history, but all
agree in representing the men of their time as weak
and puny and short-lived, compared with men of the
early ages of the world. Juvenal, in a well-known
passage, alludes to Homer's judgment, and expresses
his own : —

> " Nam genus hoc vivo jam decrescebat Homero,
>   Terra malos homines nunc educat atque pusillos." [3]

Plato, speaking of the antediluvians, says, " For
many generations, as long as the divine nature lasted
in them, they were obedient to the laws, and well
affectioned toward the gods who were their kins-
men ; for they possessed true and in every way great
spirits, practicing gentleness and wisdom in the
various chances of life and in their intercourse with
one another. . . . By such reflections, and by the
continuance in them of the divine nature, all that

---

[1] *Metamorphoses*, i. 113.

[2] *Placidus*, 4.

[3] *Satires*, xv. 69, 70. Compare Homer, *Iliad*, v. 302 *et seq.* ; Vergil, *Æneid*, xii. 900 ; Lucret., ii. 1151.

we have described waxed and increased in them ; but when this divine portion began to fade away in them, and became diluted too often, and with too much of the mortal admixture, and the human nature got the upper hand, they, being unable to bear their fortune, became unseemly, and to him who had an eye to see they began to appear base, and had lost the fairest of their precious gifts." [1]

The ancient Indian conception of the world's decadence from period to period is given in the " Laws of Manu." [2] Of the four great ages of the life of the present universe, we are living in the last and worst. In the first *yuga* all men were holy ; in the present all are utterly corrupt and vile. In the first they were tall and long-lived ; in each succeeding age they have grown dwarfed and feeble.

Similar to the Indian was the Iranian belief as reflected in the Bundahish. Here the duration of the universe is represented as filling four world-periods of three thousand years each. During the first of the four all is pure and sinless, but at its close the Evil One declares war against Ahura Mazda, the holy God, which war is destined to fill the three last ages. During the first of the three, the Evil One is unsuccessful; during the second, good and evil are exactly balanced ; while in the last, which is our own, evil obtains, and till the destined overthrow at the very end maintains supremacy. [3]

The conception which we are noticing is as old as it is universal. Berosus, reporting the earliest tra-

[1] *Critias,* 120.
[2] *Laws of Manu,* I. 68–86.
[3] *The Bundahish,* chapters i., xxxi., xxxiv.

ditions of Chaldæa, represents the first men as of
extraordinary stature and strength, and as retaining
in lessening degree these characteristics until some
generations after the Flood.[1] "Among the Egyptians," says Lenormant, "the terrestrial reign of the
god Râ, who inaugurated the existence of the world
and of human life, was a Golden Age, to which they
continually looked back with regret and envy: to
assert the superiority of anything above all that imagination could set forth, it was sufficient to affirm
that 'its like had never been seen since the days of
the god Râ.' The same idea is found again in the
Egyptian account of the succession of the terrestrial reigns of the gods, the demi-gods, heroes, and
men, as collected from the fragments of Manetho,
and corroborated by the testimony of native texts."[2]
In China, too, the catholic ethnic faith in a primeval
Golden Age was not lacking, so that everywhere
the eldest traditions — be they Shemitic, Aryan, or
Turanian — support, confirm, and illustrate the representations of the Bible touching the extraordinary
pristine vitality of Edenic nature and of antediluvian man. So overwhelming is the evidence that
this universal belief of antiquity is a reminiscence of
primitive reality, that one who expressly disclaims a
personal belief in the superior stature of the early
men nevertheless asserts that "the universality of
the popular belief attests its very ancient origin,"
and adds that "it may unhesitatingly be ranked
among those originating at a time when the great
civilized peoples of a remote antiquity, still cluster-

[1] *Fragments Cosmogoniques de Bérose.* Ed. Lenormant. Frag. 17.
[2] *Beginnings of History,* pp. 67, 73, note. See the entire chapter
and the authorities there quoted. Also chapters vi. and vii., particularly pp. 351 *et seq.*

ing about the cradle of the race, enjoyed a contact sufficiently close for some common traditions." [1]

The bearing of this unanimous verdict of ancient tradition upon the problem of the location of Eden is obvious. The traditions of the whole ethnic world, not less than the record in Genesis, require that the cradle of the race be placed in the one spot on earth where the biological conditions are the most favorable possible. According to all procurable data, that spot at the era of man's appearance upon the stage was in the now lost " Miocene continent," which then surrounded the Arctic Pole. That in that true, original Eden some of the early generations of men attained to a stature and longevity unequaled in any countries known to postdiluvian history is by no means scientifically incredible. On the contrary, the exceptional biological conditions of that land and the remarkable consensus of all tradition respecting the vigor of early giant races combine to form a fresh illustration of the principle that the more incredible things an hypothesis explains, the more irresistibly credible the hypothesis itself becomes.

[1] Lenormant, *Beginnings of History*, p. 354. The author continues, "To-day we have scientific proof that such belief [in the extraordinary stature of the early men] has no real foundation, but is simply a product of the imagination." But his alleged scientific proof is purely negative, consisting of the fact that the human skeletons which paleontologists have so far found — *none of which are from the high North* — are only of ordinary size. "As far back as we can trace the vestiges of mankind, up to the races who lived in the Quaternary period side by side with the great mammifers of extinct species, it may be proved that the medium height of our species has never exceeded its existent limits." If other early species of mammifers were gigantic in comparison with their nearest living representatives of to-day, why may not the mammifer man have illustrated the same law ?

Back in that far-off foretime, even in the lower latitudes, life was remarkably luxuriant. The paleontologists almost exhaust the resources of language in the effort to describe it. Thus, on a single page, Professor Alleyne Nicholson, of St. Andrew's University, says: "The life of the Miocene period is *extremely abundant*, also *extremely varied* in its character. . . . The marine beds have yielded *numerous* remains of both vertebrate and invertebrate sea-animals, . . . *an enormous number* of plants. . . . The remains of air-breathing animals are also *abundantly* found. . . . The plants of the Miocene period are *extraordinarily numerous*. . . . The plant-remains . . . indicate an *extraordinarily rank and luxuriant* vegetation," etc.[1] Figuier gives the following illustration : "The Lycopods of our age are humble plants, scarcely a yard in height and most commonly creepers ; but those of the ancient world were trees of eighty or ninety feet in height."[2] But we have before seen that the mother-region of all these abounding and varied floral and faunal types was within the Arctic Circle, and from their amazing exuberance in low latitudes we may form some conception of the yet superior potencies of life which were at work in that more highly favored circumpolar seed-plot of the whole earth.

In our last chapter it was suggested that the Tree in the midst of Paradise may have been as lofty as one of the giant Sequoias of California. The comparison was not made at random. In the Miocene remains in Britain, conifers are especially numerous. And "the most abundant of these is a *gigantic* pine,

---

[1] *Ancient Life-History of the Earth.* New York ed., 1878 : p. 308.
[2] *The World before the Deluge*, p. 134.

the *Sequoia Couttsiæ*, which is very nearly allied to
the huge *Sequoia gigantea* of California. A nearly
allied form, *Sequoia Langsdorfii*, has been detected
in the Hebrides." [1] From the latitude of the Sequoia grove in Mariposa County, California, to that
of the Hebrides is a long stride toward the Pole;
but we are not left to mere inference when we raise
the question whether the original starting-point of
this gigantic tree-species may not have been still
higher in the Arctic regions. The Miocene fossils
of the highest attainable Arctic latitudes tell their
own story. Limited as have been the explorations
among these fossils, as Sir Charles Lyell remarks,
"more than *thirty species* of Coniferæ have been
found, *including several Sequoias allied to the gigantic Wellingtonia* of California. . . . There are also
beeches, oaks, planes, poplars, walnuts, limes, and
even a magnolia, two cones of which have lately
been obtained, proving that this splendid evergreen
not only lived, but ripened its fruit, within the Arctic Circle. Many of the limes, planes, and oaks
were large-leaved species, and both flowers and
fruits, besides immense quantities of leaves, are in
many cases preserved. . . . Even in Spitzbergen,
within 12° of the Pole, no less than *ninety-five* species of fossil plants have been obtained." The vigor
of the vegetable life of the Miocene age in these
Arctic regions impresses the veteran geologist as
"truly remarkable."

We have a right, then, not only to draw a conclusion from the "abundant" and "extraordinarily rank
and luxuriant vegetation" of the Arctic regions in
Miocene time, but also to learn a special lesson from

[1] Nicholson, *Life-History*, p. 309.

the gigantic forms which linger on our Western coast. Had the book of Genesis described one of the trees of Eden as three hundred and twenty feet in height and thirty feet in diameter at the base, not only all the Voltaires of modern history, but also — until the discovery of California — all naturalists of the advanced anti-Christian variety, would have made no end of sport over the unscientific or mythical " Botany of Moses." But the *Sequoia gigantea* is a living, indisputable fact. Though not the oldest of the Coniferæ, it illustrates some of the earlier possibilities of vegetable life. It tells the botanist that growths once realized in great abundance are dying out, and unless perpetuated by human care are soon to disappear from our globe forever. Its last surviving representatives in the state of nature, preserved to our day by certain fortunate local conditions and by their own inherent longevity, are witnesses respecting a far-off world, — witnesses whose testimony the most incredulous must accept. They tell of the far-away dawn of the day of man, they bear testimony to the extraordinary life which characterized their distant birth-land.[1] And if these last *individuals* of an expiring race can maintain, under unfavorable biological conditions, a vigorous life *through two millenniums of time*, who shall declare it impossible that

---

[1] During the Tertiary period the Sequoias *"occurred all around the Arctic zone"* (Asa Gray). Professor J. D. Whitney finds evidence that one of the fallen trees in Placer County was over 2000 years of age. See his *Yosemite Book;* also Engler, *Entwickelungsgeschichte der Pflanzenwelt.* Leipsic, 1879–82: chap. i. and ii. It is also noteworthy that the Australian *Eucalyptus gigantea*, the only tree which surpasses the Sequoia in height, is found precisely in that country whose belated living flora and fauna are more closely related to the northern types of the early world than are any other.

the men of the time and place of the origination of the *Sequoia gigantea* should have averaged more than six feet in stature, or attained to an age quite surpassing our threescore years and ten? As to the latter point, it would require more than the combined lives of two Methuselahs to watch the growth and death of a single tree like those of California. The thought is not the incubation of the present writer; it is what the trees themselves said to the foremost botanist of America.[1]

But the exuberance of animal life in the Miocene period is not less remarkable. We quote the same author as before: "The Invertebrate animals of this period are *very numerous.* . . . The little shells of the Foraminifera are *extremely abundant.* . . . Corals are *very abundant,* in many instances forming regular reefs. . . . *Numerous* crabs and lobsters represent the Crustacea. . . . Of Insects *more than thirteen hundred species* have been determined by Dr. Heer from the Miocene strata of Switzerland alone. . . . The Mollusca are *very numerous.* . . . Polyzoans

---

[1] "We cannot gaze high up the huge and venerable trunks, which one crosses the continent to behold, without wishing that these patriarchs of the grove were able, like the long-lived antediluvians of Scripture, to hand down to us through a few generations the traditions of centuries, and so tell us somewhat of the history of their race. Fifteen hundred annual layers have been counted or satisfactorily made out upon one or two fallen trunks. It is probable that close to the heart of some of the living trees may be found the circle that records the year of the Saviour's nativity. A few generations of such trees might carry the history a long way back. But the ground they stand on and the marks of very recent geologic change and vicissitude in the region around testify that not very many such generations can have flourished just here, at least in unbroken series." — Professor Asa Gray, LL. D., "The Sequoia and its History." *Proceedings of the American Association for the Advancement of Science,* 1872, p. 6.

are *abundant*. Bivalves and Univalves are *extremely plentiful*. . . . The Fishes of the period are *very abundant*. . . . The remains of Reptiles are *far from uncommon*. . . . The Land-tortoises make their first appearance during this period. The most remarkable form of this group is the *huge Colossochelys Atlas* of the Upper Miocene deposits of the Siwâlik Hills in India, described by Dr. Falconer and Sir Proby Cautley. *Far exceeding any living tortoise in its dimensions*, this *enormous* animal is estimated as having had a length of about twenty feet, measured from the tip of the snout to the extremity of the tail, and to have stood upwards of seven feet. . . . The accomplished paleontologists just quoted show further that some of the traditions of the Hindus would render it not improbable that this *colossal* Tortoise survived into the earlier portion of the human period. . . . The Mammals of the Miocene are *very numerous*. . . . The *Edentates* (Sloths, etc.) are represented by two *large* European forms. One of these is the *large Macrotherium giganteum*. . . . The other is the *still more gigantic Ancylotherium Pentelici*, which seems to have been *as large as, or larger than, the rhinoceros*. . . . We may also note here the first appearance of true 'whalebone *Whales*,' two species of which, resembling the living 'Right Whale' of the Arctic seas, and belonging to the same genus, have been detected in the Miocene beds of North America. . . . The great order of the Ungulates, or hoofed quadrupeds, is *very largely developed* in strata of the Miocene age, various new types making their appearance here for the first time. . . . We meet for the first time with representatives of the family *Rhinoceridæ*, comprising the only existing rhi-

noceroses. . . . The family of the Tapirs is represented, . . . some of which were quite diminutive in
point of size, whilst others attained *the dimensions
of a horse.*   Nearly allied to this family, also, is the
singular group of quadrupeds which Marsh had described under the name of *Brontotheridæ.*   These
extraordinary animals, typified by *Brontotherium*
itself, agree with . . . and differ from the existing Tapirs. . . . *Brontotherium gigas* is said to be nearly
as large as an elephant, whilst *Brontotherium ingens*
appears to have attained *dimensions still more gigantic.*   The well-known genus *Titanotherium* would
also appear to belong to this group. . . . The family
of the Horses appears under various forms in the
Miocene, but the most important and best known of
these is the Hipparion. . . . Remains of the Hipparion have been found in various regions in Europe
and in India; and from the *immense quantities of
their bones* found in certain localities, it may be safely
inferred that these Middle Tertiary ancestors of the
Horse lived, like their modern representatives, in
great herds. . . . Amongst the even-toed Ungulates
we for the first time meet with examples of the *Hip-
popotamus,* with its four-toed feet, its massive body,
and huge tusk-like lower teeth. . . . The true Deer,
with their solid bony antlers, appear for the first time
here. . . . Perhaps the most remarkable of these
Miocene Ruminants is the *Sivatherium giganteum*
of the Siwâlik Hills in India.   In this extraordinary
animal there were two pairs of horns. . . . If all
these horns had been simple, there would have been
no difficulty in considering Sivatherium as simply a
gigantic four-horned Antelope. . . . It is to the Miocene period that we must refer the first appearance

of the important order of the *Elephants* and their allies (*Proboscidians*). . . . Only three generic groups of this order are known, namely, the extinct *Deinotherium*, the equally extinct Mastodons, and the Elephants ; and all these three types are known to have been in existence as early as the Miocene period, the first of them being exclusively confined to deposits of this age. . . . The most celebrated skull of the Deinothere is the one which was exhumed from the Upper Miocene deposits of Epplesheim, in Hesse-Darmstadt, in the year 1836. This skull was four and a half feet in length, and indicated an animal *larger than any existing species of the Elephant.* . . . Whilst herbivorous quadrupeds, as we have seen, were *extremely abundant* during Miocene times, and often attained *gigantic dimensions*, beasts of prey (*Carnivora*) were *by no means wanting;* most of the existing families of the order being represented. . . . Weasels and Otters were not unknown, . . . whilst the great Cats of subsequent periods are more than adequately represented by the *huge* 'sabre-toothed' Tiger. . . . Amongst the *Rodent* Mammals . . . *all the principal living groups* were differentiated in Middle Tertiary times. . . . Lastly, the Monkeys existed during the Miocene period *under a variety of forms.* . . . The *Dryopithecus* is referable to the group of 'Anthropoid Apes.' . . . *Dryopithecus* was also *of large size, equaling Man in stature*, and apparently living amongst the trees and feeding upon fruits." [1]

It would be easy to heighten the impression of this vigor and luxuriance of animal life in Tertiary and Post-tertiary times by studying the huge bird-

[1] Nicholson, *Life-History*, pp. 311 *et seq.*

tracks of the Connecticut sandstone, or the enormous skeletons of the *Dinornis giganteus* and the
Dinornis elephantopus, or the eggs of the *Æpiornis
maximus,* — eggs "measuring from thirteen to fourteen inches in diameter." [1] We might consider the
Diprotodon, which "in size must have many times
exceeded the dimensions of the largest of its living
successors, since the skull measures no less than
three feet in length." [2] Or we might rehabilitate
the "colossal" *Megatherium Cuvieri,* whose "thigh-
bone is nearly thrice the thickness of the same bone
in the largest of existing Elephants." [3] Or, again,
visiting the Jurassic beds of our own Colorado, we
might contemplate the *Titanosaurus,* one of the
latest discovered of the tenants of the early world,
of which Sir John Lubbock says that it " is perhaps
the largest land animal yet known, being *a hundred
feet in length, and at least thirty feet in height,*

---

[1] The fact that fossil remains of these gigantic extinct birds have
been found only in the Southern hemisphere militates in no wise
against the doctrine that the species originated in the highest North.
For (1) birds are the best equipped of all creatures for migration to
the remotest parts of the earth. (2.) The Connecticut Valley sand-
stones, in the Northern hemisphere, preserve the tracks of birds
"which must have been of colossal dimensions," the tracks being 22
inches in length and 12 in breadth, with a proportionate length of
stride. "These measurements indicate a foot four times as large as
that of the African Ostrich." (3.) These tracks were made in the
Triassic period, while the remains found in New Zealand and adjacent
regions belong to the much more recent Post-pliocene period, thus
giving a long lapse of years for the spread or migration of the species
from the latitude of the Connecticut Valley to that of the most Southern lands. Compare Geikie : " The higher fauna of Australia is more
nearly akin to that which flourished in Europe far back in Mesozoic time than to the living fauna of any other region of the globe."
Geology, p. 619.

[2] Nicholson, *Life-History,* p. 349.

[3] Ibid., p. 350.

though it seems possible that even these vast dimensions may have been surpassed by those of the
Atlantosaurus,"[1] also a late discovery. But why
multiply illustrations? Natural history in our times
can produce no species of fishes, or of amphibians,
or of reptiles, or of birds, or — among mammals —
of marsupials, or of edentates, or of ungulates, or
of proboscidians, or of carnivores, or of apes, which
in normal dimensions are not excelled by species of
the corresponding orders and classes belonging to
Tertiary and Quaternary ages. And this being so,
it is surely possible and credible that in the same
antediluvian ages some of the varieties of the species *Bimana* may have exceeded in stature its present average, and enjoyed a corresponding vigor of
constitution. At any rate, it will be soon enough
to deny it after human remains of suitable age shall
have been found in the vicinity of the race's origin
and earlier history. So far as past findings are concerned, even Büchner, who holds that "primitive
man was inferior even in corporeal attributes to the
men of the present day," and that "the widely spread
belief in the former existence of a race of human
giants is perfectly erroneous," still has to say, "It
is true that some very ancient skeletons or parts of
skeletons have been found, which must have belonged to *comparatively large and very muscular
men*, such, for example, as the skeleton of the famous
Neanderthal man, and the human bones recently
found by M. Louis Lartet in one of the caverns of
Perigord, . . . which seem to indicate a rude but
muscular race of men."[2] Again, speaking of the

---

[1] *Nature.* London, 1881 : p. 406.
[2] *Man in the Past, Present, and Future.* Eng. tr. by Dallas, pp.
50, 51.

skeleton to which the Neanderthal skull belongs, he
says, "The ridges and crests especially which served
as points for insertion of the muscles are *very
strongly developed*, so that we may conclude that
their possessor was a *very strong and muscular
man*." [1] It may be added that Carl Vogt, one of the
earliest and most influential of Darwin's German
disciples, also conceived of "the man of the oldest
Stone Age" as "*of large stature, powerful and long-
headed*." [2]

Here it may be well to remark that the primitive
forms of animals, while often so excelling in size
the later forms of their own kind, are by no means
to be thought of as monstrosities. The proportion
of a young child's head to his body is very different
from that of an adult's. In comparison with the
grown man, his limbs and hands and feet are remarkably plump and well rounded. Had a painter
never seen and studied a human being except in the
adult and senescent stage, the infant form would
seem to him singularly abnormal. This illustration
may help to a right judgment of certain early types
of animals. For "if we take the earliest known
and oldest examples of any given group of animals,
it can sometimes be shown that these primitive
forms, *though in themselves highly organized*, possessed certain characters such as are now only seen
in the *young* of their existing representatives. In
technical language, the early forms of life in some
instances possess 'embryonic' characters, though
this does not prevent them often attaining a size
much more gigantic than their nearest living rela-

[1] *Man in the Past, Present, and Future*, p. 53.
[2] Ibid., pp. 60, 259.

tives. Moreover, the ancient forms of life are often
what is called '*comprehensive types;*' that is to say,
they possess characters in combination such as we
nowadays only find separately developed in different
groups of animals. Now this permanent retention
of embryonic characters and this 'comprehensive-
ness' of structural type are signs of what a zoölogist considers to be a comparatively 'low' grade of
organization ; and the prevalence of these features
in the earlier forms of animals is a very striking
phenomenon, *though they are none the less perfectly
organized so far as their own type is concerned.*" [1]
To put the mistake to be guarded against in another
light, it may be said that whoever considers the departures of the most ancient forms of animal life
from the allied living forms as abnormal and monstrous in many cases simply takes the types of decadence and senility by which to test and condemn
the plumper and fuller and fairer types of physical
juvenility. In like manner, the "comprehensive"
types can be called monstrous and strange only
as these terms might be applied to the " London
Times " by a man who in all his life had never seen
any other specimen of journalism than " The North
British Wool-Growers' Monthly Bulletin," or "The
Daily Price-Current of the Southampton Associated
Grocers." What the zoölogist calls the "lowest"
forms of organization are rather the *highest*, if by
"highest " we mean those forms which are most in-
clusive, *lebenskräftig*, and susceptible of evolutionary
differentiation.[2] The notion that the faunal world at

---

[1] Nicholson, *Life-History*, pp. 60, 61. Compare pp. 367-374.

[2] "The first appearance of leading types of life are rarely embryonic. On the contrary, they often appear in highly perfect and specialized forms ; often, however, of composite type, and expressing

the time of the advent of man was a world of crudi-
ties and monstrosities — a notion to which books
and magazines of popularized science have given an
almost universal currency — is therefore entirely
false.[1] In the light of profounder science, the fairest Eden of the oldest legend is, so far as primeval
zoloögy is concerned, more credible than when the
study of Paleontology was first begun.

It must not be forgotten that in all that has now
been hinted respecting the fauna of the early world
no account has been taken of more favorable and
less favorable portions of the earth. Paleontologists
are but just beginning to consider that between the
biological conditions of the Arctic regions and those
of every other portion of the globe there must have
been, in Pre-Glacial times, the profoundest and most
far-reaching difference. The growths of a region
whose day was ten months in length, and whose
night was but two, could not fail to be vastly differ-

characters afterwards so separated as to belong to higher groups. . . .
The bald and contemptuous negation of these facts by Haeckel and
other biologists does not tend to give geologists much confidence in
their dicta." — Principal J. W. Dawson, in his " Presidential Address
before the American Association for the Advancement of Science."
Science, Cambridge, Mass., Aug. 17, 1883 : p. 195.

[1] " Dr. Hooker observes, in his recent introductory essay on the
Flora of Australia, that it is impossible to establish a parallel between
the successive appearances of vegetable forms in time and their com-
plexity of structure or specialization of organs as represented by the
successively higher groups in the natural method of classification.
He also adds that the earliest recognizable cryptograms are not only
the highest now existing, but have more highly differentiated vegeta-
tive organs than any subsequently appearing, and that the dicotyledo-
nous embryo and perfect exogenous wood, with the highest specialized tissue known (the coniferous with glandular tissue), preceded
the monocotyledonous embryo and endogenous wood in date of appearance on the globe, — facts wholly opposed to the doctrine of pro-
gression." — Sir Charles Lyell, *The Antiquity of Man*, p. 404.

ent from those of the regions where, on the average, almost twelve hours of every twenty-four are spent in darkness. "Nor can we overlook the fact that the plants and shells of the Arctic region are eminently variable."[1] If, therefore, in low latitudes the forms and powers of animal life were what we have seen, who can undertake to depict its superior exuberance and variety of manifestation in that primitive polar focus from which all faunal types proceeded![2]

The Arctic rocks tell of a more wonderful lost Atlantis than Plato's. The fossil ivory beds of Siberia excel everything of the kind in the world. From the days of Pliny, at least, they have constantly been undergoing exploitation, and still they are the chief headquarters of supply.[3] The remains

---

[1] Charles Darwin, *Animals and Plants under Domestication.* New York, 1868: ii. 309.

[2] This "eminent" *variableness* of Arctic life has its bearing upon the scientific credibility of prehistoric Arctic giants. At the present day, and in our own latitudes, men occasionally appear whose stature is four or five times the height of the smallest adult dwarfs. Accordingly, if we were to assume two and one half feet as the minimum adult stature in polar regions in primeval times, *the still prevailing* range of variation would give us in those times some men from seven and one half to twelve and one half feet in height. Possibly new fossil evidence on this point is soon to be afforded us. The following is going the rounds of the daily press: " A Carson (Nev.) dispatch says, The footprints which were so much discussed in this country and Europe, and which were originally pronounced by Dr. Harkness, of the Academy of Sciences, to be those of mammoths, are now stated by him, after a year's examination, to be only those of big-footed men." See *Proceedings of the California Academy of Science*, 1882 (Aug. 7 and 27, Sept. 4, Oct. 2). Nadaillac, in *Matériaux pour l'Histoire primitive et naturelle de l'Homme.* Paris, 1882: pp. 313-321. Topinard, in *Revue d'Anthropologie.* Paris, 1883: pp. 309-320. Also Mr. Cope, in *The American Naturalist*, Philadelphia, 1883.

[3] Von Middendorff (*Reise im Norden und Osten Sibiriens*, 1848) reckons the number of the tusks which now annually come into the market as at least a hundred pairs, on which Nordenskjöld remarks:

of the mammoth are so abundant that, as Gratacap says, "the northern islands of Siberia *seem built up of its crowded bones*."[1] Another scientific writer, speaking of the islands of New Siberia, northward of the mouth of the river Lena, uses this language: "Large quantities of ivory are dug out of the ground every year. Indeed, some of the islands are believed *to be nothing but an accumulation of drift-timber and the bodies of mammoths and other antediluvian animals frozen together*."[2] So full of these remains is the soil of these high Arctic regions that the Ostyaks and other ignorant tribes have an idea that the mammoth is an underground animal ploughing his way through the earth like a mole, and that he still lives in his subterranean passages. Nor would there seem to be anything so remarkably novel in the theory we have advocated in this book, according to which the submergence of the primeval home of mankind and the introduction of the great Ice Age are connected with the Deluge: for when, nearly two hundred years ago, the Russian ambassador, Evert Yssbrants Ides, made his bold, three-year overland journey to China, he in the high North found and reported this precise traditionary belief.[3]

"From this we may infer that during the years that have elapsed since the Russian conquest of Siberia, useful tusks from more than 20,000 mammoths have been collected." In a note the same writer expresses the opinion that Von Middendorff's estimate is quite too low, and says that a single steamer on which he sailed up the Yenisej in 1875 was on that single trip taking more than one hundred tusks to market. *The Voyage of the Vega*, p. 305.

[1] "Prehistoric Man in Europe." *The Am. Antiquarian and Oriental Journal.* Chicago, 1881 : p. 284.

[2] *Johnson's Cyclopædia, sub voce.*

[3] "The old Russians living in Siberia were of opinion that the mammoth was an animal of the same kind as the elephant, and that before the Flood Siberia had been warmer than now, and elephants had then

Summing up the present chapter, then, we have only to say that whoever accepts the conclusion to which the preceding lines of argument have conducted us will find no longer a stumbling-block in the latest revelations of Geology touching the extraordinary life-energies of far-off ages, and in the hoary myths which tell of giants and Titans and demigods in Earth's early morning. On the contrary, fossil form and ethnic myth and sacred page will all be found uniting in a common story.

lived in numbers there ; that they had been drowned in the Flood, and afterwards, when the climate became colder, had frozen in the river mud." Nordenskjöld, *Voyage of the Vega*, p. 305.

CHAPTER VIII.

REVIEW OF THE ARGUMENT.

Now if Water be the Best, and Gold be the most precious, so now to the farthest bound doth Theron by his fair deeds attain, and from his own home touch the Pillars of Heracles.[1] Pathless the things beyond, pathless alike to the unwise and the wise. Here will I search no more : the quest were vain. — PINDAR (MYERS).

IN Part Second, at the very beginning of our discussion, attention was called to the two classes of tests which the hypothesis of an Arctic polar site for Eden must of necessity meet : first, the tests which would apply alike to all the ordinarily proposed sites in temperate and inter-tropical latitudes; and second, the tests which would be inseparable from the aspects and adjustments of Nature at the Pole. In the first class seven were enumerated, and at the close of Part Fourth we saw how surprisingly and convincingly all of the seven had been met. In the second class seven others were particularized as " new features " introduced into the problem of the site of Eden by the very nature of our hypothesis. They were all of so peculiar and extraordinary a character, and they so modified the requirements to be made of all corroborative human tradition, that nothing short of the truth of the intrinsically improbable hypothesis could save it

---

[1] " Atlas gave to Heracles the κόσμου κίονας which contained all the secrets of Nature." Rawlinson's *Herodotus*, vol. i., p. 505 n. Compare below, Part VI., ch. ii. Also Jonnès, *L'Océan*, pp. 121, 107, *et passim.*

from obvious and ridiculous failure at each successive point. In the present Part we have now brought
together the facts, or at least a portion of the facts,
which go to demonstrate that the hypothesis of a
Polar Paradise, *and no other*, can meet and satisfy
each one of these new and more difficult requirements. Speaking after the manner of the mathematicians, though of course with due remembrance
of the nature of the reasoning employed, it may be
said that we have first solved our problem, and then,
by a new process and with changed elements, proved
and verified our answer. Whoever would see how
strikingly complete and cogent this verifying process is should turn back to the second chapter of
Part Second and carefully collate the seven " new
features " there enumerated with the facts of the
first seven chapters of the present Part. The result
of such a collation upon any candid mind can hardly
be doubtful.

In the writer's firm-grounded conviction, then,
LOST EDEN IS FOUND. To no one of his readers
can its true site be more surprising than it was at
first to him. Every antecedent probability seemed
in array against it. First of all, in such problems
every new hypothesis is inherently unlikely in direct proportion to the number of hypotheses previously propounded and found wanting. Where
had more been advanced by the learned and ingenious than here? Again, from its nature the hypothesis greatly aggravated the conditions and requirements of the problem itself. And if, during
centuries of discussion, no sublunary site had been
found which could meet the simple conditions of
Genesis, how unlikely that with new and far more

extraordinary conditions added a place could be found corresponding! Again, in order to its verification, the hypothesis required that a wholly new interpretation of mankind's oldest cosmological ideas and traditions should be propounded and verified, — an interpretation unanimously forbidden by the consensus of modern scholarship in almost every department of historical and archæological research. How supremely unlikely that any such undertaking could be crowned with success !

Happily, human events do not fall out according to our short-sighted human likelihoods. Even the thoughtless man sees it, and exclaims, " It is always the impossible that happens ! " The more reverent soul, who discerns in all history a higher than human agency, and in whose eyes Nature itself is supernatural, must least of all be daunted by the unpromising first appearances of any clue to truth. His conceptions of the actual are larger than those of mere believers in nature, and thereto are adjusted his conceptions of the probable. Identifying himself with that personal Power which everywhere makes for truth no less than for righteousness, he is ever expecting the otherwise unexpectable, and for the same reason ever looking upon each new truth attained, not as a personal achievement, but simply as one more proof and precious pledge of pupilhood.

In the progress of the studies here summed up many curious things have come to light, one of which may appropriately be mentioned in this place. Archæologists are well aware that more than one hundred years ago, in his " Lettres sur l'Atlantide de Platon," 1779, and " Lettres sur l'Origine des Sciences," 1777, the learned and ingenious Jean

Sylvain Bailly advocated the view that the primitive cradle of civilization was in Siberia, under the 49th or 50th degree of latitude. In the latter of the works named there occurs a noteworthy passage in which the author, rhetorically fixing the birthplace of mankind at the very Pole, remarks upon the "singular conformity" of such a starting-point, both with all the phenomena of civilization and with the indications of mythology. In the same breath, however, as if startled by his own temerity, he reassures his readers by announcing that his suggestion is "only a philosophic fiction," and that it "lacks the support of history."[1] Is it too much to say that the support of history has now been furnished?[2]

Though our hypothesis needs no further confirmation, it would be perfectly easy to develop a new and striking line of evidence from the light which it throws on the origin of the erroneous preconceptions which in the past have either perpetually suggested false theories, or else occasioned the conviction that the problem was insoluble. Thus, after what we have learned as to the posture of worshipers in all ancient nations, it is easy to under-

---

[1] "Au reste, si j'ai tracé la marche de l'homme né sous le pôle, s'avançant vers l'équateur, inventant toutes les différentes mesures de l'année, par les circonstances physiques des différentes latitudes, ce n'est qu'une fiction philosophique, singulière par sa conformité avec les phénomènes, remarquable par l'explication des fables ; fiction qui surtout n'a rien d'absurde en elle-même, et à laquelle il ne manque que d'être appuyée par l'histoire : " pp. 255, 256.

[2] Since the announcement of his results the writer has received letters from three plain, unschooled Bible-students, who appear to have anticipated, each in his own way, the conclusions of this book. One of them, Mr. Alexander Skelton, a machinist and blacksmith, of Paterson, N. J., obtained a hearing, it seems, in the *New York Tribune,* in 1878, and his argument, though brief, is remarkably comprehensive and cogent.

stand that the primitive Garden "in the Front-country" must have been in the North. But since in the Post-Glacial ages this Front-country was naturally associated with the East, and all investigators, Jewish, Christian, and Mohammedan, were trying to find some Oriental region of Paradisaic climate, with a central Tree and a quadrifurcate River by which the primitive Gan-Eden might be identified, we have in this preliminary misconception reason enough for their failure age after age.

Again, in reviewing the results of the theologians, we saw that not a few of the more modern had, like Luther, been repelled and disgusted by the apparently senseless and contradictory representations of the earlier fathers and church-teachers, in some of which Paradise was placed in heaven, and yet apparently on earth, and anon perhaps midway between heaven and earth; as high, in fact, as the moon. In view of such representations we cannot be surprised that a keen-witted satirist like Samuel Butler, in enumerating the rare accomplishments of Hudibras, should have said, —

> " He knew the seat of Paradise,
>   Could tell in what degree it lies ;
>   And, as he was disposed, could prove it
>   Below the moon, or else above it."

Our study of the prehistoric Paradise-mountain, standing upon the earth at the Arctic Pole and lifting its head "to the orbit of the moon," brings instant light into all this confusion. The mountain *is* at once in heaven and on earth. And it is interesting to note that late mediæval theologians, despite their meagre opportunities for historical research, traced this conception to just that apostle who, according to ecclesiastical tradition, as special "Apostle of India," had best opportunity to learn of the East-Aryan Meru, and to report this peculiar and venerable tradition of Paradise.[1] Moreover, as we have seen, there were in several Asiatic religions two Paradises, a celestial and a terrestrial, connected by a pillar, or bridge, up and down which holy souls could pass. When, therefore, an ancient writer is found alluding in one place to Paradise as on earth and in another to Paradise as in heaven, the confusion is not in his own mind, but merely in that of his reader.

Here, too, a good word can be put in for poor Cosmas Indicopleustes, — the man who has had the honor of being more ignorantly and contemptuously abused by modern scientists than any other cosmographer of early Christian ages. Doubtless it is easy to ridicule his rude representation of the universe, but who will assure us that, thirteen or fourteen centuries hence, it may not be equally easy to ridicule the speculations of Herschel as to the form of the Cosmic Whole? However this may be, the foregoing chapters have given a new significance to the thought of the monk "who sailed to India," showing us that his "Mountain" to the North of the known countries of his day was none other than Mount Meru, the legendary heaven-supporting culmination of the Northern hemisphere. His location of Eden, so far as the verdict of science is yet rendered, is at least as well supported as Häckel's

---

[1] "I have found it in some most ancient books that Thomas, the Apostle, was the author of the opinion . . . that Paradise was so high as to reach to the lunar circle." — Albertus Magnus, *Summa Theologiæ,* Pars II., Tract. xiii., qu. 79.

in lost "Lemuria," or Unger's in a mid-Atlantic "Atlantis." Most remarkable of all, just NORTH *of the Arctic Ocean boundary of Europe* — not in the *West*, as sometimes falsely represented [1] — he locates "*the land where men dwelt before the Flood.*" [2] If our conclusions are correct, Cosmas was the earliest known geographer who gave to the Christian world a true account of the original seat of the post-Edenic antediluvian world. Thus those who have so long made him their pet illustration of the ignorance and unscientific spirit of " Christian" teaching may yet see occasion to revise their judgment, and to transform a portion of their ridicule into praise.

The same principles which explain the strange world of Cosmas explain also the strange conception of the Earth which we found in the letters of Columbus. According to this latter, it will be remembered, the historic hemisphere was true to the spherical figure, but the hemisphere of his far West explorations rose to a lofty eminence at the equator, in what he supposed to be Asia, but which afterwards proved to be the northern part of South America. This gave to the Earth the figure shown in the adjoining cut, — a figure which he compared to that of a nearly round pear.[3] At first view this con-

---

[1] E. g., by Donnelly, *Atlantis*, p. 96.

[2] " Terra ultra Oceanum ubi ante Diluvium habitabant homines." Cosmas Indicopleustes. *De Mundo*, lib. iv. Montfaucon, *Collectio Nova*, tom ii., Tabula i., opp. p. 188.

[3] " It is probable that this idea really dates from the seventh century. We may read in several cosmographical manuscripts of that epoch that the earth has the form of a cone or a top, its surface rising from south to north. These ideas were considerably spread by the compilations of John of Beauvais in 1479, from whom, probably, Columbus derived his notion." Flammarion, *Astronomical Myths*,

ception seems altogether arbitrary, and even whimsical; but if we go back a century or two to Dante's Earth, we find a globe still more eccentric, one on which the Paradise - mount has slipped down full 30° below the equator, as shown in

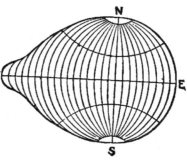

The Earth of Columbus.

the following figure. A fundamental datum for its construction is found in the description of the

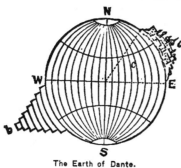

The Earth of Dante.

a. City of Jerusalem. *b.* Mountain of Purgatory. *c.* Inferno within the Earth.

Mountain of Purgatory, respecting whose location it is said, " Zion stands with this Mountain in such wise on the earth that both have a single horizon and diverse hemispheres." [1] A commentator on this says, "When the Divina Commedia was written, Jerusalem was believed to be the exact

p. 296. See also G. Marinelli, *La Geografia e i Patri della Chiesa.* Roma, 1882.

[1] Come ciò sia, se il vuoi poter pensare,
    Dentro raccolto immagina Siòn
    Con questo monte in su la terra stare,
    Sì che ambo e due hanno un solo orizzon,
    E diversi emìsperi.
                  (*Purgatorio*, Canto iv., 67–70.)

centre of the habitable hemisphere; the other was conceived to be covered with water. Out of this ocean the mountain of the poet's Purgatory rises up, like the Peak of Teneriffe, from the bosom of the waves, and is exactly opposite to Mount Zion, so that the two become the antipodes of each other. The mathematicians in their measurement of Dante's Hell proceeded in this wise: An arc of thirty degrees was measured from the meridian of Jerusalem westward as far as Cuma, near Naples, and here, at the '*Fauces Averni*' of Vergil, it pleased them to locate its dreary entrance. Another arc of thirty degrees was next measured from the same meridian eastward, so that both together made up a portion of the earth's circumference of about 4330 English miles, the chord of which would be equal to its semi-diameter. This was made the base of their operations, so that with the world's centre for its apex . . . the Inferno became as broad as it was deep. At this centre of gravity, firmly wedged in everlasting ice, the grim monarch of these dolorous realms is placed." [1]

A more recent editor remarks, "Dante's Purgatory is figured as an island mountain whose summit just reaches to the first of the celestial spheres, that of the Moon. . . . It is exactly at the antipodes of Jerusalem, and its bulk is precisely equal and opposite to the cavity of Hell. . . . On the summit of the mountain is the Earthly Paradise, formerly the Garden of Eden." [2]

---

[1] Henry Clark Barlow, *Contributions to the Study of the Divina Commedia.* London, 1864: pp. 169, 170.

[2] A. J. Butler, *The Purgatory of Dante.* London, 1880: Prefatory Note. Compare Witte's genial lecture on "Dante's Weltgebände," in his *Dante-Forschungen,* Bd. i., pp. 161–182.

Upon the correctness of "the mathematicians" above mentioned, the present writer is not prepared to pass judgment,[1] but no careful reader of the Divine Comedy can fail to see that its "Mount Zion" and the Purgatorial "*Montagna malagevole, altissima et cinta de mare*," are simply unrecognized "survivals" of prehistoric thought, — antipodal world-mountains once situate at the poles, but here relocated to suit the demands of sacred mediæval cosmology. They are the Su-Meru and Ku-Meru of India figuring in Christian poetry. In Lord Vernon's illustration of this curious cosmos, a Hindu pundit would almost certainly think he had a Puranic *mappe-monde*.[2] That after the Paradise-mount has thus declined, first to the latitude of Central Asia, then to the equator, and finally to the pendant position in which Lord Vernon places it, directly under the City of God, with a hypogene central Inferno between, — that after such translocations it should so long have eluded the recognition of all Paradise-seekers is surely little wonder.[3]

[1] Dante's instructor in the natural sciences was Brunetto Latini, who was born A. D. 1230 and died 1294. He is paid an affectionate tribute in the *Inferno*, xv. 85. He wrote a work of which *Li Livres dou Tresor*, Paris, 1863, is an Old-French edition. In it (lib. i., part iii., c. v.) the author ably advocates the doctrine of the spherical figure of the earth. Dante's references to the author and to his work have been carefully collected and presented in a learned paper in the *Jahrbuch der Deutschen Dante-Gesellschaft*, Bd. iv., pp. 1–23.

[2] See the "Figura universale della Divina Commedia," p. xxx. of vol. i. of *L'Inferno di Dante Alighieri da G. G. Warren Lord Vernon.* London, 1858.

[3] Flammarion's picture (*Myths of Astronomy*, p. 311) corresponds quite closely to Lord Vernon's, only the exactly *south polar* position of the mountain is made, if possible, more unequivocal by inserting the words "Southern Hemisphere," and making the pendant mount

Our Arctic Eden, therefore, by explaining the origin of the cosmological conceptions of ancient Chaldæa and Egypt and India, explains at the same time the origin of the most eccentric and apparently senseless conceptions of mediæval and modern cosmographers, and presents what may properly enough be called the philosophy of the errors and misconceptions and fancies of previous searchers after Paradise. It is much that an hypothesis meets all the requirements of a given problem ; it is more that it does this better than any other hypothesis ; it would seem to be past all question when it so illuminates and enriches the very data of the problem that every previous solution falls away of itself, the philosophy of its origin and of its inadequacy being patent and unquestionable.

its precise culmination point beneath. See, further, S. Günther on "Die Kosmologische Anschauungen des Mittelalters," in *Die Rundschau für Geographie und Statistik*, Bd. iv.

PART SIXTH.

THE SIGNIFICANCE OF OUR RESULTS.

But as when one lights a candle to look for one or two things which they want, the light will not confine itself to those two objects, so methinks, in seeking after these two, the Universal Deluge and Paradise, and in retrieving the notion and doctrine of the Primeval Earth upon which they depended, we have cast a light upon all Antiquity. — THOMAS BURNET.

I have laid it down as an invariable maxim constantly to follow historical tradition, and to hold fast by that clue even when many things appear strange and almost inexplicable, or at least enigmatical; for in the investigation of ancient history, the moment we let slip that thread of Ariadne, we can find no outlet from the labyrinth of fanciful theories and the chaos of clashing opinions. — F. VON SCHLEGEL, *Philosophy of History.*

Le mythe du jardin d'Éden n'est point une fiction; il nous donne, sous une forme d'enfantine poésie, la première page de l'histoire morale de humanité, de cette histoire qui a pour documents non plus simplement quelques silex plus ou moins taillés, mais toute cette survivance d'une vie divine dans l'âme humaine, manifestée par ses aspirations et ses douleurs, et par cet universal sentiment de la déchéance, qui palpite dans toutes les mythologies et est l'inspiration dominente de toutes les religions. — E. DE PRESSENSÉ.

Der Tempel des Heidenthums ist ein uralter Bau, aber ein Bau der nicht aus dem Heidenthum stammt und nicht von den Heiden selbst errichtet ist. Die Mythen-Inschriften und heiligen Legenden dieses Tempels enthalten ursprünglich die Urgeschichte der Welt und des Menschengeschlechtes, und die Verheissungen welche demselben im Anfange geworden sind. — LÜKEN.

CHAPTER I.

THE BEARING OF OUR RESULTS ON THE STUDY OF BIOLOGY AND TERRESTRIAL PHYSICS.

How seemed this globe of ours when thou didst scan it !
When in thy lusty youth there sprang to birth
All that hath life, unnurtured, and the planet
Was Paradise, the true Saturnian Earth !
Far toward the Poles was stretched the Happy Garden,
Earth kept it fair by warmth from her own breast ;
Toil had not come to dwarf her sons and harden ;
No crime (there was no want !) perturbed their rest.
        EDMUND C. STEDMAN, The Skull in the Gold Drift.

The solution of the problem of Life may come from an unexpected quarter.—
JOHN FISKE.

IF the alleged facts and the conclusions of the foregoing chapters shall be accepted as correct, it is plain that in finding the true answer to one of the longest standing and most baffling of the problems of Biblical theology we have at the same time found one of those central key-truths, acquaintance with which affects a great many other kinds of knowledge. Indeed, it is not too much to say that the acceptance of this alleged truth upon its appropriate evidences, must affect men's estimate of the *sources* of knowledge. For if the sacred traditions of mankind, when once rightly interpreted, are discovered to be in astonishing harmony with each other, and to yield results which our most advanced sciences, working in the most varied fields of research, singularly conspire to verify, this discovery cannot fail to give new significance to history in all its departments and in all its teachings. But apart from this general effect of a verification of ancient testimony, our precise conclusion as to the location of the cradle of the human race has a most evident and important connection with all physical, paleontological, archæological, philological, mythological, ethnological, and "culture-historical" speculation, — in a word, a most evident and important connection with about every problem which in a marked degree attracts and occupies our modern thought.[1] In the present Part it is proposed to notice the relation of our facts and conclusions to a few of these fields of study, and first of all, in the present chapter, their bearing upon the study of biology and terrestrial physics.

In Part Third and in the seventh chapter of Part Fifth and elsewhere, we have already had various illustrations of the fascinating and authenticating light which the biological sciences can throw upon the study of prehistoric traditions. Possibly the reader, if devoted to this kind of study, has wondered why a field of illustration so rich has not oftener been utilized by writers upon antiquity. But however important this bearing of biological upon prehistoric studies may be, it should not be forgotten that the counterpart bearing of the study

---

[1] Even psychological research may be found to have a profound interest in our result : " Here the question arises how far it [the juggler's mind-power over matter] may be affected by, or dependent upon, electrical and magnetic phenomena and surroundings and climatic influences, since it flourishes at its best, both in the Old World and in the New, as one approaches the regions of the Arctic Circle, and enters the lands of the aurora and midnight sun." G. Archie Stockwell, M. D., "Indian Jugglery and Psychology," in *The Independent*, New York, Sept. 27, 1883, p. 1221.

of the earliest traceable thoughts and beliefs of mankind upon biology and upon the most fruitful study of biology is not a whit less important. This is a point of utmost moment to the fields of knowledge concerned and also to the general theory of personal and organized culture ; yet it is a point most infrequently brought under the consideration of thoughtful readers.

It is an unfortunate and ominous fact that the average biologist of the present day sees nothing worthy of his professional attention back of the present century. The intellectual history of the human race has not the slightest interest for him or value for his work. Ages on ages of human observation and thought and speculation touching the problems of life are to him as if they had never been. If he acquaints himself with them in the slightest degree, it is usually only for the sake of amusing his hearers with what he considers the grotesque and absurd ideas of former times, and impressing them with the contrast which latter-day " science " presents. For all that his race has done until just before his own immediate teachers began, he has little more than pity and contempt.

Now, in any department of human learning, such an attitude of mind is certainly to be deplored. Its effects are detrimental in every aspect. In proportion as it prevails among any class of intellectual workers, in just that proportion does that class become isolated from the one collective and historic intellectual life of humanity. In this way the collective intellectual life suffers, and yet more do the isolated workers suffer. Humanity, conscious of an intellectual history, naturally comes to pay little attention to these men who deny it, or take no interest in it.　On the other hand, any class of men who ignore the history of the human mind and begin all true history and all true science with their own achievements, by this very procedure place themselves outside that spiritual fellowship in which all forms and fragments of knowledge find unity and mutual supplementing.　The circle of their intellectual sympathies and tastes is narrowed.　With the loss of broad sympathies and tastes they are in danger of losing even the capacity to discern and appreciate any kind of truth outside the limited range of their own specialized field of professional research. So far has this perilous tendency already gone that it is a difficult thing in any country to find a celebrated biologist whose publicly advocated theory of education for his own field of labor does not quietly ignore, or actively antagonize, the broadening historical and humanistic studies which alone can qualify a man for intelligent sympathy with all good learning.　Unless the tendency can in some way be checked, there is positive danger lest the special cultivators of biology and the natural sciences become as narrow and isolated and influenceless a guild of experts as are the antiquarian-catalogue makers of modern Europe.[1]

[1] A few years ago Mr. John Stuart Mill, in an address before a Scotch university, put forth a defense of the claims of classical studies to a place in the regular university curriculum. For this one crime he was recently editorially assailed and vilified through several columns of an American organ of natural science, and despite the fact that he was notoriously a disbeliever in Revelation, and was a professed admirer of Comte's atheistic evolutional sociology, the dreadful charge is brought forward: "He was in the Golden-Age, Paradise-Lost dispensation of thought, in which the notions of the early perfection of mankind and the superiority of the ancients were

In studies like the one which has thus far engaged us lies the best possible corrective for this one-sidedness. In this field are found stimulation for the student's curiosity, facts for his understanding, arguments for his reason, play for his imagination. And all the time his study of Nature and his study of Man are mutually helpful to each other. He now has Nature and her life before him in *two* forms : first, as she has entombed herself in the great cemetery of the rocks ; and secondly, as she has pictured herself in historic and even prehistoric human thought. If the former gives her with greater tangibility, it is only the tangibility of the mouldering skeleton. It is the latter which shows her alive and filled with all life's meanings. Each is important in its place, both being reciprocally corrective and mutually complementary.

As yet the biologist has not profited by ancient conceptions of Nature as he should have done. How long and slow has been the progress of the botanist up to this latest conception that all the life-forms of the vegetable kingdom proceeded originally from one centre, and that at the Pole ! The ancient Iranian myth of "the tree of all seeds," from which proceeded "the germs of all species of plants" that ever grew, and which, moreover, was located at the

contrasted with the degeneracy of the moderns ; and so completely was his intellect possessed and perverted by this view that he was disabled from appreciating the immense and epoch-making influence of the modern doctrine of evolution." "The Dead-Language Superstition," *Popular Science Monthly*, New York, 1883, p. 703. Such naturalists are too unlettered to know their own party leaders, or to be aware of the fact that it is precisely to biology that Mill pays the splendid tribute of declaring that among all departments of human knowledge it " affords as yet the only example of the true principles of rational classification."

North Pole, ought long ago to have suggested to him the truth as to the genetic unity of the vegetable kingdom and also as to its pristine centre of distribution. The same may be said of the zoölogist and the suggestiveness of the myths of the same people respecting "the primeval ox" and the *Gosh,* "the personification of the animal kingdom." [1]   In these survivals of ancient culture we have the forms in which prehistoric zoölogy expressed the unity, the monogenesis, and the north polar origin of the entire fauna of the earth.

It is now, perhaps, too late for the biologist to gain from these particular myths the instruction which generations ago they could have given him. By slower and more painful methods this beautiful polocentric conception of the vegetable, animal, and human worlds has at last been reached. The problems of earliest floral and faunal and ethnic distribution have shut men up to its acceptance. But if the discovery of the accordant significance of these ancient myths has been equally delayed, we may at least indulge the hope that the unexpected agreement of the prehistoric conception with that of latest science will inspire in candid students of Nature a new and higher respect for the primeval teachings and beliefs of mankind. Meantime let it not be forgotten that there are other myths, of equal antiquity and possibly of wider prevalence, the significance of which for the progress of biology may to-day be as great as ever was that of the tree of all seeds.

Notice, for example, this curious fact: that while in ancient East Aryan thought the gods on Mount

[1] Darmesteter, *The Zend-Avesta,* Part ii., p. 110.

Meru are of prodigious stature the proper tenants of the adjacent regions are somewhat less, though still gigantic ; and they seem to dwindle regularly in size from Varsha to Varsha, until we reach Bhârata, the Varsha which borders upon the equatorial ocean and is peopled with ordinary men. And as if the inhabitants of Hades, being still farther to the South, must be by some law of nature still smaller than men, Prince Satyavân's soul, when led away to Yama's abode, is described in the Mahâbhârata as only "a thumb in height." A striking gradation, every one will say. Beginning with beings sometimes represented as miles in height, it ends on the borders of the Land of Death with disembodied spirits whose stature is only a thumb's length. But this conception of the range of the kingdom of generated and mutable life was not limited to the ancestors of the Hindus. In the most ancient Greek thought the proper habitat of the Pygmies was near the equatorial Ocean-river ; farther northward was the abode of men ; still farther proceeding, one came into the region of giants ; while in polar Olympos the gods were so colossal that in his fall prostrate Arês "covered seven acres."[1] Traces of the same remarkable adjustment are found in other mythologies.[2] Possibly this far-off prehistoric conception has some significance, some lesson for the biology of to-day.

What should this lesson be if not that in all our

---

[1] *Iliad*, xxi. 407. In keeping herewith the more than gigantic Poseidon passes with four strides from Thracian Samos to Ægæ. *Il.*, xiii. 20.

[2] "The idea of the soul as a sort of 'thumbling' is familiar to the Hindus and to German folk-lore." — E. B. Tylor, *Primitive Culture*, i. 450 n.

researches into the origin and sustaining conditions
of life the phenomena of the highest North should
be taken into account? Too long have those who
busy themselves with these investigations been
turning their attention to the ice-cold abysses of the
"deep sea," hoping in some "bathybius" clot of the
sunless ocean-bottom to find the protoplasmic power
which has transmuted inorganic matter into micro-
cosms of organic life. In no such region of cold and
darkness should this search be made.[1] Let life's
beginnings and life's feeding forces be looked for
where its supreme vigor and exuberance have been
seen, — at the pristine centre whence the types and
forms of life have spread victoriously through the
world ; let them be studied at the Pole.[2]

On this subject as conservative an authority as

[1] "As we descend from the shore into deep water, the temperature
becomes lower and lower the deeper we go, until we come to a stratum or zone of water about 32°–36° Fahrenheit, where circumpolar
or Arctic life alone abounds. . . . The water of the ocean all over the
globe below a depth of one thousand fathoms is of an Arctic temperature." — Packard, *Zoölogy*, p. 665.

[2] Since the above was written, a distinguished specialist in deep-
sea dredging has borne the following striking testimony : " With regard to the constitution of the deep-sea fauna, one of the most
remarkable features is the general absence from it of Paleozoic
forms, excepting so far as representatives of the Mollusca and Brach-
iopoda are concerned ; and it is remarkable that amongst the deep-
sea Mollusca no representatives of the *Nautilidæ* and *Ammonitidæ*,
so excessively abundant in ancient periods, occur, and that *Lingula*,
the most ancient Brachiopod, should occur in shallow water only."
Professor H. N. Moseley, F. R. S., Biological Address before British
Association in 1884. *Nature*, August 28, 1884, p. 428. The same
high authority adds, " With regard to the origin of the deep-sea
fauna there can be little doubt that it has been derived almost entirely from the littoral fauna," — agreeing herein with Professor Sven
Loven in his "splendid monograph," *Pourtalesia*, Stockholm, 1883.
The funeral sermon of the *bathybius* theory of the origin of life has
already been preached, and the text of the sermon was Job xxviii. 14.

Principal Dawson recently remarked: "It is not impossible that in the plans of the Creator *the continuous summer sun of the Arctic regions* may have been made the means for the introduction, or at least for the rapid growth and multiplication, of new and more varied types of plants." [1]

In this true centre what new and interesting aspects the problems of life immediately take on! [2] Here we have a regnancy of sunlight such as we never dreamed of in our lower zones. Here we have

[1] " The Genesis and Migration of Plants," in *The Princeton Review*, 1879, p. 292.

[2] The following, from a recent newspaper, suggests some of the new lines of desirable investigation : —

" The Norwegian plant-geographer, Schubeler, a short time ago called attention to some striking and surprising peculiarities manifested by vegetation in high latitudes, which he ascribed to the intensive light-effects of the long days. Most plants in these regions produce much larger and heavier seeds than in lower latitudes. Grain is heavier in the North than in the more Southern latitudes ; the increase of weight being due to the assimilation of non-nitrogenous substances, while the protein products have no part in it. The leaves of most plants grow larger in the higher latitudes, and at the same time take on a deeper, darker color. This fact has been observed not only in most of the wild trees and shrubs, but also in fruit trees and even in kitchen-garden plants. It has further been observed that the flowers of most plants are larger and more deeply colored, and that many flowers which are white in the South become in the far North violet."

So potent and irrepressible are the powers of life in highest Arctic latitudes that neither darkness nor the indescribable cold avail against them. The algic flora well illustrates this statement. According to a writer in *Nature*, Oct. 30, 1884, nearly all Arctic algæ live several years, and, in order that they may be able to effect the work of propagation and nourishment, their organs are in operation during the dark as well as the light season. Whilst wintering at the northernmost part of Spitzbergen in 1872–73, Professor Kjellman observed, in the middle of the winter — viz., at a time when the sun was lowest, and the darkness, therefore, most intense — that a considerable development and growth of the organs of nourishment took place, while, as regards the organs of propagation, he found that a tension and a direction of terrestrial magnetism with whose biological significance we are utterly unacquainted. Here we have electric forces which pour their currents through every grass-blade, and tip the very hills with lambent flame.[1] Shall not such absolutely exceptional biological conditions and energies be found to yield some exceptional biological result? Is not this a more hopeful field for the study of the origin of life than the dark and almost congealed recesses of the deep sea? The old theologians were accustomed to call Adam and Eve

---

it was just at this season that they were most developed. Spores of all kinds were produced and became mature, and they developed into splendid plants. The Arctic algæ, therefore, present the remarkable spectacle of plants which develop their organs of nourishment, and particularly their *organs of propagation*, all the year round, even during the long Polar night, growing regularly at a temperature of between —1° and —2° C., and even attaining a great size at a temperature which never rises above freezing-point. As to "mother-region," the result at which Professor Kjellman arrived was that the algæ flora of the Arctic Ocean is not an immigrant flora, but that its origin lay in the Polar Sea itself. This theory is, he believes, proved by the fact that the Arctic algæ flora is rich in endemic species. There are many species found both in the Northern Atlantic and the Pacific Oceans, a large percentage of which reaches very far north in the Arctic Sea, and which have attained a high degree of development there, being characteristic algæ of the Arctic Ocean; and that these species have been originated there, and gradually spread to the other two oceans is, as he believes, more than probable. How little our zonal diversities of climate affect the question of the possibility of a universal distribution of a north polar flora, or even fauna, is well illustrated in the following: "A remarkable fact associated with the ocean temperature is that forms of animal life belonging to the Arctic seas have been dredged up from the Antarctic Ocean at depths of two thousand fathoms, and may have passed from pole to pole through the tropics [in deep-sea currents] *without having been subjected to a greater variation of temperature than some five degrees or so.*" Gen. R. McCormick, *Voyages of Discovery in the Arctic and Antarctic Seas.* London, 1884: vol. i., p. 354.

[1] *The Arctic Manual*, p. 739.

the "*Protoplasts;*" in their ancient polar home it is possible that science may yet discover the divine secret of all "*protoplasm.*"

Again, our new interest in one of the terrestrial polar regions gives fresh significance to the contrasts between the two.[1] Within ten years our most eminent American geologist has said, "I find no explanation in the present state of science, wherefore most of the dry land of the globe should have been located about the North Pole, and of the water about the South. Physicists say that it indicates greater attraction and therefore a greater density in the solid material beneath the southern ocean. But why the mineral ingredients should have been so gathered about the South Pole as to give the crust there greater density is the unanswered query. It may be that magnetite is much more abundantly diffused through the Antarctic crust than the Arctic. This is only one of many possibilities, and it is at present without a satisfactory fact to stand upon beyond the general truth that iron was universally present."[2]

But the diversity of the two Poles is as great and as perplexing to the biologist as to the physical geographer. "The researches made show that the two polar regions differ greatly. The seas of the

[1] "The higher mean temperature of the Northern compared to the Southern hemisphere is clearly proved and universally acknowledged." Professor Hennessy on "Terrestrial Climate" in *Philosophical Magazine and Journal of Science*. London and Edinburgh, 1859: p. 189. On the Northern hemisphere's greater length of spring and summer see Malte-Brun, *System of Universal Geography*. Boston, 1834: vol. i., p. 14. Also Mansfield Merriman, *The Figure of the Earth*. New York, 1881: p. 76. The disparity of mean temperature is now believed to be less than was formerly supposed.

[2] Professor Dana, in *American Journal of Science*, 1875, vol. xxi.

Arctic teem with animal life.   Land animals, such as the bear, wolf, reindeer, musk-ox, and Arctic fox, are scattered over the frozen surface of the land where they find the means of sustenance. The air is peopled with innumerable flocks of birds; a hardy vegetation extends close up to the Arctic Circle, and beyond it, in mosses, lichens, scurvy-grass, sorrel, small stunted shrubs, dwarfed trees, and in summer beautiful flowers.   In the Antarctic, on the contrary, vegetation ceases at a certain limit, trees terminating at about 56° S. latitude.   Animal life abounds in the seas, but though birds exist in great numbers and in varieties unknown in the Arctic, no quadrupeds are found upon the land." [1]

With this we may compare the already cited language of Sir Joseph Hooker: "Geographically speaking, there is no Antarctic flora except a few lichens and seaweeds." [2]

Would it not seem as if the South Pole must have been covered by "the barren sea" at the period when floral and faunal life, starting at its Arctic centre, began its conquering marches over all the Earth?   Or is there rather some marked difference in the biological value of the poles themselves? [3]

But polar biological research involves antecedent Polar Exploration and a wider and more system-

---

[1] C. P. Daly in *Johnson's Cyclopædia*, Art. "Polar Research."

[2] *Nature*, London, 1881, p. 447.

[3] The latter explanation would seem to be favored by the experiments of Dr. Ferdinand Cohn, who found that a positive electrode would hinder the development of micrococcus "*in bei weitem höherem Grade als die negative.*" *Beiträge zur Biologie der Pflanzen.* Breslau, 1879: p. 159.   It is also known that eggs may be hatched quicker at one pole of a magnet than at the other.

atic study of Terrestrial Physics.[1] Herein lies a fresh and novel impulse to reinvest on every side the still uncaptured citadel of the Arctic Pole. Long ago could Maury write, " As science has advanced, men have looked with deeper and deeper longings toward the mystic circles of the Polar regions. There icebergs are framed and glaciers launched ; there the tides have their cradle, the whales their nursery ; there the winds complete their circuits, and the currents of the sea their round; there the aurora is lighted up, and the trembling needle brought to rest ; there, too, in the mazes of that mystic circle, terrestrial forces of occult power and of vast influence upon the well-being of man are continually at play. Within the Arctic Circle is the pole of the winds and the poles of cold, the pole of the earth and of the magnet. It is a circle of mysteries ; and the desire to enter it, to explore its untrodden wastes and secret chambers, and to study its physical aspects has grown into a longing. Noble daring has made Arctic ice and snow-clad seas classic ground. It is no feverish excitement nor vain ambition that leads men there. It is a higher feeling, a holier motive : a desire to look into the works of creation, to comprehend the economy of our planet, and to grow wiser and better by the knowledge." If such a passion for discovery could be kindled in the presence of the older and more abstract problems, what ought to be the result when to these are added the possibility of solving at least some of the mysteries of Nature's Life, and the certainty of standing where Human Life began !

[1] See APPENDIX, Sect. VII.: "Latest Polar Research." Also Andree, *Der Kampf um den Nordpol.* 4 Aufl., Bielefeld, 1882.

CHAPTER II.

THE BEARING OF OUR RESULTS ON THE STUDY OF ANCIENT LITERATURE.

And the Greeks, who surpassed all men in ingenuity, appropriated to themselves the greater part of these things, exaggerating them, and adding to them various ornaments which they wove into this foundation in every style, in order to charm by the elegance of the myths. Hence Hesiod and the famed cyclic poets drew their theogonies, their gigantomachies, their mutilations of the gods, and in hawking them about everywhere they have supplanted the true narrative. And our ears, accustomed to their fictions, familiar to us for several centuries past, guard as a precious deposit the fables which they received by tradition, as I remarked when I began to speak; and, rooted by time, this belief has become so difficult to dislodge that to the greater number the truth appears like a story told for amusement, while the corruption of the tradition is looked upon as the truth itself. — PHILO OF BYBLOS.

SUMMING up the most probable results of all his investigations, Darwin states as his opinion that man must be considered as "descended from a hairy quadruped, furnished with a tail and pointed ears, probably arboreal in his habits, and an inhabitant of the Old World."[1]

According to Häckel, this *Homo primigenius* was a blackish, woolly-haired, prognathous, ape-like being, with a long, narrow head. His body was entirely covered with hair, and he was unable to speak.

In reading most fashionable writers upon ancient mythology and literature, one would think that they conceived of the writers of the Vedic Hymns and the authors of the myths of classic literature as very early and but slightly developed descendants of this hairy *Homo Darwinius.* Thus, according to Mr.

[1] *Descent of Man,* Pt. II., ch. 21.

Keary, at the time that the myth of the Cyclops originated, "men *really believed* that the stormy sky was a being and the sun his eye."[1] Indeed, it might almost appear, from another passage in the same book, that at the period when this Cyclops-faith was reached men had arrived at quite an advanced stage as compared with the earlier one, when as yet they knew too little to look up at the sky at all, and had an idea that the branches of the trees extended quite to heaven. "The power of gazing upward to heaven," he says, "came to us not all at once, but gradually, through lapse of time. Savages are said scarcely ever to raise their eyes, and their heads are naturally inclined with a downward gaze, so that it must be an effort for them to look at the sky and the heavenly bodies. Primeval man lived upon roots and berries, or on the lesser animals and the vermin which he gathered from the soil, and so habit as well as nature kept his eyes fixed upon the ground. We need not therefore wonder if, in their half-glances upward, our forefathers had not leisure to observe that the tree-top was *not really* close against the sky. They may well have deemed that the upper branches hid themselves in infinitely remote ethereal regions."[2]

The work which such men make in interpreting ancient literature and thought is strange enough. The ascription to Agni of the same supreme worship which the bard has just paid to Varuna or Mitra is explained as due to the extreme " shortness of the memory " of early men.[3] Only a knowledge of

---

[1] *Outlines of Primitive Belief.* 1882 : p. 27.

[2] Ibid., p. 58.

[3] Ibid., p. 115.

a most limited portion of the earth's surface can be conceded to any of the ancient nations. The early Aryans sing of the Ocean and of ships of an hundred oars, but it must not for a moment be supposed that they had ever seen or heard of the real Ocean ; they had simply originated in their imaginations a mythical one.[1] In such hands the immortal Iliad becomes merely " a tale of land-battle, the theatre of whose action is limited to the two shores of the Ægæan, the known world of the Greek." [2] Though the Homeric poems betray in various places an acquaintance with astronomy, and actually name various constellations, yet, when the question is raised as to how the poet conceived of the return of the sun during the night from the West to the East, even Mr. Bunbury silences us, telling us that in Homer's day nobody had ever thought of such a question ! [3]

Illustrations of this worse than mediæval ignorance and distortion of ancient thought and language could be multiplied to almost any extent. But as some selection must be made, it may perhaps be best to confine ourselves to three or four points in a field comparatively familiar to all readers likely to peruse these pages, — the field of Homeric cosmology. If we succeed according to our expectation we

[1] Ch. Ploix, "L'Océan des Anciens," *Revue Archéologique,* 1877, vol. xxxiii., pp. 47–54.

[2] Keary, *Primitive Belief,* p. 296.

[3] " How the sun was carried back to the point from which it was to start afresh on its course, it is probable that no one in his day ever troubled himself to inquire." (!) *Hist. Ancient Geography,* vol. i., p. 34. This does not well accord with the statement of Bergaine : " Le séjour et l'état du soleil quand il a disparu sont des questions qui préoccupent *vivement* les poëtes védiques." *La Religion Védique,* tom. i., p. 6.

shall make it plain that those interpreters of Homer whose conceptions of Greek culture are derived from current Darwinistic anthropology rather than from the poems themselves, demonstrate, by the number and character of their exegetical entanglements, the entire incorrectness of their fundamental assumption.[1]

1. The question just touched upon, the Movement of the Sun, is as good as any with which to begin, and by which to show the embarrassments into which accepted interpreters have continually fallen in consequence of denying to the ancients a knowledge of the spherical figure of the Earth.

Opening Keightley, we find the customary assertion that "according to the ideas of the Homeric and Hesiodic ages the Earth was a round, flat disk, around which the river Ocean flowed." Then he says that "men, seeing the sun rise in the East and set in the West each day, were naturally led to inquire how his return to the East was effected." He alludes to the fact that "in the Odyssey, when Helios ends his diurnal career, he is said to go under the Earth;" but he adds that "it is not easy to determine whether the poet meant that he then passed through Tartaros back to the East during the night." The "beautiful fiction of the solar cup or basin," he thus describes: "If, then, as there is reason to suppose, it was the popular belief that a lofty mountainous ring ran round the edge of the Earth, it was easy for the poets to feign that on reaching the western

[1] In W. Helbig's new work, *Das Homerische Epos von den Denkmälern erläutert*, Leipsic, 1884, we have some symptoms of a new and better type of Homeric archæology. The author holds that in Homer's day there were evidences of "lost arts," and in the treasures found at Mycenæ he sees the products of a pre-Homeric civilization.

stream of Ocean Helios himself, his chariot and his horses, were received into a magic cup or boat, made by Hephaistos, which, aided by the current, conveyed him during the night round the northern part of the earth, where his light was only enjoyed by the happy Hyperboreans, the lofty Rhiphæans concealing it from the rest of mankind. They must also have supposed that the cup continued its course during the day, compassing the earth every twenty-four hours." Of this fiction, however, Keightley confesses, "neither Homer nor Hesiod evinces any knowledge." After quoting various later poets, therefore, he concludes as follows : " From a consideration of all these passages it may seem to follow that the ideas of the poets on this subject were very vague and fleeting. Perhaps the prevalent opinion was that the Sun rested himself and his weary steeds in the West, *and then returned to the East.*" [1] By what passage, however, whether *via* the North or underneath the supposed " flat disk " of the Earth, Keightley makes no further effort to determine.

The difficulty in the way of supposing that in Homer's thought the nocturnal sun passed underneath the flat Earth-disk, through Tartaros, back to the East, is that the poet invariably represents this Underworld as forever unvisited by sunlight. In view of this, and of the ominous silence of Homer as to any winged cup sailing round the earth to the North, some interpreters warn us against expecting any consistency of thought in poetry so primitive.[2]

---

[1] *Mythology*, pp. 47-50. Here, as usual, Keightley closely follows Völcker. For the "mountainous ring " see Ukert's map.

[2] " Of popular views and conceptions one must not demand con-

Schwenck goes so far in this direction as to suggest that the island Aiaiè is a creation of the imagination in the far West, called forth for the express purpose of giving the mind a kind of resting-place, where it can leàve the sinking Helios without troubling itself with inconvenient speculations as to how he is to get back to the Orient at the appointed hour. He says: " The Homeric poetry could not allow the Sun and the daylight to rest during the night in the Homeric Hades, for in that case Hades would have been illuminated. It therefore supposes an island afar off at the end of the world, where Helios and Dawn, after they have passed over across the heavens, repose at night, and whence, after this repose, they in the morning again ascend the sky. An exact explanation as to how they come westwardly to this island and then in the morning rise in the East lies aloof from the poetry, for in Homer nothing of systems is to be found, and only each object taken by itself is correct and clear." [1]

Assume once a spherical Earth, and all these difficulties of the interpreters are at an end. East and West touch each other. Mr. Gladstone, before abandoning fully the flat-earth theory, came as near the truth as he possibly could and not hit it, when, speaking of Helios, he wrote: " The fact of his sporting with the oxen night and morning goes far to show that Homer did not think of the Earth as a plane, but round, perhaps, as upon a cylinder, and

sistency or completion. They go up to a certain point, apprehend only a part, and this only as it appears at first blush ; they leave one side all conclusive reflection, and are unconcerned about contradictions since *they* are *not conscious of any.*" — J. F. Lauer in *Anhang to Ameis's Odyssey*, x. 86.

[1] Cited in Ameis, *Odyssey, Anhang*, xii. 4.

believed that the West and East were in contact." [1]
He mistook, however, in suggesting Thrinakia as
the place of contact. It was rather on the meridian
of Aiaiè, for we are expressly told that

ὅθι τ' Ἠοῦς ἠριγενείης
οἰκία καὶ χοροί εἰσι καὶ ἀντολαὶ Ἠελίοιο.

" There are the abodes and dance-grounds of Aurora, there the risings of the Sun." [2]

Nor could anything be more natural than that the
poet, conceiving of the world of living men as
Homer did, and sending out his thoughts eastward
and westward in search of the meeting-place of evening and morning, should fix upon the meridian opposite his own, the very place and only place where
his eastward-journeying thought and his westward
journeying thought would of necessity meet. His
eastern hemisphere would naturally extend round
eastward until it met the edge of the hemisphere
extending round westward. On that farthest off meridian,[3] therefore, he made the old day give place to
the new, eve to morn. That was the doubtful line on
which Odysseus and his companions were no longer
clear: " where was East and where was West, where
Helios went behind the Earth or where he rose
again." [4]

2. The false assumption that Homer's Earth is
flat has created all the noted controversies connected
with his representations of the location of Hades.
This question has divided Homeric interpreters into
more than a dozen differing camps. Their mutually

---

[1] *Juventus Mundi*, p. 325.

[2] *Odyssey*, xii. 3, 4.

[3] That the son of Odysseus by Kirkè should have been named Teleg-
onos, "*the far-away begotten*," thus becomes peculiarly significant.

[4] *Odyssey*, x. 189-192.

contradictory solutions of the problem would be the laughing-stock of the opposers of classical studies, were these latter only sufficiently acquainted with the world's scholarship to be aware of their existence. To review and solve the question in this place would detain the general reader too long, but in the Appendix, Section sixth, the assertions here made will be found abundantly verified.

3. The same flat-earth assumption is further responsible for all the difficulties which interpreters have found in representing the Ocean, and in general the Water System of the Earth, in accordance with the Homeric data.

These difficulties have been neither few nor small. Four of them we will here notice. And, first, that growing out of the statement that from deep-flowing Ocean "flow all rivers and every sea, and all fountains and deep wells." [1] Völcker pronounces this "hard to explain." He says, "An immediate in-streaming of the Ocean into the sea can scarcely be meant, partly because sea-water and ocean-water do not unite, partly because Homer knows of no such in-streamings in the Phasis and at the Pillars of Hercules, and the origination of rivers in this way would not be thinkable." [2] Other writers, devoted to the illustration of ancient thought, seem not to have stopped to inquire whether rivers flowing up-stream from the Ocean to the hills were thinkable or not, and have gravely set before the youthful student diagrams constructed on this plan as the true representation of Homeric thought! [3]

[1] *Iliad*, xxi. 196.
[2] *Homerische Geographie*, § 49.
[3] See the older Classical Atlases. "According to Homer," says

A second embarrassing question has been this:
"If the Ocean-stream surrounded and constituted
the outermost boundary of the Earth-disk, what sustained the Ocean-stream itself and constituted its
further shore?" As Völcker says, "Who on the
further side held in the billows of the vast World-
river, that they did not flow off into the empty
spaces of heaven? Was it a narrow strip of the
inner Earth, or was it formless chaos, or the descending rim of the sky, or the inner power of the waters
themselves?" [1] Buchholz says, "By what the Ocean
itself was in turn bounded remains unclear. The
child-like imagination of the Homeric age contented
itself with that confused *halbverschwommene* conception." [2] The most natural answer, especially
from the point of view represented by Buchholz,
who, with Ukert and others, claims that the Homeric heaven was literally metallic, would seem to
be Völcker's third supposition, namely, that the rim
of the metallic sky constitutes the outer limit of the
Ocean-stream. [3] This would correspond, also, with
the general notion that the circular disk of the earth
"divided the hollow sphere of the universe into two
equal parts." [4] It would also exactly correspond to

Theodore Alois Buckley, in his translation of the *Iliad*, "the Earth is
a circular plane, and Oceanus is an immense stream encircling it,
from which the rivers *flow inward*," — of course, therefore, up-hill.

[1] *Hom. Geog.*, § 49. Compare Keightley: "As it was a stream it
must have been conceived to have a further bank to confine its
course." *Mythology of Greece*, p. 33.

[2] *Homerische Realien*, I. 1, p. 55.

[3] In his earlier work, *Die Mythologie des Japetischen Geschlechtes*,
Giessen, 1824, p. 60, Völcker distinctly represents this as the ancient
Greek conception: "*Wo der Himmel sich wahrhaft an den Okean
schliesst und dem kühnen Schiffer das letzte Ziel geworden.*"

[4] Keightley, *Mythol.*, p. 29.

Flach's curious and elaborate representation of the Hesiodic world in his recent work on the Hesiodic cosmogony.[1] Still further it would seem best to accord with Homer's language describing the heavenly constellations as bathing in the Ocean. On the other hand, however, such a supposition would be incompatible with the Homeric representation that the farther shore presented a suitable landing-place, and especially a landing-place situated, like that of Odysseus, in the Underworld. Moreover, it would be incompatible with the current notion that the Homeric heaven was supported upon mountain pillars *standing on the Earth inside* the Ocean-stream, like Mount Atlas in western Libya.[2] Again, therefore, the question returns, "Given a flat Earth surrounded by the Ocean-river, what constitutes the farther shore, and how can the mariner who lands upon it speak of himself as in the Underworld?" The learned Völcker leaves the subject with the unsatisfying observation, "The poet has not answered our questions."

A third embarrassment dwelt upon by the same advocate of the flat-earth theory is that, as he understands Homer, Hellas was the centre of the circular Earth-disk, and not more than "ten or eleven days' sail" from the Ocean in any direction; and yet the poet makes it eighteen days' sail by the shortest route from Ogygia to the land of the Phæacians, and at least another in the same direction to

[1] Hans Flach, *Das System der Hesiodischen Kosmogonie.* Leipsic, 1874. (Diagram prefixed.)

[2] Maury, *Histoire des Religions de la Grèce Antique.* Paris, 1857: vol. i., p. 596. In like manner Bunbury, *History of Ancient Geography*, vol. i., p. 33, represents the solid Homeric vault as resting on the outermost edge of the circular earth just *inside* the Ocean-stream.

Hellas, and yet Ogygia is the navel or centre of the sea. "These," says he, "are insurmountable difficulties for him who would measure with the compasses. Rather should we learn from this example what folk-faith and folk-tales are. Where there is no agreement we should not create one by main force. The Earth is circular and Hellas is its centre; that was the popular faith. But the situation of the Ocean and the extent of the Earth are at the same time such fluctuating ideas, and all any way extended voyages seem to the poet to extend to such a terrific distance, that it may well happen to him to overpass all bounds out in that realm where were, so to speak, the most terrific of all distances."[1] Thus the nodding Homer is again caught in contradiction, and to accommodate his exaggerated and terrific distances even Gladstone at first felt constrained to change the figure of the Earth-disk itself, and to present it as a vast parallelogram more extended from North to South than from East to West.[2]

The fourth difficulty involved in the current interpretation is that experienced in harmonizing the poet's representations of the Ocean, as commonly understood, with his representations of the movements of the sun, as commonly understood. The sun at evening certainly ceases to be visible to men. According to the Homeric representation he returns to the flowing of the Ocean.[3] His bright light sinks in it.[4] At his rising it is also from the Ocean

[1] *Hom. Geographie,* § 50.
[2] See his map. Comp. *Juventus Mundi,* p. 493.
[3] *Iliad,* xviii. 240.
[4] *Iliad,* viii. 485.

that he begins to mount the sky.[1] Yet his setting
is also described as a going εἰς ὑπὸ γαῖαν, under or
behind the Earth.[2] How now, with a flat circular
disk for the Earth, and with a circumfluent Ocean in
the same plane, and with an eternally dark and un-
sunned Hades just beyond the Ocean-river to the
westward, can these data be harmonized? If we attempt to conceive of the Sun as literally sinking in
the ocean and hiding his light beneath its waters, he
has not gone εἰς ὑπὸ γαῖαν, but rather " in under" the
Ocean. Moreover, the old difficulty reappears as to
how he shall get round into the East in time for his
rising again. Furthermore, if he is the whole night
concealed under the waves of the Ocean, descending
into it in the far West at his setting and ascending
out of it in the far East at his rising, how can we
arrange for his rejoicing himself night and morning
with his oxen on the island of Thrinakia?[3] But
we cannot abandon this whole supposition, and let
the Sun set *beyond* and *behind* the Ocean-stream, for
that would be in the western Hades, where he never
shines. Nor yet, again, can we say that he descends
to the surface of the Ocean simply, and then, in his
" cup," or otherwise, moves round to the Orient by
way of the North, for then, the Ocean being in substantially the same plane as the abode of men, they
would not be overspread with darkness, but would
enjoy, if not the spectacle of " the midnight sun,"
at least the full light of a sun moving round the

---

[1] *Iliad*, vii. 422 ; *Odyssey*, xix. 433.

[2] *Odyssey*, x. 191.

[3] *Odyssey*, xii. 380. The only diagram based upon this conception
which I remember to have seen is in the rare and curious work by
Johannes Herbinius, *Dissertationes de admirandis mundi Cataractis.*
Amstel. 1678 : p. 13.

22

horizon. On this supposition, too, Hades, just **west** of the river, would also be equally illuminated. *Inside* the Ocean-stream he certainly does not hide himself in the ground, for that would be incompatible with all the passages associating his rising and setting with the Ocean. But if he cannot be conceived of as setting on the hither side of the stream, nor on the farther side, nor yet as resting on the Ocean, nor yet as hiding beneath it, what possible conception of the matter remains ?

All this trouble is the natural result of one false assumption, — the assumption that Homer's Earth is a flat disk. Assume that it is a sphere, and every one of these difficulties vanishes. Then, in causing the Sun to descend to the Ocean in which lies Aiaiè the poet makes the bed to which the king of day retires the same as that from which in the morning he rises again. At the same time, from the poet's standpoint and from the standpoint of the lands inhabited by the poet's countrymen, each setting of the Sun was a going " behind the earth," to reappear on the opposite side. This view of the movement of Helios solves every perplexity ; and if Homer had the knowledge of the Earth and Heavens involved in the view, we may be sure he also knew as well as we do in what sense the Ocean is the source of all springs and rivers, and for what reason the equatorial Ocean never runs away for the lack of an ultra-terrestrial shore.

4. The same hermeneutical myopia which has thus minified and misconceived every feature of Homer's cosmography has introduced and maintained the now universal dogma that in the Homeric poems " Olympos is always the Thessalian mountain " of

that name.[1] All our youth are taught that "the early poets believed that the gods actually lived upon the top of this mountain separating Macedonia and Thessaly. Even the fable of the giants scaling heaven must be understood in a literal sense; not that they placed Pelion and Ossa upon *the top* of Olympos to reach the still higher *heaven,* but that they piled Pelion on the top of Ossa and both on the *lower slopes* of Olympos to scale the summit of Olympos itself, the abode of the gods."[2] To settle the question negatively as well as positively, revered German erudition solemnly declares, "The gods of Homer *never* live in heaven."[3] Such dogmatism challenges a fresh investigation of the question.

Taking up this subject, Keightley remarks that if we were to follow the teachings of Comparative Mythology we should have to locate the abode of Homer's gods in the heights of heaven. His language is: "Were we to follow analogy, and argue from the cosmology of other races of men, we would say that the upper surface of the superior hemisphere was the abode of the Grecian gods."[4] He goes on to allude to the conceptions of the Scandinavians and some other peoples, and adds, "Hence we might be led to infer that Olympos, the abode of the Grecian gods, was synonymous with heaven, and that the Thessalian mountain and those others which bore the same name were called after the original heavenly hill."

It is a pity that the learned author could not have

---

[1] Ameis and Hentze, *Ilias,* i. 44.
[2] Smith's *Classical Dictionary,* Art. "Olympus."
[3] Völcker, *Homerische Geographie,* pp. 9, 12.
[4] *Mythology.* Fourth Edition. London, 1877: p. 34.

accepted this very sensible conclusion; but he did not. Rejecting the admitted intimations of Comparative Cosmology, he says, "A careful survey, however, of those passages in Homer and Hesiod in which Olympos occurs will lead us to believe that the Achæans held the Thessalian Olympos, the highest mountain with which they were acquainted, to be the abode of their gods."

The only passage specially referred to by Keightley, as establishing this view, is the Iliad, xiv. 225 *seq.*, where the language employed is not at all inconsistent with the idea that, in descending from the summit of Olympos, Hera descended from the northern sky. More elaborate is the argument of Völcker,[1] but its logical cogency is by no means admissible.

The true Homeric conception of the abode of the gods is far loftier, grander, and more poetic than that given us by such interpreters. According to the poet's real representation, that abode is "the wide heaven," — not the atmospheric heaven, οὐρανὸν ἐν αἰθέρι καὶ νεφέλῃσιν, for this is a special possession of Zeus (Iliad, xv. 192); it is the upper sky,

---

[1] *Homerische Geographie und Weltkunde,* pp. 4-20. Copied by Buchholz, *Hom. Realien,* I. § 12. Professor Blackie's reasoning is entirely subjective: "In a spiritual religion, like Christianity, the word heaven will always be kept as vague as possible; in an imaginative and sensuous religion, like the Greek, it must be localized. A Zeus with human shape and members must sit on a terrestrial seat; and the only seat proper for him is the highest mountain in the country to which he belongs. Now, as the original seat of the Greeks, when they rested from their long journey by the Caspian and Euxine westward, was the plains of Macedonia and Thessaly, the necessary locality for the throne of the Supreme God and the council of the Immortals was Olympos, the extreme east end of the long Cambunian range separating Thessaly from Macedonia, to the north of the Peneios and the defile of Tempe." *Homer and the Iliad.* Edinburgh, 1866: vol. iv., p. 174.

the celestial dome in which sun, moon, and stars wheel silently around the Pole. To the early Greek, as to the early Perso-Aryan, it was easy to conceive of this celestial dome as a heavenly mountain, vast, majestic, of unearthly beauty, and peopled with glorious beings invisible to mortals. And this heavenly mountain he called Olympos. The Thessalian mount, the Bithynian, and all the dozen others of the same name [1] were sacred only so far as they symbolized and commemorated their heavenly original. In the Odyssey, xi. 315, it is plain that Homer speaks of the Thessalian Olympos along with other Thessalian mountains; [2] but in general he means by Olympos the heights of the northern heaven viewed as the proper abode of the gods. [3]

The proofs of the incorrectness of the current

[1] Heyschius professed to have knowledge of fourteen mountains bearing the name of Olympos.

[2] To all who deny that heaven was to Homer the abode of the gods this passage presents insurmountable difficulties. To place Ossa upon Olympos, then upon Ossa Pelion, in order, by means of the three, to climb up into an abode situated on the top of the undermost of the three, is the problem! No wonder that Völcker thinks Homer has been overpraised for his knowledge of localities and of the arrangement of mountains : "Der Olymp muss auf jeden Fall zu unterst kommen, und die Folgerung aus dieser Stelle für die Homerische Localkenntniss und Grundlage der Wirklichkeit in Anordnung der Berge müssen wir dahin gestellt sein lassen." *Hom. Geog.,* p. 9. Truly amusing is the haughty remark under which Hartung beats a retreat : "Warum aber sollte ein Gelehrter über solche Wiedersprüche sich Scrupel machen da die religiöse Vorstellung sich niemals daran gestossen hat?" *Die Religion und Mythologie der Griechen,* Th. iii., 6. But one German, and he a Swiss, seems to have apprehended the inevitable implication of this passage : "Jedoch war dem Griechen wohl bewusst, dass die Götter nicht eigentlich und wirklich auf dem Olymp wohnten, wie aus der Beschreibung des Kampfes des Otus und Ephialtes gegen die olympischen Götter hervorgeht." Rinck, *Die Religion der Hellenen.* Zurich, 1853 : voi. i., p. 207.

[3] Compare Pictet, *Les Origines.* Paris, 1877 : tom. iii., p. 225.

interpretation appear on almost every page of the Homeric poems. The designation of the gods by the formula οἳ οὐρανὸν εὐρὺν ἔχουσιν occurs twice in the Iliad and sixteen times in the Odyssey, but the expressions "who possess the wide heaven," in Odyssey, xix., line 40, and "who possess Olympos," line 43, are plainly identical in meaning.[1] So in the Iliad, "the immortals who possess the Olympian mansions" and "the gods who possess the wide heaven" are unquestionably interchangeable phrases.[2] Hence also "the Olympians," "the Uranians," and "the Epouranians" are names of the same beings.[3] In Hesiod's Theogony the expression ἐντός Ὀλύμπου, "within Olympos," occurs no less than three times.[4] To translate it according to the current interpretation of Homer is to locate the palace of Zeus in the heart of an earthly mountain and to transform the "*Lichtgestalten*" of his heavenly court into Trolls.

In book twenty-four of the Iliad, verse ninety-

---

[1] Comp. xii. 339; also the Homeric Hymn, *In Apollinem*, ii. 320, 334. In the *Iliad*, viii., lines 393 and 411, the selfsame portals are called now "gates of heaven," now "gates of Olympos."

[2] Book i. 18; ii. 13, 30, 484; v. 383, 404, *et passim*. See Völcker, *Homerische Geographie*, p. 13 (§ 9).

[3] Book i. 399, xx. 47, and often; i. 570; v. 373, 898, etc.; vi. 129, 131, 527. Compare i. 497 :—

Ἠερίη δ᾽ ἀνέβη μέγαν οὐρανὸν Οὔλυμπόν τε.

A similar identification occurs in Hesiod, *Theogony*, v. 689. See L. Preller, "Daher der Himmel und der Olymp auch ganz gleichbedeutend gebraucht werden können." *Griechische Mythologie*. Leipsic, 1854: vol. i., p. 48.

[4] Lines 37, 51, 408. The interpreters of Hesiod have found this so great a *crux* that Göttling and Paley make it a ground for questioning the genuineness or antiquity of the passages. See also Schoemann, *Die hesiodische Theogonie ausgelegt und beurtheilt*. Berlin, 1868: p. 303. Yet Pfau, in Pauly's *Real-Encyclopaedie*, Art. "Olympos," affirms that we find in Hesiod "exactly the same conceptions of Olympos" as in Homer.

seven, we are told that Iris and Thetis were impelled up "*to heaven*" (ἐς οὐρανὸν). But the moment
the Father of gods and men begins discourse,
he says, "Thou hast come *to Olympos*, O goddess
Thetis;" and in verse one hundred twenty-one the
bard resumes, "Thus he spoke; nor did the silver-
footed goddess Thetis disobey, but rushing im-
petuously, she descended down from the tops of
Olympos."[1]

One of the most vivid of the pictures of Olympian
life in the whole Iliad is that portraying (book xv.
14 ff.) the punishment of Hera by Zeus. In the
literal translation of Buckley, it is thus rendered:
"O Hera, of evil arts, impracticable, thy stratagem
has made noble Hector cease from battle, and put
his troops to flight. Indeed, I know not whether
again thou mayst not be the first to reap the fruits
of thy pernicious machinations, and I chastise thee
with stripes. Dost thou not remember when thou
didst swing from on high, and I hung two anvils
from thy feet, and bound a golden chain around thy
hands, that could not be broken? And thou didst
hang in the air and clouds, and the gods commis-
erated thee throughout lofty Olympos; but standing around, they were not able to release thee; but
whomsoever I caught, seizing, I hurled from the
threshold *of heaven* till he reached the earth, hardly
breathing."

Although the words "of heaven" are supplied by
the translator, the contrast required by the expres-

---

[1] Similar cases occur; *Iliad*, i. 195, 208, compared with 221; v.
868 with 869; xix. 351 with 355; xx. 5 with 10; *Od.*, xi. 313 with
316; xx. 31 with 55; also 103 with 113. It is astonishing that Faesi
can say that the case in the text is the only one found in the
Iliad. *Odysee, Einleitung*, p. xvii.

sion "reached the earth" compels the supply in order to make good sense.

In book first Hephaistos gives his own account of this same hurling out of heaven. He says, "Be patient, my mother, and although grieved restrain thyself, lest with my own eyes I behold thee beaten, being very dear to me; nor then, though full of grief, should I be able to assist thee, for Olympian Zeus is difficult to be opposed. For upon a time before this, when I desired to assist thee, having seized me by the foot, he cast me down from the heavenly threshold (βηλοῦ θεσπεσίοιο).[1] The whole day was I hurled, and at the setting of the sun I fell on Lemnos, and but little of life remained in me."

Nothing can well be plainer than that this whole scene is conceived of as occurring high in the vault of heaven. To locate it on any "many-peaked mountain" every way embarrasses the imagination.[2] Moreover, Lemnos is not situated under Thessa-

[1] "Heavenly threshold" is Buckley's rendering of this term, though he elsewhere distinguishes Olympos from heaven, as in note on book xvi. 364. In ancient cosmology the "door of heaven" was situated at the North Pole of the sky. Khândogya-Upanishad, xxiv. 3, 4, 7, 8, 11, 12. *Sacred Books of the East*, vol. i., Pt. I., pp. 36, 37. For the rabbinical usage see Eisenmenger, *Entdecktes Judenthum*, Bd. ii., p. 402.

[2] Thus Völcker, after reminding the reader that "there can be no doubt that the gods are here represented as on Olympos, and not where Hera hung ἐν αἰθέρι καὶ νεφέλῃσιν," exclaims very naturally, "Where now is the end of the rope made fast?" He immediately adds as his answer, "Ohne Zweifel περὶ ῥίον Οὐλύμποιο! — Without doubt around the peak of Olympos!" No wonder he places an exclamation point after such a masterpiece of interpretation. Possibly the French savant, M. Boivin, who to explain *Od.*, vi. 40 ff., contended that Homer conceived of Olympos as an *inverted* mountain, having its snowy top near the earth and its snowless and rainless roots in heaven, caught his idea from Völcker's exegesis of this passage!

lian Olympos, nor could the word κάππεσον describe Hephaistos's motion in space from the one to the other. So irresistible, indeed, is the right interpretation that Keightley, unconscious of his inconsistency, elsewhere says, "The favorite haunt of Hephaistos on earth was the isle of Lemnos. It was here he fell when flung *from heaven* by Zeus for attempting to aid his mother Hera." [1] In like manner Professor Geddes, with a forgetfulness equally entertaining, writes of Zeus "hurling Hephaistos over the *celestial battlements*," and of his being "able to draw gods and earth and sea aloft *into the sky*." [2]

The not less famous passage in the opening lines of book eighth is even more conclusive: "Whomsoever of the gods I shall discover, having gone apart from the rest, wishing to aid either the Trojans or the Greeks, disgracefully smitten shall he return to Olympos; or, seizing, I will hurl him into gloomy Tartaros, very far hence, where there is a very deep gulf beneath the earth, and iron portals, and a brazen threshold,[3] as far below Hades as heaven is from earth; then shall he know by how much I am the most powerful of all the gods. But come, ye gods, and try me, that ye may all know. Having suspended a golden chain from heaven, do all ye, gods and goddesses suspend yourselves therefrom; yet would ye not draw down from heaven to earth your supreme counselor Jove, not even if ye labor ever so much: but whenever I, desiring, should

---

[1] *Mythology*, p. 97.

[2] *The Problem of the Homeric Poems*, p. 133.

[3] Here is the Underworld door and threshold corresponding to the upper, north polar one from which Hephaistos was hurled down to earth. Compare also Hesiod's description.

wish to pull it, I could draw it up together, earth, and ocean, and all; then, indeed, would I bind the chain around the top of Olympos, and all these should hang aloft. By so much do I surpass both gods and men."

Comment is unnecessary. Until the whole of a thing can be suspended upon and supported by a part of itself, no interpreter can make the top of Olympos in this passage signify the top of a mountain in Thessaly.[1]

If any further evidence can be needed to show that no mountain of earth can meet the requirements of the language of the Iliad respecting Olympos, it is surely afforded in the passages already alluded to where suppliants, addressing the gods as "Olympian," are said to stretch forth their hands toward "the starry heavens." An example of this is the following : " But the guardian of the Greeks, Gerenian Nestor, most particularly prayed, stretching forth his hands to the starry heaven : ' O Father Zeus, if ever any one in fruitful Argos, to thee burning the fat thighs of either oxen or sheep, supplicated that he might return, and thou didst promise

---

[1] The heroic manner in which Professor Geddes accepts this grave alternative and shifts his own embarrassment to the shoulders of the poet is somewhat discouraging to interpreters who have an inclination to find a rational meaning in their author. He says, "The manner in which this ῥίον Οὐλύμποιο is referred to in a concrete form shows that it was not only a visible but [also a] commanding object in the poet's landscape ; so much so that it *embarrasses his physical speculations and conceptions of the Cosmos* [sic], since it is made the pinnacle on which the world of sea and land is to be suspended by the golden chain. The ῥίον *here*, however, *must be a part of the veritable mountain, not any idealized Olympos.*" (!) Wm. D. Geddes, LL. D., *The Problem of the Homeric Poems.* London, 1878: p. 257. This is as bad as the exclamatory arbitrariness of Völcker, on the same passage, *Geog.*, § 11.

and assent, be mindful of these things, O Olympian, and avert the cruel day.' " [1]

Nor is the language of the Odyssey less opposed to the prevailing interpretation. Here Olympos is metaphorically spoken of precisely as we speak of heaven: "For Olympos hath given me grief" (iv. 722). Again, in a memorable passage, it is depicted in terms which plainly belong to no sublunary sphere: "Thus having spoken, blue-eyed Athenè departed to Olympos, where they say is forever the firm seat of the gods; it is neither shaken by the winds, nor is it ever bedewed by the shower, nor does the snow approach it; but a most cloudless serenity is spread out, and white splendor runs over it, in which the blessed gods are delighted all their days. To this place Athenè departed when she had admonished the damsel." [2]

In book xx. 30, Athenè descends "from heaven" (οὐρανόθεν καταβᾶσα), while in line 55 her return is described as "to Olympos." So in line 103 Zeus thunders

ἀπ' αἰγλήεντος 'Ολύμπου

ὑψόθεν ἐκ νεφέων,

but in line 113 the same thundering is described as

ἀπ' οὐρανοῦ ἀστερόεντος.

As in the Iliad, so in the Odyssey, suppliants address their prayers toward "the starry heaven;" [3]

---

[1] Book xv. 371, 375. Comp. x. 461; iii. 364; vii. 178, 201; viii. 365; xvi. 232; xix. 257; xxi. 272; xxiv. 307, etc.

[2] Book vi. 40. On p. 65 of his *Mythology*, Keightley quotes this passage as apparently somewhat inconsistent with his view, but nevertheless renews his assertion that "the Greeks of the early ages regarded the lofty Thessalian mountain named Olympos as the dwelling of their gods." Compare Völcker: "In nearly all poets such contradictions are found." *Geog.*, p. 6.

[3] *Odyssey*, ix. 527, and elsewhere.

and the gods who possess Olympos are called ὑπερθε μάρτυροι, or the "witnesses on high." [1]

So unmistakable is this language and the entire usage of the Odyssey that various recent writers, not emancipated from the traditional view as respects the Iliad, have yet perceived and admitted the identity of Ὄλυμπος and the upper οὐρανός in the former work. Among German scholars, Faesi [2] and Ihne [3] have expressed themselves in this sense, and prominent among the Scotch, Professor Geddes. [4] The latter says, "There is nothing in the Odyssey which obliges us to think of *Mount* Olympos." Testimony from such a quarter is of course all the more convincing.

In Homeric thought, then, the abode of the gods was where we should antecedently expect to find it, namely, in the heights of heaven. Considered with reference to the august sovereign of gods and men,

[1] *Odyssey*, xiv. 393, 4.

[2] Note on *Iliad*, i. 420, and in *Einleitung* to the *Odyssey*, p. xvii.

[3] Smith's *Dictionary of Biography*, Art. "Homer," p. 510.

[4] *Op. cit.*, §§ 155, 156, pp. 260–263. Professor Geddes' elaborate argument to prove that "the Olympos of the Achilleid" is "a veritable mountain, and that in Thessaly" is entirely inconclusive. The use of ἀγάννιφος no more necessitates a literal interpretation than does a poet's application of the term "snowy" to a living bosom, or "fleecy" to the clouds. So πολύπτυχος proves nothing at all to his purpose, since Euripides — never having read the Professor's instructive statement, "The epithet πολύπτυχος, *applicable only to mountains*, is a sufficient barrier to prevent the identification with οὐρανός" — applies it again and again to many-strata-ed Ouranos. Even the Professor's one only evidence not by his own concession merely "presumptive," to wit, the "great simile" of the *Iliad*, book xvi. 364, tells against rather than for him, for the ἀπ' Οὐλύμπου νέφος cannot possibly come αἰθέρος ἐκ δίης into the atmospheric οὐρανὸν where clouds move, unless Olympos be where the divine ether is, high above the atmospheric heavens. Völcker's treatment of the passage is so absurd that Geddes does not even attempt to follow it. *Hom. Geog.*, § 13.

the polar sky-arch was a palace, the royal residence, the δῶμα or δόμος of Zeus.[1] Viewed with reference to its tints, steel-blue and gold, it was described as metallic, σιδήρεος, χάλκεος and πολύχαλκος, terms which metallic interpreters like Voss and Buchholz and Bunbury have pushed to absolute literalness.[2] Conceived of as an ethereal height, it was pictured as a heaven - high mount, "snowy" as its own white clouds. Then to the climbing imagination, mounting height above height in the vain attempt to reach the summit, the mountain became αἰπύς (Il., v. 367, 869; xv. 84); μακρός (Il., i. 402, and in ten other passages); πολυδειράς (Il., i. 499; v. 754; viii. 3); and πολύπτυχος (Il., viii. 411; xx. 5). This last description, "the Olympos *of many layers, or thicknesses*," is peculiarly expressive. Instead of signifying the "ridges" of a mountain or range of mountains, as Geddes and so many before him have affirmed, it

---

[1] The house of Hephaistos in Olympos is plainly styled "starry." *Iliad*, xviii. 370, comp. with 146, 148. Moreover, Aristotle, or whoever wrote the "Letter of Aristotle to Alexander on the System of the World," in one passage expressly identifies *Ouranos* and *Olympos*, saying that for diverse etymological reasons we call the outermost circumference of heaven by both names. See Flammarion, *Astronomical Myths, or History of the Heavens*, p. 156. Even Völcker, in first laying down the thesis which has so misled all his successors ("dass Uranus und Olympus nie als synonym bei Homer gebraucht werden"), frankly confesses that this is "gegen die bisher allgemein gehegte Meinung;" that is, "contrary to the opinion hitherto generally held." *Homerische Geog.*, p. 4. With gods of Homeric size, a single one of whom required *seven acres* for his couch, the idea of placing the whole Olympian Court and *Götterleben* on the sharp, narrow, clearly visible peak in Thessaly is ridiculous.

[2] Buchholz (*Hom. Realien*, Bd. i. 1, p. 3) declares the metaphorical interpretation "*zu gekünstelt*," for those early times, and roundly asserts that, "according to the idea of the Homeric Greek, heaven is *eine metallene Hohlkugel.*" He should have added that to the same infantile mind Aphroditè was a solid gold image (*Odyssey*, viii. 337), and the voice of Achilles (*Iliad*, xviii. 222) a brass projectile.

pictures that world-old conception of a firmament, not single-storied, but with heaven above heaven, to the "third," or the "seventh," or the "ninth." These heavens were conceived of by Homer himself as in layers one above another, like the curved *laminæ* (πτυχαί) of a shield.[1] And what adds to the fitness of the comparison and to the fitness of the cosmic adornment of Achilles' shield is the fact that to the *omphalos* of a shield there corresponded the central and ever-abiding *Omphalos* of the Skies.

5. Finally, our larger and more rational interpretation of Homeric ideas beautifully explains "the tall Pillars of Atlas," and solves the multiform perplexities of the ruling authorities on this question.

In approaching the study of this subject several questions occur to every thoughtful beginner, the answers to which he can nowhere find. For instance : How can Homer speak of the Pillars of Atlas, using the plural, when elsewhere in the early Greek mythology the representations always point to only one ? Again, if there is but one, and that in the West, near the Gardens of the Hesperides,[2] what corresponding supports sustain the sky in the East, the North, and the South? Or, if Atlas's Pillar

---

[1] See Homer's own τρίπτυχος, *Il.*, xi. 353, in just this sense. Compare the marvelous description in Plato's *Republic*, 616. Depuis had caught the right idea when he penned the words, "*l'Olympe, composé de plusieurs couches sphériques.*" *Origine de Tous les Cults*, tom. i., p. 273. So a recognition of the fact that the nine subterranean, or south polar, Mictlans, or abodes of the dead, of the Aztecs were simply the counterparts of their nine celestial, or north polar, Tlalocans, or heavens, instantaneously clears up the long-standing difficulties of the interpreters of that mythology. See Bancroft, *Native Races*, vol. iii., pp. 532-537.

[2] Hesiod, *Theogony*, 517. Atlas pflegt immer mit den Hesperiden genannt zu werden. Preller, *Griechische Mythologie*, vol. i., p. 348.

is only one of many similar ones supporting heaven around its whole periphery, how came it to be so much more famous than the rest? Or, if Homer's plural indicates that all of them belonged to Atlas, how came the idea of one Pillar to be so universally prevalent? If the support of heaven was at many points, and at its outermost rim, how could Hesiod venture to represent the whole vault as poised on Atlas's head and hands?[1] Again, if it is the special function of Atlas, or of his Pillar, to stand on the solid earth and hold up the sky, he would appear to have no special connection with the sea: why, then, should Homer introduce the strange statement that Atlas "knows all the depths of the sea"? This certainly seems very mysterious. Again, if the office of the Pillar or Pillars is to prop up the sky, they of course sustain different relations to earth and heaven. They bear up the one, and are themselves borne up by the other. Yet, singularly enough, Homer's *locus classicus* places them in exactly the same relation to the two.[2] Worse than this, Pausanias unqualifiedly and repeatedly asserts that, according to the myth, Atlas supports upon his shoulders "both earth and heaven."[3] And with this corre-

---

[1] *Theogony*, 747. Moreover, how could one limited being have charge of so many and so widely separated pillars? "It can scarcely be doubted that the words ἀμφὶς ἔχουσιν, *Odyssey*, i. 54, do not mean that these columns surround the earth, for in this case they must be not only many in number, but it would be obvious to the men of a myth-making and myth-speaking age that a being stationed in one spot could not keep up, or hold, or guard, a number of pillars surrounding either a square or a circular earth." Cox, *Mythology of the Aryan Nations*. London, 1870: vol. i., p. 37 n.

[2] "For that both heaven and earth are meant, not heaven alone, is proved by various poetic passages, and by other testimonies." — Preller, *Griechische Mythologie*, vol. i., p. 348.

[3] Book v. 11, 2; 18, 1. One interpreter makes the profound sug-

sponds the language of Æschylus.[1] But what sort
of a poetic imagination is this which represents a
mighty column as upholding not only a vast super-
incumbent weight, but also, and at the same time,
its own pedestal? Is this a specimen creation of
that immortal Hellenic genius, which the whole modern world is taught almost to adore?

Turning to the authorities in textual and mythological interpretation, our beginner finds no help.
On the contrary, their wild guesses and mutual
contradictions only confuse him more and more.
Völcker tells him, with all the assuring emphasis of
leaded type, that "in Atlas is given a personification
of the art of navigation, the conquest of the sea by
means of human skill, by commerce, and the gains of
commerce." [2] Preller instructs him to reject this
view, and to think of this mysterious son of Iapetos
as a "sea-giant representing the upbearing and supporting almightiness of the ocean in contrast with
the earth-shattering might of Poseidon." [3] The classical dictionaries only perplex him with multitudinous puerilities invented by ignorant Euhemeristic
scholiasts, — stories to the effect that the original
Atlas was merely the astronomer who first constructed an artificial globe to represent the sky ; or
that he was a Northwest African, who, having ascended a lofty promontory the better to observe the
heavenly bodies, fell off into the sea, and so gave

gestion that in Homer's passage the γῆν is " added by a zeugma " !
Merry and Riddell, *Odyssey*, i. 53.

[1] *Prometheus Bound*, 349, 425 *seq.*

[2] *Mythologie des Japetischen Geschlechts*, p. 49 *seq.* Followed by
K. O. Müller, Keightley, Anthon, and many others.

[3] *Griechische Mythologie*, vol. i., pp. 32, 348. Followed by Faesi
and called by Professor Packard "the usually accepted."

name both to the mountain and to the Atlantic Ocean. Schoemann does not profess a positive and certain understanding of the matter, but suggests that the mysterious Titan was in all probability "originally a gigantic mountain-god" of some sort.[1]

Bryant at first makes Atlas a mountain supporting a temple or temple-cave, called *Co-el*, house of God, whence "the Cœlus of the Romans," vol. i., p. 274. In the next volume, however, he says that "under the name of Atlas is meant the Atlantians." And quoting the Odyssey, he translates thus : " *They* [the Atlantians] *had also long Pillars, or obelisks, which referred to the sea, and upon which was delineated the whole system both of heaven and earth ;* ἀμφὶς, *all around, both on the front of the obelisk and on the other sides.*"[2]

If our investigator asks, as did an ancient grammarian, how Atlas could stand on the earth and support heaven on his head, if heaven was so far removed that an anvil would require nine days and nights in which to fall through the distance, Paley kindly explains that "the poet's notion doubtless was that Atlas held up the sky near its junction with earth in the far West."[3] In this case, of course, a reasonably short giant would answer the purpose. If, after all his consultations of authorities, our youth is still unsatisfied, and to make a last effort for light turns to the illustrious Welcker, he learns as an im-

---

[1] G. F. Schoemann, *Die hesiodische Theogonie ausgelegt.* Berlin, 1868 : p. 207.

[2] *Analysis of Ancient Mythology.* London, 1807 : vol. ii., 91.

[3] *The Epics of Hesiod*, p. 229. On the other hand, another English interpreter would give us a giant with shoulders as broad as the whole heaven, and translate ἀμφὶς ἔχουσιν "which support at either side ; *i. e.,* at the East and West." Merry and Riddell, *Odyssey*, i. 53.

portant final lesson that when an ancient author says "heaven and earth," it is not for a moment to be supposed that he literally means "heaven and earth," and that, if they had remembered this, writers on mythology would have spared themselves "a vast amount of brain-racking and ineffectual *pro-and-contra* pleading." [1] With this as the sole outcome of all his researches, may not a beginner well despair of ever getting any knowledge of the meaning of the myth, if, indeed, he can still imagine it to have had a meaning?

Here, as everywhere, the truth at once explains and removes all the difficulties which a false and groundless presupposition has created.

Once conceive of the Homeric world as we have reconstructed it, and how clear and beautiful the conception of the Pillars of Atlas becomes! They are simply the upright axes of earth and heaven. Viewed in their relation to earth and heaven respectively, they are two; but viewed in reference to the universe as an undivided whole, they are one and the same. Being coincident, they are truly one, and yet they are ideally separable. Hence singular or plural designations are equally correct and equally fitting. Transpiercing the globe at the very "navel or centre of the sea," Atlas's Pillar penetrates far deeper than any recess of the waters' bed, and he may well be said to "know the depths of the whole sea." Or this statement may have reference to that primordial

---

[1] "Viel Kopfbrechens und vergeblichen Hin-und Herredens hat der Ausdruck des Pausanias gemacht ἐπὶ τῶν ὤμων κατὰ τὰ λεγόμενα οὐρανόν τε ἀνέχει καὶ γῆν, der auch bei dem Gemälde von Panänos (5, 11, 2) wiederkehrt: οὐρανὸν καὶ γῆν ἀνέχων παρέστηκε, indem man οὐρανὸν καὶ γῆν buchstäblich verstehen zu müssen glaubte." — *Gr. Götterlehre*, vol. i., pp. 746, 747.

sea in which his Pillar was standing when the geogonic and cosmogonic process began. In this sense
how appropriate and significant would it have been
if applied to Izanagi![1]

Again, the association of Atlas with the Gardens
of the Hesperides, so far from disproving our interpretation, actually affords new confirmation, since
Æschylus, Pherecydes, and the oldest traditions
locate the Hesperides themselves, not in the West,
but in the extreme North, beyond the Rhiphæan
Mountains, in the vicinity of the Hyperboreans.[2]
In fact, there are very strong reasons for believing
that these Gardens of the Hesperides were nothing
other than the starry gardens of the circumpolar
sky; that therefore the Hesperides were called
the "Daughters of Night," and that the great ser-

---

[1] Compare the Vedic statement, "He who knows the Golden Reed
standing in the waters is the mysterious Prajapati." Muir, *Sanskrit
Texts*, vol. iv., p. 21. Garrett, *Classical Dictionary of India*, Art.
"Skambha." Still another explanation is suggested by the *Rig-Veda*,
x. 149: "Savitri has established the earth by supports; Savitri has
fixed the sky in unsupported space; Savitri, the son of the waters,
knows the place where the ocean supported issued forth." Muir,
Sanskrit Texts, vol. iv., p. 110 (comp. Ludwig's German version). According to this, he would be conceived of as knowing the depths of
the whole ocean, because its celestial springs are about his head, and
its lowest depths at his feet. — Since the foregoing was first printed
the author has met with the remarkable diagram, published four hundred years ago in the *Magarita Philosophica*, in which Atlas is represented as a venerable man, with his feet at the inferior and his head
at the superior Pole of the heavens, precisely according to our interpretation. A reproduction of it can be seen in Flammarion, *Astronomical Myths*, p. 150. See, moreover, Aristophanes, *Aves*, 180 foll.,
for the significant etymology of πόλος.

[2] Preller, *Griechische Mythologie*, vol. ii., p. 149. Völcker, *Mythologische Geographie*, pp. 133 *seq.* Wolfgang Menzel, *Die vorchristliche
Unsterblichkeitslehre*, vol. i., p. 98. On "*la Colonne dite Boréale*,"
spoken of by a Greek geographer B. C. 275, see Beauvais, *Revue de
l'Histoire des Religions*. Paris, 1883: p. 711 n. Comp. p. 700.

pent which assisted the nymphs in watching "the golden apples" was none other than the constellation Draco, whose brilliant constituent *Alpha*, the astronomer's Thuban, was, less than fifty centuries ago, the Pole-star of our heaven.[1]

Once more, our interpretation perfectly harmonizes the passages which represent Atlas as a heaven-supporter with those which represent him as equally supporting earth. More than this, it reveals the curious fact that Homer's description of the tall Pillars of Atlas identifies them with the axes of earth and heaven so unmistakably that, in order to blunder into the common mistranslation of it, it was first necessary to invent, and get the lexicographers to adopt, a span-new special meaning for the words ἀμφὶς ἔχειν, — a meaning necessitated by no other passage in the whole body of Homeric Greek. Homer's beautifully explicit language is, —

ἔχει δέ τε κίονας αὐτὸς
μακράς, αἳ γαῖάν τε καὶ οὐρανὸν ἀμφὶς ἔχουσιν.

"Who, of his own right, possesses the tall Pillars *which have around them earth and heaven.*" [2] Nowhere in Homeric, if indeed in any ancient Greek, does the expression mean "*to prop asunder.*" [3]

Finally, as to the supposed difficulty of imagining a heaven-upholder so tall that it would take a brazen anvil nine days and nights to fall from his head to his feet, if Professor Paley had remembered Sandalfon, the Talmudic Atlas, he would hardly have

[1] Gustav Schlegel, *Uranographie Chinoise.* La Haye, 1875 : pp. 506, 507, 685.

[2] Compare *Odyssey*, xv. 184.

[3] Buttmann (*Lexilogus,* English translation, 5th ed., pp. 94–104) is no more successful in showing such a meaning than are the older dictionary-makers.

thought it necessary to locate the Hesiodic one on the edge of the earth where the sky is low. Of Sandalfon, Rabbi Eliezer has said, "There is an angel who standeth on earth, and reacheth with his head to the door of heaven. It is taught in the Mishna that he is called Sandalfon; he exceedeth his companions as much in height as one can walk in five hundred years, and that he stands behind the chariot [Charles's Wain] and twisteth or bindeth the garlands for his Creator."[1]

Atlas's Pillar, then, is the axis of the world. It is the same Pillar apostrophized in the Egyptian document known as the great Harris Magic Papyrus, in these unmistakable words: "O long Column, which commences in the upper and in the lower heavens!"[2] It is, with scarce a doubt, what the same ancient people in their Book of the Dead so happily styled "the Spine of the Earth."[3] It is the Rig-Veda's *vieltragende Achse des unaufhaltsam sich drehenden, nie alternden, nie morschwerdenden, durch den Lauf der Zeiten nicht abgenutzten Weltrads, auf welchem* ALLE WESEN STEHEN.[4] It is the Umbrella-staff of Burmese cosmology, the Churning-stick of India's gods and demons. It is the Trunk of every cosmical Tree.[5] It is the shadowless Lance of Alex-

---

[1] Eisenmenger, *Entdecktes Judenthum*, Bd. ii., p. 402 (Eng., vol. ii., p. 97). In all ancient cosmologies "the door of heaven" is at the North Pole. *Sacred Books of the East*, vol. i., pp. 36, 37.

[2] *Records of the Past*, vol. x., p. 152. Other references to the Heaven-supporting Pillar may be seen in Brugsch, *Thesaurus Inscriptionum Ægyptiacarum*, i. 82, 83, 87, 177 *et passim*. Comp. fig. opposite p. 175, and fig. No. 12, p. 124.

[3] Chap. cxlii.

[4] *Rig Veda*, i. 164. Grassmann and Ludwig.

[5] Ludwig, in his version of the *Veda*, finds repeated occasion for the use of the expression "*Stengel der Welt.*"

ander ; the tortoise-piercing (earth-piercing) Arrow of the Mongolian heaven-god ; the Spear of Izanagi ; the Hacha de Cobre on which the heavens of the Miztecs rested.[1] It is the Cord which the ancient Vedic bard saw stretched from one side of the universe to the other.[2] Is it not the Psalmist's "Line" of the heavens which "is gone out through" the very "earth" and on "to the end of the world"? It is the Irminsul of the Germans, as expressly recognized by Grimm. It is the Tower of Kronos. It is Plato's Spindle of Necessity. It is the Azacol of the North African Sunis. It is the Ladder with seven lamps in the rites of Mithra. It is the Talmudic Pillar which connects the Paradise celestial and the Paradise terrestrial.

In the foregoing discussions of Homeric cosmology we have had a sufficient exhibition of the cause and cure of current — malpractice shall we call it? — on the part of interpreters of Homeric poetry. Their baseless assumptions and blunders have been renewed and multiplied in nearly every field of archæology, — Assyrian, Egyptian, Hebrew, Persian, Indian. Whithersoever "modern research" has gone it has carried with it, as a kind of first principle and rule of interpretation, the assumption that the early nations cannot possibly have known anything about the world, beyond what undeveloped tribes and peo-

---

[1] F. Gregorio Garcia, *Origen de los Indios del Nuevo Mundo.* Madrid, 1729 : p. 337. Here, the "pole-axe" of ignorance has supplanted the pole-axis of ancient science. Bancroft, *Native Races*, vol. iii., p. 71. Compare the "Golden Splinter" of Manco Capac. Réville, *Hibbert Lectures*, 1884 : p. 131.

[2] *Rig Veda*, x. 129, 5.

ples would of necessity observe within their own contracted boundaries. The inconsistencies of ignorance and of half-knowledge and of an undisciplined, "child-like" imagination are therefore to be expected at every step. Even the squarest contradictions must not surprise. Indeed, in respect to Homer, the learned Sengebusch has actually formulated the universal proposition that the results of investigations in different departments of Homeric study "will *always* be found to contradict each other."[1] In view of the accepted modern results of investigation into Homer's cosmology one is tempted to justify the proposition, only qualifying it in a mild degree, as follows: The results of all Homeric investigations based upon the assumption that Homer was too "primitive" a man to know where the sun sets will always be found self-contradictory.

Against all such barbarizing misinterpretation of ancient literature it is high time that a protest should be heard. Long enough has the beauty and the breadth of ancient thought, in poetry and myth and even in word-building, been obscured and hidden by this conceited assumption of the modern teacher. It was bad enough when the old grammarians, assuming that Homer could have had no idea of other than the nearest waters, mutilated the grand proportions of the Odyssey to fit the voyagings of its hero into the western basin of the Mediterranean, or, worse yet, into the Euxine.[2] But this, after all, was an altogether pardonable offense

---

[1] Hoffmann, *Homerische Untersuchungen*, vol. i., p. 30.

[2] Mr. W. J. Stillman, in the *The Century Magazine* for 1884, has just resketched in this antiquated fashion "The Track of Ulysses," confessing, however, that for his location of the all-decisive Ogygia "there is no evidence : " pp. 562, 563. See his map.

compared with the currently accepted procedure of
scholars, who, brought up apparently on magazines
of popular science, and imagining that Columbus
was the first man to whom the idea ever occurred
that the earth is round, approach the study of antiquity merely as the study of an older department of
barbarian folk-lore. Surely it is time to investigate
the great creations of ancient mind in a different
spirit.[1] It is nothing short of deplorable to consider
the mass of senseless argument and false explanation annually crowded into the memories of successive classes of academic and collegiate youth, — arguments and explanations which neither to teacher
nor taught have even the poor merit of intelligently
illustrating the evils of wrong principles of classical
hermeneutics. The discussions and results of the
present treatise have at least disclosed a conceivable
beginning of human history, according to which the
early generations of men can hardly have failed to
acquire that knowledge of the mechanism of the
heavens which all the oldest traditions of the race
ascribe to them.[2] And if, in consequence of the

---

[1] " Je tiefer Dr. Schliemann bei Troja grub, desto höhere Cultur
liess sich aus den Funden erschliessen ; so können auch wir sagen, je
älter die Nachrichten sich zeigen, desto grössere Bildung der Vorfah-
ren verrathen sie." Anton Krichenbauer, *Beiträge zur homerischen
Uranographie*, Wien, 1874, p. 13. Comp. 68, 69 *et passim*. The
statement has reference to astronomical science among the earliest
Greeks.

[2] "Among the Jews there are traditions of a very high antiquity
for their astronomy. Josephus says : ' God prolonged the life of the
patriarchs that preceded the Deluge, both on account of their virtues
and to give them the opportunity of perfecting the sciences of geom-
etry and astronomy, which they had discovered ; which they could
not have done if they had not lived 600 years, because it is only after
the lapse of 600 years that the *great year* is accomplished.'

" Now, what is this great year or cycle of 600 years ? M. Cassini,

acceptance or even the discussion of the proffered results, the eyes of scholars shall at last once more be directed to the study of the great literary and other art-works of ancient mind in a new and more modest spirit, the gains which are sure to accrue therefrom will be neither few nor small.

the director of the Observatory of Paris, has discussed it astronomically. He considers it as a testimony of the high antiquity of their astronomy. 'This period,' he says, ' is one of the most remarkable that have been discovered ; for if we take the lunar month to be 29 days, 12 h. 44 m. 3., we find that 219,146½ days make 7,421 lunar months, and that this number of days gives 600 solar years of 365 days, 5 h. 51 m. 36 s.' If this year was in use before the Deluge, it appears very probable, it must be confessed, that the patriarchs were already acquainted to a considerable degree of accuracy with the motions of the stars, for this lunar month agrees to a second, almost, with that which has been determined by modern astronomers." — Flammarion, *Astronomical Myths.* Paris, p. 26.

CHAPTER III.

THE BEARING OF OUR RESULTS ON THE PROBLEM OF THE ORIGIN AND EARLIEST FORM OF RELIGION.

The more I search into the ancient history of the world, the more I am convinced that the cultivated nations commenced with a purer worship of the Supreme Being; that the magic influence of Nature upon the imaginations of the human race afterward produced polytheism, and at length entirely obscured spiritual conceptions of religion in the belief of the people. — A. W. VON SCHLEGEL.

La prétendue évolution de la vie sauvage, telle que la décrit l'école naturaliste en la considérant comme le premier degré du développement de l'humanité, a deux grands défauts: elle part de trop bas, et elle s'élève trop haut; car il lui est impossible d'expliquer les progrès qu'elle constate dans l'humanité, une fois qu'elle la fait débuter par la bestialité complète. — E. DE PRESSENSÉ.

THERE is another class of investigations of re-markable present interest, — investigations lying partly in the anthropological and partly in the theological field of research, — on which the discussions and results of the present treatise have a most important bearing. They are the questions which relate to the Origin, the Primordial Form, and the true History of Religion.

Such light is greatly needed at the present time. As we have seen, all the most ancient traditions of the race represent mankind as having commenced existence in a divine fellowship, and as having lost this holy and blessed estate only through sin. This view of the Origin of Religion has prevailed from the beginning of traceable history among all nations of the earth, varying only to such slight extent as would permit polytheistic peoples to conceive of the primeval divine fellowship polytheistically, and the monotheistic peoples monotheistically. To a monotheist it is significant that several of the ancient nations, representing widely differing races, as for example the Egyptians, the Persians, and the Chinese, seem to have been more monotheistic in their earliest traceable conceptions of religion than in their later and latest creed and practice. But without dwelling upon this, it may be stated as a broad and impressive fact that, with the exception of a few speculative authors, nearly all of whom have lived since the middle of the last century, the solid traditional belief of the whole human family in every age of the world has been that man began his existence pure and sinless, and in conscious and intelligent divine communion.[1] *This is the pan-ethnic no less than the Biblical doctrine of the Origin and First Form of Religion among men.*

It was remarked a moment ago that at the present time new light is greatly needed on this question. The need is special for the reason that for about a hundred years past certain speculative minds, oblivious of the early history of mankind, ignoring the sacred books of all nations, despising the consentaneous convictions of all peoples, and more or less ridiculing the very idea on which religion itself is based, — namely, the idea of the existence and action of extra-human and super-human personalities, — have undertaken to set aside the view which we have above described as the pan-ethnic doctrine of the Origin of Religion, and to substitute

[1] Compare Lenormant, *Beginnings of History*, ch. ii. The Duke of Argyll's *Unity of Nature*. London, 1884 : chapters xi., xii., and xiii.

for it some other explanation, so framed as to make it appear that religion originated from man himself, apart from any divine manifestation, or teaching, or impulse whatsoever. The result has been a succession of crude speculations, inadequate in their premises and contradictory in their respective conclusions. Professing unusual philosophic candor, aided by the interest which always attends novel attempts to set aside the beliefs of ages ; adapting themselves to every class of readers, and especially to all the successively ruling fashions in non-religious and irreligious current speculation, these writers have at last not only wrought a perfect confusion in this portion of the Philosophy of Religion, but have furthermore so degraded and bestialized their readers' conception of primitive humanity, and so outraged all probability in their descriptions of primitive savagery, that even from biological and sociological sides a strong reaction has already set in.

It will be instructive briefly to review the history of these speculations, and to note the successive stages of ever-deepening error and the mutual contradiction of their much-admired results.

The first of them of any note was David Hume, the English deist and champion of philosophic doubt. In his " Natural History of Religion " (published in 1755), he lays down this as his first and fundamental proposition : " Polytheism was the primary religion of mankind."

His first argument in support of this thesis is an appeal to the evidence of post-christian history. He puts it thus : —

" It is a matter of fact, incontestable, that about 1700 years ago all mankind were polytheists. The

doubtful and skeptical principles of a few philosophers, or the theism — and that not entirely too pure
— of one or two nations, form no objection worth regarding. Behold, then, the clear testimony of history.
The farther we mount into antiquity the more do we
find mankind plunged into polytheism. No marks, no
symptoms, of any more perfect religion. The most
ancient records of the human race still present us
with that system as the popular and established
creed. The North, the South, the East, the West,
give their unanimous testimony to the same fact.
What can be opposed to so full an evidence?"

The force of this passage consists almost exclusively in its cool positiveness of dogmatic assertion. Plainly, the condition of the majority of mankind 1700 years ago affords no just criterion by
which to judge of the condition of the race thousands of years before that. Indeed, to any believer
in historic evolution of any sort, it would seem antecedently certain that the condition of men several
thousand years after the commencement of their existence must be very different indeed from their
primitive condition. But, furthermore, he grants
that 1700 years ago the prevalence of polytheism
was, after all, not universal; there were "one or
two nations" of theists, and even philosophers in
other nations, who doubted the truth of polytheism.
It was absurd, therefore, to talk of "the *unanimous*
testimony" of North and South, East and West.

The second point urged by Hume is the improbability of the supposition that "a barbarous, necessitous animal, such as man is, on the first origin
of society," a being "pressed by such numerous
wants and passions," should have had either the

disposition, or the capacity, or the leisure, so to study "the order and frame of the universe" as immediately to be led "into the pure principles of theism." He grants that a careful and philosophic consideration of the unity and order of the natural world is sufficient to conduct one to an assured belief in the being of one Supreme and Almighty Creator, but he says, "I can never think that this consideration could have an influence on mankind when they formed their first rude notions of religion." Assuming that the first men must necessarily have been "an ignorant multitude," he says, —

"It seems certain that, according to the natural progress of human thought, the ignorant multitude must first entertain some groveling and familiar notion of superior powers before they stretch their conception to that perfect Being who bestowed order on the whole frame of nature."

The force of this argument it is difficult to see. It all rests upon two assumptions: first, the assumption that the first men were the lowest barbarians, — to use his own words, "barbarous, necessitous animals;" and, secondly, the assumption that there was, apart from the philosophic study of nature, no other way in which they could have obtained a belief in the existence of the Creator. As no religionist of any age has ever admitted these assumptions, and as Hume adduces no particle of proof for either of them, this part of his argument is surely quite unworthy of a professed philosopher.

His next and last point is the impossibility of the loss of the monotheistic faith if it had once been reached by the earliest men. He says, —

"If men were at first led into the belief of one superior Being by reasoning from the frame of nature, they could never possibly leave [have left] that belief in order to embrace polytheism ; but the same principles of reason which at first produced and diffused over mankind so magnificent an opinion must be [have been] able, with greater facility, to preserve it. The first invention and proof of any doctrine is much more difficult than the supporting and · retaining of it."

Here our author appears to even poorer advantage than in either of his former arguments. In the first place, as before, he ignores the possibility of supposing a knowledge of God by means of a divine self-manifestation, thus covertly misrepresenting or evading the only point in debate. In the second place, the assertion that if the first men had attained to a pure theism they never could have left it and become polytheists should be compared with his own later assertions in Section viii. of the same treatise, where he describes what he himself calls the "Flux and Reflux of Polytheism and Theism." This section opens thus : —

"It is remarkable that the principles of religion have a kind of flux and reflux in the human mind, and that men have a natural tendency to rise from idolatry to theism, and to sink again from theism into idolatry."

The author then states his well-known theory of the origin of polytheism as the first form of religion, and his theory of the rise of monotheism out of polytheism. But when a people have thus reached a belief in a God possessed of "the attributes of unity and affinity, simplicity and spirituality," there comes — so he declares — a natural relapse into polytheism. The explanation of this is given in these words : —

"Such refined ideas [as those of pure monotheism], being somewhat disproportioned to vulgar comprehension, remain not long in their original purity, but require to be supported by the notion of inferior mediators or subordinate agents, which interpose between mankind and their supreme deity. These demi-gods, or middle beings, partaking more of human nature, and being more familiar to us, become the chief objects of devotion. . . . But as these idolatrous religions fall every day into grosser and more vulgar corruptions, they at last destroy themselves, and by the vile representations which they form of their duties make the tide turn again toward them."

Thus monotheism and polytheism are, to Hume, two opposites, between which the human mind forever oscillates. This being so, it is plain that this oscillation is grounded in reason, or it is not. If it is grounded in reason, then primitive men may have reasoned their way into monotheism as their first religious faith, and still have relapsed into polytheism as the natural and rational reaction. On the other hand, if the oscillation is not grounded in reason, then, as by his own account all later religious states of mankind have been unreasonable, the *first* may have been altogether different from what Hume would have considered rational; that is, may have been a state of pure monotheism.

Such was Hume's attempted demonstration of the primitiveness of polytheism, and the whole of it.

Five years later, in 1760, De Brosses, one of Voltaire's correspondents, published his crude but noteworthy book on "The Worship of Fetiches; or, Parallel of the Ancient Religion of Egypt with the Present Religion of Nigritia." This was the writer who first gave currency to the word "fetichism," and who first postulated it as the invariable antecedent of polytheism. De Brosses, however, was a professed believer in primeval divine revelation, and he made the Hebrews an exception to his general claim that all ancient nations began with fetichism, rose thence to polytheism, and tended thence toward monotheism. In the early part of the present century, however, Auguste Comte, ignoring any primeval revelation, elevated De Brosses' generalization into an absolute law of historic development. He gave the greater plausibility and influence to it by representing this law of theological progress as only part of a yet broader social law, according to which humanity, having traversed this "theological stage" in the manner indicated, passes next through a "metaphysical" one, and finally attains the "scientific" stage of atheistic positivism.

In Germany, in 1795, Hume's opinion found an able representative in G. L. Bauer, of Altdorf, and ten years later we see Meiners, in his "Universal History of Religion," repeating and enforcing the notion of the absolute primitiveness of fetichism. The rationalistic and pantheistic tendencies of German speculation about this time were, of course, favorable to any new theory which discredited the Biblical one, and thus it came to pass that before the middle of the present century the De Brosses theory, in its completer Comtean form, became al-

24

most universally adopted. Speaking of its prevalence, Professor Max Müller says:—

"All of us have been brought up on it. I myself certainly held it for a long time, and never doubted it till I became more and more startled by the fact that, while in the earliest accessible documents of religious thought we look in vain for any very clear traces of fetichism, they become more and more frequent everywhere in the latter stages of religious development, and are certainly more visible in the later corruptions of the Indian religion, beginning with the Atharvana, than in the earliest hymns of the Rig Veda."[1]

For many years our works on primeval history have been saturated with this idea. Even professedly Christian writers upon the History of Religions, and upon Comparative Theology, have largely fallen in with the prevailing notion. As one has well said, "The very theory has become a kind of scientific fetich, though like most fetiches it seems to owe its existence to ignorance and superstition."

For some time past, however, this long dominant dogma of naturalism has been losing credit with all careful students of the world's religions, and indeed with the more thorough professional ethnologists. In his recent work, "The Hibbert Lectures on the Origin and Growth of Religion,"[2] Max Müller, himself for a long time, as we have seen, a believer in the theory, publicly challenges its correctness. In Lecture second, after rapidly sketching the rise and remarkable prevalence of the theory, he exposes,

---

[1] *Origin and Growth of Religions.* London and New York, 1879: p. 58.

[2] Reviewed by C. P. Tiele, in *Theol. Tijdschrift,* for May, 1879.

with much acuteness and with his usual wealth of illustrative facts, the indiscriminateness with which the term fetichism has been currently used, and the worthlessness of evidence upon which Comte and others have relied. He sets forth, respectfully but strongly, the inadequacy of their psychological explanation of the origin of fetichism, and shows that even the West African fetich-worshipers hold at the same time other views properly polytheistic, or, in some cases, even monotheistic. Summing up his own conclusions, he says, —

" The results at which we have arrived after examining the numerous works on fetichism from the days of De Brosses to our own time may be summed up under four heads : —

" First. The meaning of the word fetich has remained undefined from its first introduction, and has by most writers been so much extended that it may include almost every symbolical or imitative representation of religious objects.

" Second. Among people who have a history we find that everything which falls under the category of fetich points to historical and psychological antecedents. We are therefore not justified in supposing that it has been otherwise among people whose religious development happens to be unknown or inaccessible to us.

"Third. There is no religion which has kept itself entirely free from fetichism.

" Fourth. There is no religion which consists entirely of fetichism." [1]

So able an *exposé* of the shortcomings of the fetichistic philosophy of the origin of religion, com-

[1] *Origin and Growth of Religions*, p. 115.

ing from the pen of a scholar so widely and deserv-
edly revered, cannot fail to produce in the world of
general readers and second-hand writers a profound
and wholesome impression. Probably the work will
fail of becoming "epoch-making" solely in consequence of something for which the author is not responsible, namely, the fact that in discussing to-day
this dogma of primitive fetichism one is really dealing with an issue which in advanced circles is already dead. Even Mr. Andrew Lang, perhaps the
most antagonistic of all Professor Müller's review-
ers, is not himself willing to make fetichism the
"first 'moment' in the development of religion." [1]
Ten or fifteen years earlier the polemic would have
done many times the good it can now. During this
period a decided change has taken place. There remained a decade or two ago a further step, and but
one further step, for the advocates of the naturalistic
view of the origin of religion to take. Hume had
made polytheism the primitive faith ; Comte thought
to go back of this, and to postulate a still more rudimentary form as antedating polytheism. It remained to go back of fetichism, and predicate of the
first men *absolute atheism.* This various recent authors have done, prominent among whom, in England, is Sir John Lubbock. In chapter iv. of his
work, miscalled "The Origin of Civilization, and the
Primitive Condition of Man," [2] he classifies "the first
great stages of religious thought" as follows : —

First. *Atheism ;* "understanding by this term not

---

[1] *Custom and Myth.* London, 1884 : pp. 212-242.

[2] The first edition was published in 1870. Later echoes are heard
in Mortillet, *Le Préhistorique.* See the *Revue de l'Histoire des Religions.* Paris, 1883 : p. 117.

a denial of the existence of a deity, but an absence of any definite ideas on the subject."

Second. *Fetichism.* In the state of primeval atheism men were " not without a belief in invisible beings." They especially believed in human shadows, ghosts, and the people seen in dreams, etc., though these spirits were not conceived of as immortal, or as possessing any supernatural powers. They were feared only because they were supposed to have power and disposition to inflict disease, or otherwise to injure men yet in the flesh. Now, inasmuch as it was believed that by means of the fetich these evil spirits could be controlled and coerced to the will of the worshiper, fetichism, viewed in its relation to religious development, is pronounced by Lubbock " a decided step in advance." Viewed in itself, " it is mere witchcraft."

Third. *Totemism,* or Nature-worship. This our author nowhere clearly distinguishes from fetichism. In this stage of religious progress, " the savage does not abandon his belief in fetichism, from which, indeed, no race of men has yet entirely freed itself, but he superinduces on it a belief in beings of a higher and less material nature. In this stage everything may be worshiped, — trees, stones, rivers, mountains, the heavenly bodies, plants, and animals."

Fourth. *Shamanism.* " As totemism overlies fetichism, so does Shamanism overlie totemism." Here the gods are conceived of as far more " powerful than men," as " of a different nature," as residing far away, and as " accessible only to the Shamans," who are " occasionally honored by the presence of the deities, or are allowed to visit the heavenly regions." This in its turn is pronounced "a considerable advance" over the preceding stage of religious thought.

Fifth. *Idolatry*, or Anthropomorphism. Here "the gods take still more completely the nature of men, being, however, more powerful. They are still amenable to persuasion; they are a part of Nature, and not creators. They are represented by images or idols."

Sixth. To the sixth stage no name is given; but it is described as one in which "the deity is regarded as the author, not merely a part, of Nature. He becomes for the first time a really supernatural being."

Seventh. In this last and highest stage, which he also leaves unchristened, morality becomes "for the first time associated with religion." [1]

We will not stop to criticise in detail this extremely confused and ill-named classification, or the assumptions on which it rests. Its most characteristic feature is its postulation of universal primitive atheism as antedating every form of religious development in our race. So far as he rested this dogma either upon the affirmed absence of all religious beliefs and usages among the lowest savages of to-day, or upon the principle that the religious conceptions of a people are always in exact proportion to its degree of civilization, his refutation quickly began. The next year after the publication of his work, in a learned treatise on "Primitive Culture," E. B. Tylor challenged several of Lubbock's authorities for the statement that non-religious tribes have been found, while in his new work on "The Human Species,"

[1] Chaps. iv.–vi.

1879, the learned and able Professor of Anthropology in the Paris Museum of Natural History, Quatrefages, went yet further, not only maintaining with Tylor that no atheistic tribe of savages has yet been discovered, but also expressly denying the proposition that elevation of religious conceptions invariably corresponds to the elevation of a people in the scale of general civilization or knowledge of the arts. The fact that these objections to the hypothesis of primitive atheism came, not from theologians, but from scientific men, — from fellow-students in the fields of anthropology and ethnology, — gave them, with many, all the greater weight.[1] The careful reader, however, cannot fail to see that the only difference between Lubbock and some of his critics is merely one of name, and not of thing; that the alleged primitive state which he calls atheistic exactly answers to what Tylor and Darwin would describe as the earliest form of animistic religion, and to what Herbert Spencer would call the first rudimentary beginnings of ghost and ancestor worship. Nor can we fail to see that the consistent Darwinian evolutionist *must* place the beginnings of human history so near the plane of the brute-life as to make it almost certain that its first stage was truly non-theistic, if not, indeed, altogether non-religious.

Precisely at this point notice should be taken of the elaborate work of Otto Caspari, of Heidelberg, entitled "Die Urgeschichte der Menschheit, mit

[1] Professor Roskoff has done Mr. Lubbock the honor to take up every tribe and people, in the extended list which the latter had claimed as non-religious, and to exhibit in every case evidence of their religious character. See his work, *Das Religionswesen der rohesten Naturvölker*. Leipsic, 1880.

Rücksicht auf die natürliche Entwickelung des frühe-
sten Geisteslebens" (" The Primitive History of Mankind, with Respect to the Natural Evolution of the
Earliest Spiritual Life)." This two-volumed treatise
was issued at Leipsic in 1872, and reached a second
edition in 1877. A very large portion of it is devoted to the exposition of the author's view of the
origin and natural evolution of religion in the early
history of the race. This view is characterized
by an originality and elaborated with an ingenuity
which render the book as fascinating to the student
as the most absorbing romance. The author is a
pure and professed evolutionist, but instead of attempting to solve his problem with Lyell and Broca
from the data of Paleontology, or with Darwin and
Häckel from the data of Zoölogy, or with Huxley
and Bastian from the data of Biology, or with Müller and Noiré from the data of Philology, or with
Prichard and Peschel from the data of Ethnology,
or with Tylor and Lubbock from the data of Cul-
ture-History, or with Waitz and Topinard from the
data of General Anthropology, he approaches it and
grapples with it as a problem for that higher and
broader science to which all of the above are tribu-
tary, — the science to which its German originators
have given the name *Völker-Psychologie* (Ethnic or
Anthropic Psychology). He cannot consider the
problem solved until, beginning with the psychological facts of brute-life, we are able to represent to
ourselves the successive steps and stages by which
the originally animal mind slowly evolved all the
spiritual and religious conceptions, emotions, habits,
and ideals of the historic and actual human race.
His own attempt to do this is not free from arbitrary

assumptions or inconsistencies, but, as a whole, it is a marvel of subtile analysis and constructive ability. In contrast with it the expositions of Hume and Lubbock appear as clumsy and grotesque as the early theories of geology, described in Goldsmith's "Book of Nature," now look to the modern student.

One of the oldest of the anti-supernaturalist explanations of the origin of religion is that which ascribes it to the ignorant and superstitious fears of earliest men.

"Primus in orbe deos fecit timor,"

wrote Petronius, and Lucretius' fuller exposition of the same notion is familiar. No such explanation satisfies Caspari. He cannot conceive how fear could ever become that compound of reverence and love which is of the essence of religion. Fear simply prompts the brute to shun, as far as may be, the object feared. Equally unsatisfactory is the notion that the heavenly bodies and the sublimer phenomena of nature inspired the awe and curious questionings out of which religion could have grown. The primitive man, like the anthropoid brute, took no notice of the remote and lofty. Nothing had interest for him save that which was perceived to be vitally related to him in the struggle for existence. The range of his conceptions and of his sympathies was limited to the objects which were his allies or his enemies in this perpetual battle. Religion, therefore, is not to be traced to any inworking of nature, or of natural objects upon the human mind. It had a deeper and yet more obvious genesis in natural human relationships. The first and root form of all piety was filial piety. The first object of truly religious regard was *the parent.* This reverential and affectionate regard of the consciously ignorant, weak, and dependent child for the indefinitely wise, strong, and helpful father or mother is essentially religious. At an extremely early date it must have become extended from the parent to the all-defending and all-regulating tribal chieftain, and to the aged and experienced counselors of the rude primeval communities. The natural tendency of uncivilized men to gesture-language must have produced habitual forms of rendering homage, — the germ of which we may observe in the homage paid by the bees to their queen, — and thus parents, chieftains, and sages were the first objects of religious reverence and homage among men. As yet men had no conceptions of nature as a whole, no intellectual interest in stars, or trees, or animals, no mental provocation to worship anything else than "*the ethically exalted*," as it appeared in the narrow circle of the family and tribal life. There was no thought of an unseen world, no idea of souls, no proper conception even of death. The dead man was supposed to be simply asleep, or in a long swoon. Being self-evidently helpless for the present, like a sick member of the family, he called out natural pity and care. Food and drink were placed in readiness against his awakening. If he had to be left behind, he was put in a cave to protect him against wild beasts, and his weapons were left for his use.

On the basis of this naïve conception of things the rise of animal worship first becomes conceivable. The beast which has devoured a man, living or dead, is now as much man as beast. The man has not ceased to be ; he has simply blended his life in that of the beast, and become a "man-beast." The ferocity of the new compound is easily mistaken for an angry wish on the part of the late man to take vengeance on his relatives or associates for not having more effectually protected him from the devouring animal. But if the "man-beast" is human enough to remember and avenge such real or supposed neglects on the part of his late friends, he must be human enough to recognize and appreciate any wellmeant attempts to appease his anger and propitiate his favor. Hence a natural basis, not for universal animal worship, but for the worship of the more common carnivora, and these Caspari endeavors to show were the first that attained such distinction.

Here, also, is found the origin of cannibalism. A man has killed his foe. If he leaves him merely dead he will some time come to life again as bad as ever. If haply before this some wild beast devour him, he will then become a ferocious and malevolent "man-beast," — a worse enemy than before. There is no way of making the victory final and secure, except by eating him up one's self. Then the life and valor of the slain become life and valor to the slayer. Even the eating of others than foes is in this way made intelligible. As the Fan Negroes are said to eat — " with a certain tenderness " — the bodies of their wives and children, so the primitive man, seeking the safest possible place for the body of his dead friend, may have thought it a far friendlier act to eat him up than to leave him to take his chances at the hand of worms underground, or beasts of prey above it. Between the two motives, the desire to appropriate the vital forces of the foe and the wish to do the best possible thing for the unwakable friend, our author thinks that anthropophagy became in the first age of the world almost universal. The very piety of the surviving toward the dead contributed to the dissemination of the revolting custom.

Our limits will not permit an equally full account of the remaining stages by which religion grew to be what it has been and is in the world. Suffice to say that possible millenniums from the beginning of human history " toward the end of the Stone Age," there occurred the greatest revolution in human thought and belief and life which the race has yet witnessed. This was brought about by the rise and adoption of the belief that trees and men and beasts — in fine, all natural objects — are possessed of invisible, impalpable, vital principles, souls. That which produced and supported this strange, new notion was a discovery which, estimated by the breadth and profoundness of its influence, must be placed at the head of all others, — the discovery, namely, of the art of kindling fire. This mysterious and novel power of evoking what seemed a bright and living being from the realm of the invisible, by means of the "fire-drill," half bewildered even the priestly caste, in whose hands the awful secret lay. Their attempts to use it led to Shamanism and a sincere magic. By means of the observed vital heat of living things and the coldness of the dead the new element was quickly identified with the inner essence of life itself, and the new art the more commended to universal attention by means of its beneficent applications in the hands of the Flamens, or Fire-priests, to the purposes of healing. The same identification of heat and life soon associated phallus and fire-drill, and introduced the strange and apparently monstrous aberration of phallic worship. Under these new ideas it was only natural that sun and star and lightning flash should come to have a new significance for man, and make their impress on religion. Animal worship was profoundly modified in ways ingeniously set forth. The simple oblations of the earlier period give place to sacrifices to fire, and to the heavenly bodies. So strong is the desire to become transformed into white, flaming spirits, and to be joined to the supernal fellowship of such, that men bring themselves as offerings, and seek transfiguration in the holy altar flames. Hence human sacrifices; hence also incremation of the dead. In time, the idea of the soul takes on greater and greater definiteness; so also the idea of the immaterial supersensual gods. The long-continued stimulation of the imagination renders myth-constructions possible. Some of the great priesthoods of history invent hieroglyphic and alphabetic writing, and in time there naturally follow sacred books, cosmogonies, codes of religious laws, etc., etc. The magic wand of the first fire-bringer has at last created a spiritual and unseen counterpart to the world which is seen. In this enchanted world we live to-day; the lowest of us showing our faith by superstitious fetichism, the highest of us by attempts at a purely spiritual worship. That highest Christian conception, "God is light, and in Him is no darkness at all," is simply the culmination of a mode of thinking which started ages ago with the spark which some savage prehistoric flint-chipper struck out of the flinty stone.[1]

[1] Very similar to Caspari's view is that set forth by Professor J. Frohschammer in his late work, *Die Genesis der Menschheit.* München, 1883: pp. 68-381.

The brevity of this sketch of Caspari's theory renders it impossible to do full justice to the skill and plausibility with which he has elaborated it. Still less have we space for that detailed review which would be needed were we to undertake a refutation of the scheme in part or whole.

In striking opposition to the theory of Caspari stands that of Jules Baissac, elaborated in his " Origines de la Religion." [1] He, too, begins with primitive animality, and proposes to trace the rise and natural evolution of religion from that far-off starting-point of the human race. But, instead of magnifying the initial influence of a pure domestic life in Caspari's truly German method, Baissac — in a manner characteristically French, shall we say ? — starts with a deification of mere maternity, conceived of as self-originating and self-sufficing. This form of religion prevailed during the remote period anterior to the time when it was discovered that males had any participation in the procreation of the species. The religious symbols of that far-off age were "les élévations et tumescences terrestres, naturelles ou artificielles, et les cavités souterraines ; les tumescences comme image du sein maternel en état de pregnation et les profondeurs et cavités comme ventre sacré de la divine mère. De là le culte des ballons ou montagnes à croupe arrondie ; de là le symbolisme des tumuli, des pyramides, des grottes, des puits, des labyrinthes, des dolmens." In this period all motherhood is divine, and all life and change in nature are mentally represented as a spontaneous, and exclusively female, conceiving and bringing forth.

[1] Paris, 2 tomes, 1877. Compare Baring-Gould, *Religious Belief*. New York, 1870: Part I., pp 411–414.

In the second period, which is still anterior to the idea of marriage and to the establishment of the idea of personal property or individual rights, the function of the male principle has been discovered ; and now Nature, the divine mother, is conceived of as analogous to a woman of the period, — a mother fecundated only by male energy, but by male energy from any quarter. To use Baissac's own terms, she is a " prostituée divine, ayant son symbole dans la terre ouverte à tous les germes." [1]

In the third period the two principles are brought into a relation of equality, and now the divine becomes hermaphrodite.

In the fourth the male principle is given priority, the religious symbols of maternity give place to the phallic symbols, the institutions of marriage and property arise, the power of atmospheric and celestial divinities begins to supersede that of earth-spirits. The fifth stage is marked by the entire predominance of these celestial divinities and the definite rejection of the ancient chthonian and subterranean powers. In the sixth comes the final separation of the Heaven and the Earth, the idea of creation, and the idea of an almighty and transcendent Creator of all things.

The manner in which the author elaborates this remarkable interpretation of the history and symbolism of religion, through two octavo volumes of 300 pages each, is as ingenious as it is disgusting.

Behold the savory outcome of these successive philosophic and scientific rebellions against history ! And whom of all these wise men of the West shall we follow? The first form of religion, says one of

[1] *Origines,* p. 131.

them, was an animal hallucination of the early anthropoids respecting sexual generation. No, says another, it was a genuine worship of invisible gods and goddesses, like the beautiful Olympian divinities of Greece, — a religion whose fruits in character and conduct compare most favorably with those of Christian monotheism.[1] Absurd! exclaims a third. "Polytheism" is a very high type of religion; men never could have reached that until after the invention of the fire-drill, nobody knows how many ages from the beginning. Fools all! rejoin the more thorough-going. Know ye not that primitive men were far lower than our lowest modern savages, — as incapable of any religious ideas as they were of using the integral calculus?

At the beginning of the exposition of these speculations it was intimated that their contradictory and incredible outcome had already provoked a degree of reaction even from biological and sociological writers. This reaction is too instructive to leave unnoticed.[2] It comes from men who, religiously or theologically speaking, seem in full sympathy with the rejecters of the old Biblical and pan-ethnic faith; but they find they cannot go along with these rejecters without surrendering more than any biologist or sociologist can afford to surrender if he would maintain a credible philosophy of the history of man and of human society. To a simple disciple of history the spectacle of their embarrassment and of their attempts at extrication is in an eminent degree entertaining. Indeed, the best refutation of whatever is wrong in all these new conceptions of

---

[1] Hume's above-cited *Essay*, closing sections.
[2] Compare *Revue des Deux Mondes*, April, 1880, pp. 660–665.

primordial religion will be found, not in a blind and indiscriminate polemic against them *en masse*, but in showing how every departure from the traditional conception involves the careful thinker in perplexing if not insoluble problems, and how easily all the real facts on which these proposed departures are based can be arrayed in support of the traditional conception. To this task we turn.

First, then, according to Genesis, the earliest representatives of the human race began their existence in Paradise unclad, unhoused, and possessed of none of the outward and visible signs of what is called civilization. Had Mr. Lubbock been permitted at the time to visit the spot, he would have seen — so far as Moses suggests — no printing-press, no power-loom, perhaps not even a "fire-drill" or flint "arrow-head." He would have seen no god, no Miltonic guard of angels, no Eden gates, *no temple or altar.* He would have noticed in the luxuriant tropical landscape simply a wealth of graceful animal forms, rising in manifold gradations, and culminating in two fair human figures. He would doubtless have gone his way, and reported at the next meeting of the Anthropological Society the discovery of a new Otahcite, whose naked and artless inhabitants were evidently at the bottom of the scale as respects "culture," and in the sub-fetichistic "atheistic stage" as respects religion. So doing, he would have committed no greater blunder than many of his favorite reporters have made in describing such people as the Andaman Islanders.[1]

---

[1] For the complete vindication of this statement see Sir Henry Sumner Maine, *Early Law and Custom*, London, 1883, pp. 229–231 ; Quatrefages, *The Human Species*, New York, 1879, chap. xxxv. ; and

25

According to the old conception, no less than according to the new, the arts were only gradually developed. Men were destitute of the art of metal-working and of all to which that was essential until the days of Tubal Cain. Musical instruments there were none until invented by Jubal. Everything in sacred Scripture indicates the kind of social and industrial progress for which, in connection with the beginnings of human society, one would naturally look.

So far, then, the believer in Sacred History has no occasion whatever to disagree with the believer in Natural History. Häckel and Peschel and Caspari hold, with Moses, to the monogenesis of the race, and even place their imaginary "Lemuria" just under the northern portion of the Indian Ocean, hard by one of the traditional seats of Eden. Their account of man's migrations from that centre, and of his primeval destitution of the arts, conflict with no fact recorded in Holy Scripture. Neither party can tell precisely how long the period antecedent to the rise of the first great historic civilizations of Asia, Egypt, and Greece lasted, and neither can tell how long ago it terminated, so that even in their confessed ignorances both are in accord.

But, secondly, the believer in Sacred History, Hebrew or Ethnic, cannot accept the eagerly advocated notion that the intellectual condition of the earliest men was not higher than that of the lowest savages of to-day. Ignorant of many things those earliest generations must have been, but it is equally certain

especially Roskoff, *Das Religionswesen der rohesten Naturvölker*, Leipsic, 1880, and Réville, *Les Religions des Peuples non-civilisés*, Paris, 1883, tom. i., ch. i.

that they must have been above the line which sep-
arates stationary or retrograding peoples from progressive ones.   They were men capable of investigating the powers and laws of nature, of originating
arts absolutely new in the history of the world, and
of making successive inventions which revolution-
ized the social state.

With this representation we should expect the
Darwinian, on sober second thought, to agree.   For
it is a well-known fact that our lowest savages are
dying out, while the men who peopled the world in
accordance with the law of the survival of the fittest,
at a period in the earth's history when, in important
respects, according to Darwin, the environment was
less favorable to the human struggle for existence
than now, must have been superior to these degenerating and vanishing tribes.   And as all evo-
lutionists, in enumerating the qualities which win
in the struggle for existence, lay great stress upon
superior intellectual endowments, it is only a natural inference that the native intelligence of the
earliest men was at least superior to that of the lowest modern savage.   Turning to the writers in question we find our antecedent expectations confirmed.
Thus Mr. Herbert Spencer, in one of his matur-
est works, expresses himself as follows : "There
are sundry reasons for suspecting that existing men
of the lowest types, forming social groups of the
simplest kinds, do not exemplify men as they originally were.   Probably most of them, if not all of
them, had ancestors in higher states, and among
their beliefs remain some which were evolved during those higher states. . . . There is inadequate
warrant for the notion that the lowest savagery has

always been as low as it is now. . . . That supplanting of race by race, and thrusting into corners such inferior races as are not exterminated, which is now going on so actively, and which has been going on from the earliest recorded times, must have been ever going on. And the implication is that remnants of inferior races, taking refuge in inclement, barren, and otherwise unfit regions, have retrograded." [1]

In like manner Darwin himself conceives of the first men as capable of rising in thought above the knowledge furnished by the senses, *as able to represent to themselves the unseen and spiritual.* And he expressly calls their mental faculties "high," saying, "The same high mental faculties which first led men to believe in unseen spiritual agencies, then in fetichism, polytheism, and ultimately in monotheism, would infallibly lead him, so long as his reasoning powers remained poorly developed, to various strange superstitions and customs." [2] Thus Darwin justly considers the character of the very aberrations of the human intellect in its infantile stage a striking proof of the loftiness of its powers.

Lubbock ascribes to the earliest men a like ability to conceive of the supersensual and to govern themselves largely by ideals. Though sometimes describing the primitive generations as in a state of "utter barbarism," or as having been "no more advanced than the lowest savages of to-day," this seems to occur only by inadvertence; for in the later editions of his already quoted work, "The Origin of Civilization," page 483, he expressly admits and asserts that he does not regard cannibals as repre-

---

[1] *Principles of Sociology,* pp. 106–109.
[2] *Descent of Man,* vol. i., p. 66.

sentatives of the first men.[1] On the same page he says, "It may be as well to state emphatically that all brutal customs are not, in my opinion, primeval. Human sacrifices, for instance, were, I think, certainly not so."

Caspari no less emphatically affirms that the social state of the North American Indians and of the Australians is not primitive, but a result of degeneration. He says, " We know a succession of such tribes, of which, in fact, only *ausgeartete verkommene Banden und staatliche Splitter* remain in existence, who, wild and savage, wander about in the primitive forests, miserably to perish." [2]

Tylor takes the same general ground, maintaining that the best representatives of primitive men are not the lowest but " the higher " of the uncivilized races. Thus he says, " In a study of the nature-myths of the world it is hardly practicable to start from the conceptions of the very lowest human tribes, and to work upward from thence to fictions of higher growth ; partly because our information is meagre as to the beliefs of these shy and seldom quite intelligible folk, and partly because the legends they possess have not reached the artistic and systematic shape which they attain to among races next higher in the scale. It therefore answers better

---

[1] Let us hope that it is by a like inadvertence, merely, that Professor Sayce speaks of " the savage tribes of the modern world, and *the still more savage* tribes among whom the languages of the earth took their start." *Introduction to the Science of Language*, vol. ii., p. 31. Compare p. 269, where, speaking of the mythopœic man, whom he considers a considerable advance on the primitive savage, the professor says, " He had not yet learned to distinguish between the lifeless and the living ; " " he had not yet realized that aught existed which his senses could not perceive."

[2] Vol. i., p. 113.

to take as a foundation the mythology of the North American Indians, the South Sea Islanders, and other high savage tribes *who best represent in modern times the early mythological period of human history."* [1]

In chapter ii. of the same work he presents the evidence that many of the very lowest tribes of the modern world have become what they are by degeneration.

But, thirdly, if the best representatives of the first men must be sought, not among the lowest, but rather among the higher, of the uncivilized peoples, then surely we are justified in rejecting the notion of all those writers who, since the time of De Brosses and Comte, have maintained that primitive men personified and vitalized and fetichized all natural objects about them.

On this point the author of the "Outlines of Cosmic Philosophy" is less clear-sighted than his master, Herbert Spencer. Boldly and ably as he criticises Comte in some other particulars, in this Mr. Fiske surrenders to him wholly. He says, "We may safely assert, with Comte, that the earliest attitude assumed by the mind in interpreting nature was a fetichistic attitude." [2] Spencer, however, recognizing the fact that the lower mammals, birds, and even insects are able to distinguish animate from inanimate objects, and that to deny this capacity to the first men would be to make them less and lower than animals, commits himself unreservedly to the view in harmony with that of the Biblical record. Quoting the stock examples of savages who, on

[1] *Primitive Culture,* vol. i., p. 321.
[2] Vol. i., p. 178, *et passim.*

first seeing a watch or a compass, imagined that it was alive, he shows the naturalness of the mistake, and very properly says : "We must exclude these mistakes made in classing things which advanced arts have made to simulate living things, since such things mislead the primitive man in ways unlike those in which he can be misled by the natural objects about him. Limiting ourselves to his conceptions of these natural objects, we cannot but conclude that his classification of them into animate and inanimate is substantially correct. Concluding this, we are obliged to diverge at the outset from certain interpretations currently given of his superstitions. The assumption, tacit or avowed, that the primitive man tends to ascribe life to things which are not living is clearly an untenable assumption. Consciousness of the difference between the two, growing ever more definite as intelligence evolves, must be in him more definite than in all lower creatures. To suppose that without cause he begins to confound them is to suppose the process of evolution inverted." [1]

This writer, therefore, whom Darwin in one passage calls "our great philosopher," explicitly rejects the dogma of the primitiveness and universality of animism and fetichism among the earliest men. According to him, animistic and fetichistic beliefs were not "primary beliefs ;" they were errors into which "the primitive man was betrayed during his early attempts to understand the surrounding world." "The primitive man no more tends to confound animate with inanimate than inferior creatures do" (p. 146).

[1] *Principles of Sociology*, pp. 143, 144.

Caspari, too, as we have seen, denies to fetichism a primitive character.[1] Ascribing its rise to the new ideas which the discovery of the art of fire-kindling produced, he makes the worship of "the morally exalted" (*des sittlich Erhabenen*), represented by the personal father, the tribal chieftain, and the deceased ancestor, far older, possibly thousands of years older, than any worship of fetiches. With Lubbock there is no moral element in religion until it reaches its last and highest stage. With Caspari, on the contrary, religion is essentially moral in its first emergence, and has from the first moment of its existence an actual and relatively worthy personal object. This is a prodigious scientific advance from the positions of Hume, Comte, Lubbock, and all their followers, and by postulating a high moral nature and moral life at the very beginnings of human history it renders the Biblical conception of those beginnings not only conceivable, but even antecedently probable.

Fourthly. The Bible and the sacred traditions of nearly all peoples present monogamy as the first form of marriage, ascribing all deviations from it to the ungoverned selfish passions of men. This view, Lubbock and the writers whom he has followed, McLennan and Morgan, emphatically reject. These theorists claim that among the first men the late

---

[1] Compare the like utterance of Frohshammer : "Mit Fetischismus hat das Gottesbewusstsein und religiöse Cultus nicht begonnen." *Die Genesis der Menschheit.* München, 1883 : p. 71. Also, the recent declaration of a learned Professor of Roman Law : " Die religiöse Anschauung aller Völker ist, denke ich, ausgegangen von dem Glauben an Einen göttlichen Willen, welcher über Allen und zu Oberst waltet." J. E. Kuntze, *Prolegomena zur Geschichte Roms.* Leipsic, 1882 : p. 23.

Oneida Community system of "complex marriage," or, as Lubbock calls it, "communal marriage," universally obtained. The appropriateness of the term *marriage* is very far from clear. The first communities were mere herds, in which all the women were "wives" to all the men. In McLennan's opinion "the next stage was that form of polyandry in which brothers had their wives in common ; afterward came that of the *levirate, i. e.*, the system under which, when an elder brother died, his second brother married the widow, and so on with the others in succession. Thence he considered that some tribes branched off into endogamy, others into exogamy ; that is to say, some forbade marriage out of, others within, the tribe. If either of these two systems was older than the other, he held that exogamy must have been the more ancient. Exogamy was based on infanticide, and led to the practice of marriage by capture. Lubbock, on the contrary, believes that the communal marriage, which he assumes to have been the primitive form, "was gradually superseded by individual marriage founded on capture," and that this led, first, to exogamy, and then to female infanticide, thus reversing Mr. McLennan's order of sequence. "Endogamy and regulated polyandry, though frequent," he says, "I regard as exceptional and as not entering into the normal progress of development." [1] Still different is the theory of Bachofen, set forth in his work entitled "Das Mutterrecht." Assuming sexual promiscuity as the primordial state, he considers that under this system the women, instead of being rendered more and

[1] *Origin of Civilization*, pp. 94, 95. Compare D. McLennan, *The Patriarchal Theory*. London, 1884: p. 355.

more debauched and corrupted by the practice, as we might suppose, became on the contrary, in process of time, so refined, that after a season they felt shocked and scandalized by the beastly state of things, revolted against it, and established a system of marriage with female supremacy, the husband being subject to the wife, property and descent being required to follow the female line, and women enjoying the principal share of political power.

Gradually, however, the more spiritual ideas associated with fatherhood prevailed over the more material ideas associated with motherhood. The father came to be considered the real author of life to the offspring, the mother a mere nurse; property and descent were traced in the male line, sun-worship superseded moon-worship, men absorbed all political power, — in a word, as primitive "Hetairismus" was followed by the "Mother-Law" system, so this now gave way to the modern social state.

The chief evolutionist authorities disagreeing so widely on this point, it is surely proper to look further. So doing, we find a number of at least equally respectable, scientific and speculative representatives of the evolutional school, who expressly question, if they do not openly reject, the dogma of universal sexual promiscuity as the primeval social state. Thus Herbert Spencer argues through many pages of his "Principles of Sociology" against McLennan, claiming that monogamy must be conceived of as going back to the beginning. However unsettled social and sexual relations then were, "promiscuity," he affirms, "was checked by the establishment of individual connections prompted by men's likings, and maintained against other men by force" (p. 665).

Again he says, " The impulses which lead primitive men to monopolize other objects of value must lead them to monopolize women " (p. 664). And again, " Monogamy dates back as far as any other marital relation " (p. 698). Darwin takes substantially the same view, positively discrediting the alleged sexual promiscuity of the earliest communities.[1]

In like manner another of the latest of English writers on this subject, James A. Farrer, in his book entitled " Primitive Manners and Customs," [2] emphatically rejects the notion that a brutal and forcible bride-capturing was ever universal, and denies that the customs relied upon by McLennan and others to prove its prevalence are to be viewed as a survival of such a custom. As to the absolutely first form of marriage he does not express an opinion, but the theory of primitive monogamy would better agree with his general representation than any other. The same may be said of Caspari, who, though he does not expressly postulate the priority of monogamy, yet ascribes to filial piety a rôle in the first origination of religion which seems to necessitate such a postulate.[3] So Mr. John Fiske's suggestion that the transition from the anthropoid animals to truly human beings was probably effected by the prolongation of infancy and of parental care incident to the slower evolution of a highly complex organism, and by the family life thus necessitated and brought about, is more harmonious with the doctrine of primitive monogamy than with any other. It would not be surprising, therefore, if this class of

---

[1] *Descent of Man,* vol. ii., pp. 362–367.
[2] London, 1879.
[3] See vol. i., pp. 322, 358, 367.

considerations, which we meet again in Noiré's theory of the origin of language, should gradually lead to such a reconstruction of Darwinistic sociology as will postulate monogamy as the one and only form of sexual relation by virtue of which man could have arisen out of the lower and preceding animal orders. Mr. Spencer calls Mr. Fiske's suggestion "an important" one, and he explains it in a note appended to a significant declaration respecting the biological and sociological value of monogamy (p. 630). Elsewhere, after stating that "irregular relations of the sexes are at variance with the welfare of the society, of the young and of the adults," and after ascribing the gradual dying out of the Andamanese to their promiscuity of sexual relation,[1] he says, "We may infer that the progeny of such unions (as had a degree of exclusiveness and durability) were more likely to be reared and more likely to be vigorous" (p. 669). Again, a page or two later, he uses this language : "As under ordinary conditions the rearing of more numerous and stronger offspring must have been favored by more regular sexual relations, there must on the average have been a tendency for those societies most characterized by promiscuity to disappear before those less characterized by it " (p. 671). But Spencer himself must grant that in the earliest ages, upon the whole, the race multiplied and spread from generation to generation, so that we must at least conclude from his own declaration, that the approximately monogamous societies and

---

[1] Mr. E. H. Man's recent paper on the Andaman Islanders (*The Journal of the Anthropological Institute*, vol. xii., i. 69, and ii. 13) denies the alleged sexual promiscuity, and illustrates the worthlessness of much of the evidence on which popular ethnographers rely.

unions were more numerous than the approximately promiscuous ones. Well, therefore, may Mr. Lang, our latest advocate of McLennan's theory, concede the possibility that " man *originally* lived in the patriarchal or monogamous family," and seek to content his fellow sociologists with the assurance that " *if there occurred a fall from the primitive family,* and if that fall was *extremely general,* affecting even the Aryan race, Mr. McLennan's adherents will be amply satisfied." [1]

Fifthly. The Bible represents the earliest men as capable of entertaining the conception of a supreme Divine Being, the Maker of the heavens and earth, the Creator and rightful Lord of men. It represents them as capable of realizing the moral obligation of obedience to the Creator, and as possessed of freedom to obey or to disobey. It gives us to understand that, as a matter of fact, a few then as now were faithful to their light and to their convictions of duty, while the greater part lived in conscious violation of the promptings of their own consciences. As a natural consequence immoralities multiplied : these demoralized and brutalized those who practiced them. Then demoralized and brutalized parents were followed by children less well instructed and less well endowed than they themselves had been, and so, despite exceptional men and exceptional families who were more faithful to conscience, the general demoralization went on. The song of Lamech, Gen. iv. 23, 24, is the song of a true savage, though of one who has known the law of right and duty. One can hardly read it without imagining it first sung in a kind of domestic war-dance in the hut of

[1] *Custom and Myth.* London, 1884 : pp. 246–248.

its polygamous author. He glories in his homicides, and evidently belongs to those who with savage lust and brutality "took them wives of all which they chose." He was a representative of his Cainite kindred. By the mass of these and those who intermarried with them the Father and Lord of all creatures was ignored and gradually misconceived, and at last superseded by creations of man's own disordered mind and heart, until the pure primitive religion of the righteous patriarchs became a false worship as irrational and immoral as the mass of those who gave themselves to its loathsome and cruel practices. With some populations this abnormal and immoral evolution proceeded to thoroughly unnatural and self-destructive results, such as religious prostitution, sodomy, human sacrifices, cannibalism, etc. On the other hand, then as now, fidelity to truth and goodness led its possessor to larger knowledge and to higher spiritual experiences. Then as ever the principle held good, "To him that hath shall be given." Hence alongside and within and above the historic evolution of a large portion of the race from evil to evil there was another evolution of a smaller but more vital portion from good to good. If Satan's kingdom steadily unfolded, so did also the kingdom of God. And while the one was in the direction of spiritual and physical degeneration and death, the other was in the direction of life and ultimate spiritual ascendency. Both of these partial or special evolutions were within and part of the universal evolution of the race under its preëstablished nature and conditions, one of which fundamental conditions is its immanency in the Divine. Such is the picture presented us by all the monotheistic religions of the world, and it is substantially confirmed by most of the ancient traditions of the human race.

Now in all this there is nothing inconsistent with any well-established facts or principles of science. Some authorities which Lubbock himself quotes prove not only that uncivilized tribes are capable of entertaining the theistic conception of the world, but also that not a few of them when first found actually possessed remarkably high and pure conceptions of the Supreme Spirit and of man's relation to him. Thus he cites Livingstone as saying that " the uncontaminated African believes that the Great Spirit lives above the stars." In trying to prove the absence of prayer among certain savages, he admits witnesses who show that the Esquimos, the North American Indians, and the Caribs believed in the existence of a Supreme Spirit, the " Master of Life." He even quotes the following objection to prayer made by Tomochichi, the chief of the Yamacraws, to General Oglethorpe, to wit: " That the asking of any particular blessing looked to him like directing God ; and if so, that it must be a very wicked thing. That for his part he thought everything that happened in the world was as it should be ; that God of himself would do for every one what was consistent with the good of the whole ; and that our duty to him was to be content with whatever happened in general, and thankful for all the good that happened in particular." What civilized religionist, what purest monotheist, ever apprehended or expressed this theological problem more clearly than did this Indian chief ? Lubbock quotes another author as saying that the Caribs considered the Great Spirit as endowed with so great goodness that he does not take revenge even on his enemies.[1]

So Mr. Tylor allows not only that most barbarians are able to conceive of a Creator, but also that they actually believe in one. He says : —

"Races of North and South America, of Africa, of Polynesia, recognizing a number of great deities, are usually and reasonably considered polytheists, yet their acknowledgment of a Supreme Creator would entitle them at the same time to the name of monotheists," if belief in a Supreme Deity, held to be the Creator of the world and chief of the spiritual hierarchy, were the sufficient criterion of monotheism. "High above the doctrine of souls, of divine manes, of local nature spirits, of the great deities of class and element, there are to be discerned in savage theology shadowings, quaint or majestic, of the conception of a Supreme Deity." [2]

He illustrates the prevalence of this conception by facts related of barbarous peoples in almost every quarter of the globe. Speaking of the remarkable clearness of this idea and belief among the New Zealanders, the Hawaiians, the Tongans, Samoans, and other representatives of the Polynesian race, he says : —

"Students of the science of religion who hold polytheism to be but the misdevelopment of a primal idea of divine unity, which in spite of corruption continues to pervade it, might well choose this South Sea Island divinity as their aptest illustration from the savage world." [3]

[1] *Origin of Civilization*, pp. 374, 375.
[2] *Primitive Culture*, vol. ii., p. 332.
[3] Compare Quatrefages, pp. 486–495

He quotes Moerenhout as saying : —

"Taaroa is their supreme, or rather only, God; for all the others, as in other known polytheisms, seem scarcely more than sensible figures and images of the infinite attributes united in his divine person."

He adds the following sublime native description of this Supreme God : —

" He was ; Taaroa was his name ; he abode in the void. No earth, no sky, no men. Taaroa calls, but naught answers; and alone existing he became the universe " (p. 345).

Though an outspoken opponent of the theory that polytheism arose from moral and spiritual degeneration, his own facts are so strong that for the explanation of some of them he is constrained to resort to it. Speaking of the "conceptions of the Supreme Deity in the savage and barbaric world," he says, " The degeneration theory may claim such beliefs as mutilated and perverted remnants of higher religions, in some instances no doubt with justice."

That a religion originally good and pure may degenerate and become corrupt is conceded even by Lubbock. At the close of his sketch of "the lowest intellectual stages through which religion has passed," he uses this significant language : —

" I have stopped short sooner, perhaps, than I should otherwise have done, because the worship of personified principles, such as Fear, Love, Hope, etc., could not have been treated apart from that of the *Phallus, or Lingam*, with which it was so intimately associated in Greece, India, Mexico, and elsewhere ; and which, though at first modest and pure, — as all religions are in their origin, — led to such

26

abominable practices that it is one of the most painful chapters in human history." [1]

Reading this, the disciple of history simply asks, If men could so corrupt the originally modest and pure worship of Aphrodite, why not also the originally pure worship of El?

Sixthly. The disclosure of the Arctic Eden solves all further difficulties in the Hebrew conception of the religious development of mankind.

This doctrine as to the cradle of the race concedes to the devotee of prehistoric archæology all his claims as to the lowly beginnings of every *historic* civilization developed in our postdiluvian seats of humanity. It welcomes every revelation which fossil bone, or chipped flint, or lacustrine pile, or sepulchral mound has ever made, finding in it precious illustration of those "times of ignorance" through which our expatriated race has made its passage (Acts xvii. 30; Rom. i. 18–32). It is equally ready for every conclusion of the scientific anthropologist. By his own doctrine of the power of environment, and by his own picture of Mammalian life in Tertiary and Quaternary times, it constrains him to admit that if the Eden of Genesis was at the Pole, the Biblical picture of Antediluvian Man, with his extraordinary vigor and stature and longevity, with his extraordinary defiance of the authority of God, and with his extraordinary persistence in the indulgence of self-centred passions and appetites and ambitions, is credible in the highest degree. And that nothing may be lacking to its perfect confirmation, the comparative mythologist discovers that in this new Eden he is given the master-key to his

[1] *Origin of Civilization,* p. 350.

own science, and that every great system of ancient mythology and of mythological geography must now be freshly and intelligently interpreted in the light of it. The old, old stories of a Golden Age, of the Hesperidian Gardens, of the Tree of Golden Fruit, of the Hyperborean Macrobii, of the insurrection of the Titans, of the destruction of mankind by a Flood, are history once more. Their authenticity as history is attested by new and unchangeable evidences, — by witnesses as unbribable as the axis of the earth and the pole of the heavens. No more can the investigator of the history and philosophy of religion rule out the ancient myths of humanity as senseless, or seek to interpret them as results of an inevitable " disease of language." No more can they be palmed off upon us as capricious variations of that myth of dawn, or of the sun, or of the storm, which we are told that the fancy of " primitive " men is ever weaving. They are simply blurred chapters from the neglected and abused and almost lost Bible of the Gentiles, confirming and establishing the opening chapters of our own.

Summing up, then, we see : 1. That in rejecting the historical conception of the primeval religious belief of mankind Hume took up a position which none of his own successors consider as at all tenable.

2. The further these successors have carried their revolt against history, the more have they become involved in contradiction with each other.

3. The more consistently and radically the dogma of primitive savagery has been carried out, the more inevitably has it landed its advocates in the doctrine of primitive bestiality.

4. In their eagerness to destroy the possibility or credibility of primeval monotheism, these more consistent and radical theorists have inadvertently gone so far as to render a self-consistent evolutional biology or sociology impossible.

5. In consequence hereof the more clear-sighted of the representatives of Darwinism are just now deftly re-approaching the long-scouted historic conception, by representing the first men as superior to the modern savage in intellectual endowment, by calling their powers high, by considering their judgments of natural objects substantially correct, by admitting their knowledge of the true and normal form of the family, by conceding to them a truly human appreciation of ethical excellences and obligations, by allowing to them a capacity to conceive of an almighty Supreme Spirit, the Author and rightful Governor of the world, and by recognizing that nearly all religions present clear traces of corruption. So far as principles are concerned these representations surrender their whole case. With these data Adamic Revelation becomes quite as possible and quite as credible as Abrahamic, or Mosaic, or Christian Revelation.

6. The *Anlage* for religion is no product of age-long advances in civilization and in the arts. The unclad Adam of the garden was no more incapacitated for the knowledge of his Father than was that naked second Adam, for whose advent Mary provided the swaddling-clothes. If the former seems too undeveloped to be an organ of divine revelation, the latter, the highest of all these organs, the absolute Revelator, began quite as low. If nomad Arabs of to-day can see in storm and stars sublime mani-

festations of one almighty personal Power, why could not the nomadic Abel as well? If the Gospel messenger of to-day can cause the rudest Fijian to know God and to experience a sense of divine forgiveness and favor, why may not God's earliest preachers of righteousness have produced a like effect on sincere souls before the discovery of the art of metal-working? Once let the anthropological and sociological postulates demanded even by Herbert Spencer be granted, and the ancient historic conception of Primitive Monotheism becomes both possible and eminently reasonable. As an escape from the conflicting and mutually destructive theories of the naturalistic school in its different departments, it presents, on merely speculative grounds, a positive attractiveness. Its full array of evidences, however, is simply co-extensive and identical with the evidences for the reality of Historic Revelation as a whole. Everything which goes to show that God has intelligibly revealed himself to men at all bears more or less directly upon the credibility of a Revelation "*in the beginning.*"

7. Lastly, the Arctic Eden completes the reconciliation of Biblical and secular learning in their relations to the problem of the primitive religion of men. As we have seen, both science and theology now find in this primeval *Bildungsherd* at the Pole ·the one prolific centre whence all the floral and faunal and human life-forms of the whole earth have proceeded. In an "environment" of such creatively potent, world-overflowing nature-forces as were there, any culmination of life's manifestations short of a "Golden Race" of men, kingly in stature, *Rishis* in intelligence, measuring their *Deva*-like

lives by centuries, would have been an incongruity. That a loving Creator — creating because loving — should have put himself into instant personal communion with these highest of his creatures, moral natures fashioned in his own image and after his likeness, children of his love, is to a theist, even an ethnic theist, the only credible representation. That such a lusty race should have been open to temptation on the line of apparently innocent aspiration after still higher perfections, that they should have desired to "be as gods," that they should have coveted experimental and personal knowledge of evil as well as of good, — these are suppositions which no serious anthropologist will pronounce inadmissible. That the actual revolt of such an order of moral agents from the true law and basis of its life should have carried into its subsequent historic developments consequences of profoundest import is as much a necessary implication of the law of heredity and of the established constitution of nature as it is an instinctive inference from the preconceived character of a perfect Moral Governor. Given such antediluvian men, one must pronounce the history of antediluvian religion, as reported in the oldest memories and in the most sacred scriptures of humanity, a self-attesting chronicle.

CHAPTER IV.

THE BEARING OF OUR RESULTS ON THE PHILOSOPHY
OF HISTORY AND THE THEORY OF THE DEVELOP-
MENT OF CIVILIZATION.

*It would be a valuable contribution to the Study of Civilization to have the ac-
tion of Decline and Fall investigated on a wider and more exact basis of evidence
than has yet been attempted.* — E. B. TYLOR.

*L'or fut certainement le premier métal que l'on connut. . . . Les trois ages des
poètes, l'age d'or, l'age d'airain, et l'age de fer sont une réalité, et non une fiction.*[1] — A. DE ROCHAS.

BESIDES their philosophies of religion, the apostles
of universal primeval savagery have also their Philosophy of Human History and of Social Progress.
First of all, they would have us believe that man has
existed upon the Earth hundreds of thousands of
years,[2] and that for at least the first hundred thousand years, possibly for twice or thrice this period,

[1] *Revue Scientifique*, Paris, September 22, 1883.

[2] With an impressive attempt at accuracy Professor Mortillet
says, "at least 230,000 to 240,000 years." *Le Préhistorique*, p.
627. Haeckel says, "in any case more than 20,000 years," "probably more than 100,000 years," "perhaps many hundred thousand
years." *Natürliche Schöpfungsgeschichte*, p. 595. Mr. John Fiske,
building upon Croll, thinks that "the human race has covered both
the eastern and the western hemispheres for thousands of centuries,"
and that the period during which man has possessed sufficient intelligence to leave a traditional record of himself is "only an infinitesi-
mal fraction" of the time. In one passage he fixes on the period of
"eight hundred thousand years," and at one time Lyell and others
favored the same duration. *Cosmic Philosophy*, ii. 320, 295. Compare on the other side Southall, *The Recent Origin of Man*, Phila.,
1875, and *The Epoch of the Mammoth and the Apparition of Man
upon the Earth*, Phila., 1878.

he lived like a wild beast in thickets and dens and caverns of the earth.[1] His one occupation was the struggle for existence. The very cave in which his wretched young were sheltered from the storm was continually exposed to invasion by the cave-hyena and the cave-bear, fiercer and more powerful than the modern type. His multitudinous enemies were all provided with offensive and defensive armor, — with tusk and fang, with claw and beak, with lances steeped in never-failing deadliest poisons. To every foe they could oppose an almost impenetrable hide, a mail of horny scales, a solid shell. He, by strangest anomaly, was destitute of all. He was a naked and defenseless babe in the Indian jungle of Earth's fierce and venomous carnivora. He had not a weapon, not an implement with which to shape one. Even had he had implements ever so good, he would not have known enough to fashion himself the rudest club from the branch of a tree. He had not yet "learned to look up" to where the tree branches grew. "Habit as

---

[1] "In the dim mist of bygone ages our ancestors lived the life of wild beasts in forests and caves." Élisée Reclus, *Ocean, Atmosphere, and Life,* vol. ii., p. 190. "We must assign to him the position of a savage, but of a savage as far below the buffalo-hunting Pawnee as the latter is removed from the cultivated representative of the Caucasian race." Rau, *Early Man in Europe.* N. Y., 1876: p. 162. "On such a view" as that "of the modern naturalist, *savage life itself is a far advanced condition.*" Tylor, *Primitive Culture,* vol. i., p. 37. "All our recent investigations in Europe into the state of the arts in the earlier Stone Age lead clearly to the opinion that at a period many thousands of years anterior to the historical, man was in a state of great barbarism and ignorance, *exceeding that of the most savage tribes of modern times.*" Lyell, *Principles of Geology,* vol. ii., p. 485. For a contrary view see the Duke of Argyll's chapter "On the Degradation of Man" in his *Unity of Nature.* London, 1884: pp. 374-447.

well as nature kept his eyes fixed upon the ground." As we saw in the preceding chapter, he supposed that "the branches of the trees extended quite to heaven, hiding themselves in infinitely remote ethereal regions." Indeed, according to some of these advocates, this precious "primitive man" could not distinguish a tree when he saw it. He was not at all certain that its outspreading roots and branches were not the legs and arms of a fellow-man who happened to grow in that particular way. So says a "generally-understandable-scientific lecturer" of Germany, Dr. Wilhelm Mannhardt. Let us note his exact statement: "However inconceivable it may be to us moderns, there truly was a time when people were *unable to make any conceivable distinction between a plant and a man.*"[1]

It is somewhat to be feared lest writers of this sort have been a little precipitate in rejecting so determinedly the traditional idea of extraordinary antediluvian longevity. For if the earliest generations of mankind were in truth such idiotic specimens as here represented, the great problems as to the possibility of their defending themselves against the bloodthirsty and powerful carnivora by which they were

---

[1] " Alle lebenden Wesen, vom Menschen bis zur Pflanze, haben Geborenwerden, Wachsthum und Tod miteinander gemein, und diese Gemeinschaft des Schicksals mag in einer fernen Kindheitsperiode unsers Geschlechts so überwältigend auf die noch ungeübte Beobachtung unserer Vorältern eingedrungen sein, dass sie darüber die Unterschiede übersahen, welche jene Schöpfungsstufen voneinander trennen. So unbegreiflich es uns Modernen klingen mag, hat es in Wahrheit eine Zeit gegeben, in der man keinen begreiflichen Unterschied zwischen einer Pflanze und einem Menschen zu machen wusste." *Sammlung gemeinverständlicher wissenschaftlicher Vorträge, herausgegeben von Rudolf Virchow und Franz von Holtzendorff.* Nro. 239. Berlin, 1876.

surrounded, and as to the possibility of their learning
sufficiently early how to wring a subsistence from
the unfriendly soil, must give place to the still more
perplexing and more fundamental problem as to the
possibility and credibility of primitive procreation
itself. To say nothing of the question as to the
whence of the very first of these feeble and down-
looking intelligences, it is plain that if ever they
did have successors to take up and carry forward
and upward their type of life, in some way and *at
some time within the natural life of the first individuals,* — incredible as it may be " to us moderns,"
— it must (happily for us) have dawned upon some
man's mind, or on whatever then occupied the place
of his mind, that between Daphne (or whoever was
practically the first woman) and a tree *some* distinction was discernible. And as the friends who
give us such witless ancestors are prodigal to a fault
in their allowance of ages of time whenever any
ordinary geological or zoölogical result is to be
reached without troubling a Higher Power, it seems
to a calm on-looker a very penurious and illogical,
not to say cruel, procedure to require these embry-
otic representatives of incipient humanity to create,
or rather to evolve and bring to *practicable* perfection, the high arts and sciences of intelligent per-
ception, of human as distinguished from dendrolog-
ical physiology, of gynecology and obstetrics, — all
within the few swift years of a modern human lifetime. With "two hundred and thirty thousand to
two hundred and forty thousand years " at his command, or even "many hundred thousand," we really
hope Dr. Mannhardt will see his way to reconsider
this point, and to deal with the *protistoi* of the hu-

man world in a more liberal and truly evolutionistic spirit.[1]

Happily, the apostles of what De Maistre calls the *banale* hypothesis of primeval savagery have done their worst, and doing this have shattered their own party into an indefinite number of mutually antagonistic factions, each protesting against all who happen to be more thorough-going and radical than themselves. Thus Spencer is in array against McLennan, Caspari protests against Mannhardt, Vogt endeavors to outdo Darwin, and so on to the end of the chapter. The modern Babel is worse than the ancient. To one surveying at the present time the different departments of science which relate to Man, it would seem as though in each the breakdown of the theory of primitive human brutishness and imbecility were complete, though not yet publicly proclaimed and acknowledged. A review of the situation, with authentic citations of the dissen-

---

[1] There is some evidence that the geologists are becoming increasingly skeptical as to the time-pieces relied upon by the ruling school of paleontological anthropologists. For example: "The present rates of the retrocession of Niagara, or of the deposit of Nile mud, or of stalagmite in caverns, or of the accumulations of the rocks themselves, or of the movement of glaciers, have been vainly used as natural chronometers, on the assumption that they have been going on at the same rate through all the past, and have been warranted never to stop, or to want winding up, or to go faster or slower than at the moment the observer was looking at them. Such attempts are so obviously futile that it is not a little strange to find them seriously made by men like Wallace and Mortillet." W. Boyd Dawkins, "Early Man in America." *North American Review*, Oct., 1883, p. 338. See also "The Niagara Gorge as a Chronometer," by G. Frederick Wright, in the *Bibliotheca Sacra*, and in the *Am. Journal of Science* for 1884. Still more significant is the alarmingly revolutionary "Opening Address" delivered last summer in Montreal before the Geological Section of the British Association by President W. T. Blanford, F. R. S., and printed in *Nature*, Sept. 4, 1884, pp. 440 ff.

tient and often contradictory utterances of representative leaders, would be most timely, but the task must be left to other and more competent hands. Here, foregoing all exposures of such a kind, we will simply suggest to the reader a few obviously important memoranda : —

1. Considered in the light of antecedent probabilities, there is no discoverable reason, or apology for a reason, why the first *Homines* should have been but half-witted, any more than those perfect *Nautili* which, ages earlier, with astounding skill navigated the old Silurian seas.[1]

2. Given Human beings, normally endowed at the beginning, and we see experience everywhere showing how all the savagery of past and present history could easily and naturally have originated simply from disregard of natural and moral law.

3. Given at the beginning nothing but Animal powers, and we find nothing in the whole range of experience, from the first dawn of history until now, paralleling or in any wise rendering intelligible the hypothetical biological legerdemain of Nature by which these zoölogic powers were once, *and once only,* transmuted into Human.[2]

[1] Since these pages were placed in the printer's hands the following has appeared in the scientific journals : "A discovery by Dr. Lindström in the Silurian rocks of Gotland is worthy of special notice. In beds which are said to be the equivalent of our Niagara group he has discovered a remarkably well-preserved scorpion. Dr. Thorell, one of the foremost students of Arachnida in the world, and Dr. Lindström are preparing a paper upon it, and have given it the name of *Palæophoncus nuncius.* No scorpions, nor indeed any Arachnida, have before been found fossil in beds lower than the carboniferous deposits, in which some twenty-five species have been found in this country and Europe ; *yet this Silurian example is more perfect than any specimen of a fossil scorpion from any formation.*"

[2] "That man, equally with the monad and the Conferva, owes his

4. If Paleontology presents to us certain types of life which indicate in their successions a certain progress, it must not be forgotten that the same science presents us other types, whose successions with equal clearness reveal a progressive degeneracy and an ultimate disappearance. The movement may be forward, but it *may* also be backward. "As to the class Reptilia," says Sir Charles Lyell, "some of the orders which prevailed when the Secondary rocks were formed are confessedly much higher in their organization than any of the same class now living. If the less perfect Ophidians, or snakes, which now abound on earth had taken the lead in those ancient days among the land reptiles, and the Deinosaurians had been contemporary with Man, there can be no doubt that the progressionist would have seized upon this fact with unfeigned satisfaction as confirmatory of his views. Now that the order of succession is precisely reversed, and that

origin to a protoplasmic germ, in which are contained all the possibilities of his after development, is no piece of scientific romance, but demonstrable truth. . . . All forms of protoplasm, however alike in appearance and composition science may and does declare them to be, are not identical in their potentialities. They do not, in other words, all possess similar powers of becoming similar organisms. The speck which remains an Amœba has no power of evolving from its substance a higher form of life. The protoplasmic spore of a seaweed is a seaweed still, despite its similarity to other or higher forms of plant-germs. The germ of the sponge, again, remains possessed of the powers which can convert it into a sponge alone. And the differences between such protoplasmic specks and the germ which is destined to evolve the human frame can only be declared as of immense extent, and as equaling in their nature the wide structural and functional distinctions which we draw betwixt the sponge and the man. Of such differences in the inherent nature of protoplasm under different conditions we are as yet in complete ignorance." — Andrew Wilson, Ph. D., F. L. S., *Chapters on Evolution.* London, 1883: pp. 74, 75.

the age of the Iguanodon was long anterior to that
of the Eocene palæophis and the living boa, while
the crocodile is in our own times the highest representative of its class, a retrograde movement in this
important division of the vertebrata must be admitted."[1] With this agrees the emphatic declaration of
Andrew Wilson : "A study of the facts of animal
development is well calculated to show that life is
not all progress, and that it includes retrogression
as well as advance. Physiological history can readily be proved to tend in many cases towards back-
sliding instead of reaching forwards and upwards to
higher levels. *This tendency, beginning now to be
better recognized in biology than in late years,* can
readily be shown to exercise no unimportant influence on the fortunes of animals and plants."[2] In
view of these facts of retrogression, the latest writers
on the history of life on our planet, even when professing, with the last-quoted author, to accept of
Darwin's philosophy as true, are at the same time
very generally saying, "It cannot be the whole
truth."[3]

---

[1] *The Antiquity of Man*, Philadelphia ed., p. 402.

[2] Andrew Wilson, Ph. D., F. L. S., *Chapters on Evolution*, p. 343
(italics ours). See pp. 342–365. The progress of paleontological
research is constantly bringing new illustrations to light. *Revue Scientifique*. Paris, 1884: p. 282. Even in our late age of the world
"highly specialized forms of life are in fact numerically a minority of
living beings." E. D. Cope, "On Archæsthetism," in the *American
Naturalist*. Phila., 1882 : vol. xvi., p. 468. Compare same writer
on "Catagenesis," in vol. xviii. (1884), pp. 970–984.

[3] What could be more striking and impressive than the following
fresh testimony from this field : "The flora of the whole Paleozoic
period . . . is very distinct from that of succeeding times. Still, the
leading families of *Rhizocarpeæ, Æquisetaceæ, Lycopodiaceæ, Filiceæ,*
and *Coniferæ,* established in Paleozoic times, still remain, and the
changes which have occurred *consist mainly in the degradation of the*

5. Again, by the same testimony of the rocks, life need not, of necessity, either advance or retreat ; it may stand as first originated from age to age. Says Professor Nicholson, "There are various groups, some of them highly organized, which make their appearance at an extremely ancient date, but which continue throughout geological time almost unchanged, *and certainly unprogressive. Many* of these *'Persistent Types'* are known, and they indicate that under given conditions, at present unknown to us, it is possible for a life-form to subsist for an almost indefinite period without any important modification of its structure." [1]

6. All arguments for the alleged self-evolution of the Human Race out of preceding animal races, based upon an alleged universal and uniformly progressive self-evolution of life-forms in the animal kingdom, are, in view of the above facts, arguments originating in ignorance or in fraud.

7. According to the teachers of the current agnostic anthropology and atheistic history, modern Man is the supreme product, the crowning glory, of the cosmic life-process, at least so far as our planet is concerned. Yet, by their own concessions, through all the unmeasured æons during which this being has been maturing and perfecting, the Earth has steadily been losing its life-giving warmth, its once delightful and almost equable climate has slowly

three first families, and in the introduction of new types of Gymnosperms and Phænogams. These changes, delayed and scarcely perceptible in the Permian and Early Mesozoic, seem to have been greatly accelerated in the Later Mesozoic." Principal Dawson, "On the More Ancient Land Floras of the Old and New Worlds." Paper read before the British Association in Montreal, Aug. 1884. *Nature,* p. 527.

[1] *Life-History of the Earth,* p. 371, 2.

given place to Sahara heat and Arctic cold, its once luxuriant flora has yielded to types of marked inferiority, and its degenerating fauna ceased to come up to the measure of the stature of preceding forms.[1] This is saying that one and the same secular Deterioration of Environment has devitalized and degraded all forms of life *save one*, but that, unaided and alone, it has elevated that one to the physical, intellectual, and spiritual kingship of the world.[2]

8. In proportion as the discussions and conclusions of this treatise have vindicated and illustrated the trustworthiness of the most ancient Traditions with reference to the location of the first abode of the race, in precisely the same degree have they authenticated and verified those same Traditions as trustworthy sources of information with respect to Man's primitive state, his intellectual powers, and his knowledge of the Divine.

Finally, the varying Power of Man over Nature, dwindling whensoever by vice he descends beastward, increasing whensoever by virtue he ascends

---

[1] " The Pliocene period is the declining age of the European flora, the time when the climatic conditions are definitively altered, when the vegetation gradually becomes poor and ceases to gain anything. The progress of the phenomenon is slow, but it moves along an inclined plane, on which it never stops. Those ornamental plants, those precious trees, those noble and elegant shrubs, which are now care fully trained by artificial culture in European conservatories were until then inhabitants of Europe, but they left it forever. One by one the ostracised plants take their departure, lingering here and there on the road to exile. It is this exodus that we should have to describe, if we could follow step by step the march of retrogression, and indicate species by species the progress and the result of this abandonment of our soil." — G. de Saporta, *Le Monde des Plantes avant l'Apparition de l'Homme.* Noticed in *Am. Journal of Science,* 1879, p. 270.

[2] See above, page 100, note.

Godward, is to a truly scientific and philosophic eye full of significance. The slightest study of the manifestations of this power in history inwardly convicts us of unfaithfulness, as a race, to the true law of our being. We cannot help feeling that we ought to be lords of Nature. Our actual relation to the cosmic forces is not, and in historic time never has been, the ideal and true relation. It was no narrow-minded "bibliolater" who penned the following expression of this feeling ; it was Ralph Waldo Emerson : "As we degenerate, the contrast between us and our house is more evident. We are as much strangers in Nature as we are aliens from God. We do not understand the notes of birds. The fox and the deer run away from us ; the bear and the tiger rend us. . . . Man is a god in ruins. When men are innocent, life shall be longer, and shall pass into the immortal as gently as we awake from dreams. Man is the dwarf of himself. Once he was permeated and dissolved by spirit. At present he applies to Nature but half his force. . . . Meantime, in the thick darkness, there are not wanting gleams of a better light, — occasional examples of the action of man upon Nature with his entire force. Such examples are the traditions of MIRACLES in the antiquity of all nations, the HISTORY OF JESUS CHRIST, the achievements of a principle in political revolutions, the miracles of enthusiasm, the wisdom of children. . . . *The problem of restoring to the world original and eternal beauty is solved by the redemption of the soul.*"

The above is an utterance as true and deep as it is beautiful and poetic. And here in this ancient and Biblical conception of Man's relation to Nature

27

is given the sun-clear solution of the whole controversy between the advocates of universal racial and
technological degeneration, on the one hand, and the
advocates of universal racial and technological pro-
gression, on the other. Both parties are right and
both are wrong. The one has vindicated and em-
phasized one vital class of facts ; the other, another
class equally vital. Christian thought interprets and
harmonizes them both. It shows us through all human history racial and social and technological decadence wherever men have rejected or. ignored God.
It shows us, on the other hand, racial and social and
technological progress wherever men have acknowledged and lovingly served that Divine One in whom
we live and move and have our being. Here, then,
is the law of true human progress. As Emerson
in his more Christian moods would put it, The restoration of the lost harmony between Man and his
House must begin with the *Redemption of his Soul.*

As to the primeval condition of our race, a truly
scientific mind will wish to base its conception not
on the air-hung speculations of mere theorists, but on
an immovable foundation of fact, attested and confirmed by the widest, oldest, and most incontestable
of all concurrences of divine and human testimony.
According hereto, as in its beginning light was light,
and water water, and the Spirit spirit, so in his beginning *Man was Man.* It says that the first men
could not have been *men* without a human consciousness, and that they could not have had a human consciousness without rationality and freedom.
It says that they could not have possessed conscious rationality and freedom without the percep-
tion of ethical qualities and the personal taste of

moral experiences. It boldly asserts that, according to every principle of just analogy, the notion that it took the earliest men one hundred thousand years to get an idea of the conditions of normal intellectual, and ethical, and social living is as incredible as that it took the first-born mammal one hundred thousand years to find its mother's milk. It calls attention to the fact that all the oldest historic peoples of every continent unite in the testimony that the first men had knowledge of superhuman personalities, good and evil. It dwells upon the equally universal tradition that primeval human life, while progressive in everything which accumulating human experience would of necessity improve, was yet from the first the life of decidedly super-bestial, almost god-like intelligences, as daring ultimately in evil as potent originally for good. It holds on the same authority that after centuries and possibly millenniums of such history as great natures undisciplined by virtue are ever reproducing, the social organism was incurably corrupted and the moral world-order itself defied. As Plato's Egyptian priests told Solon, "the divine portion in human nature faded out;" the purely human "gained the upper hand," and, spoiled by the very excellence of their fortune, "men became unseemly. To him who had an eye to see they appeared base, and had lost the fairest of their precious gifts. They still *appeared* glorious and blessed, at the very time when they were filled with unrighteous avarice and violence. Then the GOD OF GODS, who rules with law, and is able to see into such things, perceiving that an honorable race was in a most wretched state, and wanting to inflict punishment upon them that they might

be chastened and improved," made fresh announce-
ments of divine penalty and promise, to the end
that haply He might recall them to that earlier and
better life, when they had "despised everything but
virtue, neither were intoxicated by luxury;" when,
being "possessed of true and great spirits, they practiced gentleness and wisdom in their intercourse
with one another;" when they "were obedient to
the laws and well affectioned toward the gods." [1]
These gracious endeavors of Divine compassion
proving fruitless, the integrity of the world's rational purpose and significance could be conserved
only by penalty, and by a new moral and physical conditioning of the race. No change of moral
administration could suffice, since every wise appli-
ance of *merely moral* influence and instruction had
been exhausted. A new physical environment and
conditioning was essential to the new moral methods
which, in this critical juncture, Humanity was need-
ing. The inbringing of such a new physical environment would of itself carry to human consciences,
individual and social, the profoundest and most ef-
fectual of moral meanings. Both the physical and
the moral change came in that world-convulsion
which Plato calls "the Great Deluge of all." In it
perished what Hesiod and Ovid and so many others
called the "Golden Race" of men, — the first, the
fairest, the strongest, the longest-lived of all that
ever bore the human form divine. Under its waters
were engulfed precious accumulations of science,
the primordial creations of art, the *incunabula* of all
literature. So sore was this loss of man's costliest
possessions that either myth or truthful history has

[1] *Critias,* 120.

filled the early Shemitic world with the pathetic story that the God of gods, while arranging for the righteous judgment upon the ungodly, Himself still so compassionated the successors and heirs of its unhappy victims as to command the patriarchal minister of His will to make an indestructible monumental record of all that the progenitors of a new Humanity would need to know.[1]

The new physical conditions under which the race was placed were the conditions brought in by the Diluvian cataclysm. They involved (1) expatriation, the great Glacial Age compelling an entire abandonment of the mother-region of the human family ; (2) dispersion, the frozen and sterilized condition of even what is now the North Temperate zone rendering the struggle for the means of subsistence a most arduous and difficult one ; (3) deterioration of physical constitution corresponding to the biological conditions of the new and deteriorated environment ; and (4), as a natural consequence of the whole, an abbreviation of the normal longevity previously enjoyed. Being at the same time reduced to the lowest social unit in the way of organization, — the Family, — and being, in consequence of the poverty of Nature's provision, compelled to spread in proportion as it multiplied, the new Humanity of "the world which now is" was signally guarded against the repetition of those insolent and God-defying forms of sin in consequence of which a nemesis of cosmical proportions had overtaken the antediluvian world.[2]

[1] Josephus, *Antiquities*, i. 2, 3. Lenormant, *Beginnings of History*, p. 445. Polar "Sippara" and the "Siriad land" are one.

[2] The events described in Gen. xi. 1-9 may have occurred "*in* the Front-country" (v. 2). See above, page 221, note 1.

Such is the conception of primeval human history which the oldest traditions of the oldest nations set over against this late-born dream of "primitive savagery." It is the conception of the whole Christian world — of the whole Jewish world — of the Mohammedan world — of the ancient Greek and Roman world — of the world of the eldest Asiatic and Egyptian antiquity. It is the irrefutable *Selbstzeugniss* of the Human Race respecting facts of which it has the knowledge of a living and most interested participating witness.[1]

According to the results of this treatise the primitive seat of the world's first civilization was outside the boundaries of all lands known to recorded history. This being so, Mr. Tylor's confident challenge has for the present quite lost its force. "Where," he exclaims, — "where now is the district of the Earth that can be pointed to as the primeval home of Man which does not show by rude stone implements buried in its soil the savage condition of its former inhabitants?"[2] The "cave-men" of Europe can as little illustrate man's antediluvian condition as Robinson Crusoe's cave could illustrate Westminster Cathedral. *Postdiluvian* civilization, or barbarism, whichever one may choose to call it,

---

[1] "The men of old time . . . must surely have known the truth about their own ancestors. . . . How can we doubt the word . . . as they declare that they are speaking *of what took place in the family?*" Plato, *Timæus*, 40. It is satisfactory to note that that undervaluation of oral tradition which is inseparable from the theory that man is merely an improved beast, and which shows its natural fruit in such free-handed reconstructors of history as Professors Kuenen and Wellhausen, has proceeded so far that even rejecters of the traditional estimate of the Pentateuch and of the Old Testament are beginning to react restively against it. See APPENDIX, Sect. VII.

[2] *Primitive Culture*, vol. i., p. 60.

may be studied in "Stone Age" implements and products wherever we may find them, but never should it be forgotten that, back of all dawnings of new knowledge and new arts here revealed, lay the fuller knowledge and the more perfect arts of a favored antediluvian world.[1]

Let no one say that the profession of such an opinion betrays the prejudice of a Christian education; that it is ignoring the fruits of a century's study; that it is simply repristinating the doctrine

[1] In his late work, entitled *India : What can it teach us ?* (London, 1883) Professor Max Müller well challenges the first principles of our dominant school of " Culture-students," as follows : " What do we know of savage tribes beyond the last chapter of their history ? Do we ever get an insight into their antecedents ? Can we understand what, after all, is everywhere the most important and the most instructive lesson to learn, how they have come to be what they are ? There is, indeed, their language, and in it we see traces of growth that point to distant ages, quite as much as the Greek of Homer, or the Sanskrit of the Vedas. . . . Unless we admit a special creation for these savages they must be as old as the Hindus, the Greeks, and Romans ; as old as we ourselves. We may assume, of course, if we like, that their life has been stationary, and that they are to-day what the Hindus were no longer than three thousand years ago. But that is a mere guess, and is contradicted by the facts of their language. They may have passed through ever so many vicissitudes, and what we consider as primitive may be, for all we know, a relapse into savagery, or a corruption of something that was more rational and intelligible in former stages. Think only of the rules that determine marriage among the lowest of savage tribes. Their complication passes all understanding. All seems a chaos of prejudice, superstition, pride, vanity, and stupidity. And yet we catch a glimpse here and there that there was some reason in most of that unreason ; we see how sense dwindled away into nonsense, custom into ceremony, ceremony into force. Why, then, should this surface of savage life represent to us the lowest stratum of human life, the very beginnings of civilization, simply because we cannot dig beyond that surface ? " A hundred years hence the story that the wise men of the nineteenth century sought to reconstruct the beginnings of human history by the study of the lowest contemporary savages will be one of the choicest of popular illustrations of the folly of " ante-scientific times."

of a forgotten Goguet, and seeking to resurrect the long dead Banier. If any reader is tempted to such utterances, it is possible that an imaginary conversation may help him to juster conclusions.

Let us fancy ourselves at Cnossus, upon the shores of Crete, hundreds of years before the Christian era. A traveler has just landed, — a Greek from Athens, intent upon visiting the celebrated temple and cave of Zeus. As he is walking to the temple he falls in with two companions, the one an intelligent Cretan, the other a traveler from Lacedæmon. After due salutations they naturally discourse of the laws and institutions of the country, of their origin, and of the origin of all states and laws and civilizations. And this we may imagine is a part of their conversation : —

The Athenian : Do you believe that there is any truth in ancient traditions ?

The Cretan : What traditions ?

Ath. The traditions about the many destructions of mankind which have been occasioned by deluges and diseases, and in many other ways, and of the preservation of a remnant.

Cr. . Every one is disposed to believe them.

Ath. Let us imagine one of them : I will take the famous one which was caused by a Deluge.

Cr. What is to be remarked thereon ?

Ath. I should say that those who then escaped would only be hill shepherds, — small sparks of the human race preserved on the tops of mountains. Such survivors would necessarily be unacquainted with the arts of those who live in cities, and with the various devices which are suggested to them by interest or ambition, and all the wrongs which they contrive against one another.

Cr. Very true.

Ath. Let us suppose, then, that the cities in the plains and on the sea-coast were utterly destroyed at that time. Would not all implements perish and every other excellent invention of political or any other sort of wisdom utterly fail at that time?

Cr. Why, yes; and if things had always continued as they are at present ordered, how could any discovery have ever been made even in the least particular? For it is evident that the arts were unknown during thousands and thousands of years. And no more than a thousand or two thousand years have elapsed since the discoveries of Dædalus, Orpheus and Palamedes, — since Marsyas and Olympus invented music, and Amphion the lyre, — not to speak of numberless other inventions which are but of yesterday.

Ath. Have you forgotten the name of a friend who is really of yesterday?

Cr. I suppose that you mean Epimenides.

Ath. The same, my friend; for his ingenuity does indeed far overleap the heads of all your great men; what Hesiod had preached of old, he carried out in practice, as you declare.

Cr. Yes, according to our tradition.

Ath. After the great destruction, may we not suppose that the state of man was something of this sort. In the beginning of things there was a fearful illimitable desert and a vast expanse of land; a herd or two of oxen would be the only survivors of the animal world; and there might be a few goats, hardly enough to support the life of those who tended them.

Cr. True.

Ath. And of cities or governments or legislation, about which we are now talking, do you suppose that they could have any recollection at all ?

Cr. They could not.

Ath. And out of this state of things has there not sprung all that we now are and have : cities and governments, and arts and laws, and a great deal of vice and a great deal of virtue ?

Cr. What do you mean ?

Ath. Why, my good friend, how can we possibly suppose that those who knew nothing of all the good and evil of cities could have attained their full development, whether of virtue or of vice ?

Cr. I understand your meaning, and you are quite right.

Ath. But, as time advanced and the race multiplied, the world came to be what the world is.

Cr. Very true.

Ath. Doubtless the change was not made all in a moment, but little by little, during a very long period of time.

Cr. That is to be supposed.

Ath. At first they would have a natural fear ringing in their ears which would prevent their descending from the heights into the plain.

Cr. Of course.

Ath. The fewness of the survivors would make them desirous of intercourse with one another ; but then the means of traveling either by land or by sea would have been almost entirely lost with the loss of the arts, and there would be great difficulty in getting at one another ; for iron and brass and all metals would have become confused, and would have dis appeared ; nor would there be any possibility of ex-

tracting them; and they would have no means of
felling timber. Even if you suppose that some implements might have been preserved in the mountains, they would quickly have worn out and disappeared, and there would be no more of them until
the art of metallurgy had again revived.

Cr. There could not have been.

Ath. In how many generations would this be attained?

Cr. Clearly not for many generations.

Ath. During this period, and for some time afterwards, all the arts which require iron and brass and
the like would disappear.

Cr. Certainly.

Ath. Faction and war would also have died out
in those days and for many reasons.

Cr. How would that be?

Ath. In the first place, the desolation of these
primitive men would create in them a feeling of affection and friendship towards one another; and,
in the second place, they would have no occasion
to fight for their subsistence, for they would have
pasture in abundance, except just at first, and in
some particular cases; on this pasture-land they
would mostly support life in a primitive age, having
plenty of milk and flesh, and procuring other food
by the chase, not to be despised either in quantity
or quality. They would also have abundance of
clothing, and bedding, and dwellings, and utensils
either capable of standing on the fire or not; for
the plastic and weaving arts do not require any use
of iron: God has given these two arts to man in
order to provide him with necessaries, that, when
reduced to their last extremity, the human race may

still grow and increase. Hence in those days mankind were not very poor; nor was poverty a cause
of difference among them; and rich they could not
be, if they had no gold or silver, and such at that
time was their condition. And the community
which has neither poverty nor riches will always
have the noblest principles, there is no insolence
or injustice; nor, again, are there any contentions
or envyings among them. And therefore they were
good, and also because they were what is called
simple-minded ; and when they. were told about
good and evil, they in their simplicity believed what
they heard to be very truth and practiced it. No
one had the wit to suspect another of a falsehood,
as men do now ; but what they heard about gods
and men they believed to be true and lived accordingly ; and therefore they were in all respects such
as we have described them.

Cr. That quite accords with my views, and with
those of my friend here.

Ath. Would not many generations living on in a
simple manner, although ruder, perhaps, and more
ignorant of the arts generally, and in particular of
those of land or naval warfare, and likewise of other
arts, termed in cities legal practices and party con-
flicts, and including all conceivable ways of hurting
one another in word and deed ; although inferior to
those who lived before the Deluge, or to the men of
our day in these respects, would they not, I say, be
simpler and more manly, and also more temperate,
and in general more just? The reason has been
already explained.

Cr. Very true.

Ath. I should wish you to understand that what

has preceded and what is about to follow has been, and will be, said with the intention of explaining what need the men of that time had of laws, and who was their lawgiver.

Cr. And thus far what you have said has been very well said.

Ath. They could hardly have wanted lawgivers as yet ; nothing of that sort was likely to have existed in their days, for they had no letters at this early stage ; they lived by habit and the customs of their forefathers, as they are called.

Cr. Probably.

Ath. But there was already existing a form of government which, if I am not mistaken, is generally termed a lordship, and this still remains in many places, both among Hellenes and barbarians, and is the government which is declared by Homer to have prevailed among the Cyclopes : —

" They have neither councils nor judgments, but they dwell in hollow rocks on the tops of high mountains, and every one is the judge of his wife and children, and they do not trouble themselves about one another."

Cr. That must be a charming poet of yours ; I have read some other verses of his, which are very clever ; but I do not know much of him, for foreign poets are little read among the Cretans.

The Lacedæmonian. But they are in Lacedæmon, and he appears to be the prince of them all ; the manner of life, however, which he describes is not Spartan, but rather Ionian, and he seems quite to confirm what you are saying, tracing up the ancient state of mankind by the help of tradition to barbarism.

Ath. Yes ; and we may accept his witness to the fact that there was a time when primitive societies had this form.

Cr. Very true.

Ath. And did not such states spring out of single habitations and families who were scattered and thinned in the devastations ; and the eldest of them was their ruler, because with them government originated in the authority of a father and a mother, whom, like a flock of birds, they followed, forming one troop under the patriarchal rule and sovereignty of their parents, which of all sovereignties is the most just?

Cr. Very true.

Ath. After this they came together in greater numbers, and increased the size of their cities, and betook themselves to husbandry, first of all at the foot of the mountains, and made inclosures of loose walls and works of defense, in order to keep off wild beasts ; thus creating a single large and common habitation.

Cr. Yes ; at least we may suppose it.

Ath. There is another thing which would probably happen.

Cr. What ?

Ath. When these larger habitations grew up out of the lesser original ones, each of the lesser ones would survive in the larger ; every family would be under the rule of the eldest, and, owing to their separation from one another, would have peculiar customs in things divine and human, which they would have received from their several parents who had educated them, and these customs would incline them to order, when the parents had the element of order in them ; and to courage, when they had the element of courage in them. And they would naturally stamp upon their children, and upon their children's children, their own institutions ; and, as we are saying, they would find their way into the larger society, having already their own peculiar laws.

Cr. Certainly.

Ath. And every man surely likes his own laws best, and the laws of others not so well.

Cr. True.

Ath. Then how we seem to have stumbled upon the beginnings of legislation !

Cr. Exactly.

Ath. The next step will be that these persons who meet together must choose some arbiters, who will inspect the laws of all of them, and will publicly present such of them as they approve to the chiefs who lead the tribes, and are in a manner their kings, and will give them the choice of them. These will themselves be called legislators, and will appoint the magistrates, framing some sort of aristocracy, or perhaps monarchy, out of the dynasties or lordships, and in this altered state of the government they will live.

Cr. Yes, they would be appointed in the order which you mention. . . .

But we will not pursue the conversation farther. Is the reader indignant that he has been made to listen so long to Abbé Banier, clumsily disguised in the robes of a pretended Athenian philosopher and discoursing, all out of character, on matters which betray "the prejudices of a Christian education"? It may well be. To a reader of Lubbock and Tylor and Vogt, the sentiments of the Athenian traveler do seem singularly in accord with Holy Scripture.

But let not the innocent suffer for the guilty. It happens that our imaginary conversation is not of our imagining. It was written more than two thousand years before the birth of Abbé Banier, and by as good a pagan as the famed Athenian Plato.

On the whole, we are of the opinion that the great consentaneous Traditions of the Human Race will yet outlive a considerable number of Bachofens and Büchners and Buckles, and that if ever the burial-place of Moses shall be discovered, it will not be found to be in any of the ignominious graveyards periodically prepared for him by on-coming Professors of Hebrew eager for a stunning inaugural. Despite the ingenious "higher" criticism of to-day's ephemeral "authorities," the Biblical scholarship of the future is more likely to carry the age of the composition of the Eden story backward than forward. The documents embedded in the opening chapters of Genesis may yet prove to be, what reverent and orthodox scholars have already affirmed — fragments of the Sacred Scriptures of the Antediluvian Patriarchal Church.[1] Whether so or no, one ancient word shall evermore be verified : "The grass withereth, the flower fadeth ; but the word of our God shall stand forever."

Our treatise opened with a pathetic picture, — it must close with another. Long-lost Eden is found ; but its gates are barred against us. Now, as at the beginning of our exile, a sword turns every way to keep the Way of the Tree of Life.

[1] Moffat : *Comparative History of Religions.* New York, 1871 : vol. i., pp. 99 *seq.*

Sadder yet, it is Eden no longer. Even could some new Columbus penetrate to the secret centre of this Wonderland of the Ages, he could but hurriedly kneel amid a frozen desolation and, dumb with a nameless awe, let fall a few hot tears above the buried and desolated hearthstone of Humanity's earliest and loveliest home.

Happily for us, O Menschengeschlecht, a trusty hand has added to the third of Genesis the closing chapters of the Patmos Apocalypse. The thought of the old forever evanished Eden is henceforth bearable, for from afar we have caught the vision of a Sinless Paradise, the frostless Gardens, the Tree, and the River of the Heavenly City of God.

Ja, wenn des Nordwinds rauhes Tosen
Der Erde Gärten zugeschneit,
Dann blühen erst des Himmels Rosen
In unverwelkter Herrlichkeit.
Ja, sind wir Gäste hier zu Landen
Auf dieser kalten Winterflur,
So ist noch eine Ruh vorhanden
Dem Seufzen aller Kreatur.

KARL GEROK.

28

APPENDIX.

SECTION I. — THE EARTH OF COLUMBUS NOT A TRUE SPHERE.

(*Illustrating pp. 3–7 ; 306, 307.*)

THE following authentic account of the views entertained by Columbus respecting the figure of the Earth will be welcome to many readers : —

" I have always read that the world comprising the land and the water was spherical, and the recorded experiences of Ptolemy and all others have proved this by the eclipses of the moon and other observations made from East to West, as well as the elevation of the Pole from North to South.   But as I have already described, I have now seen so much irregularity, that I have come to another conclusion respecting the Earth, namely, that it is not round as they describe, but of the form of a pear, which is very round except where the stalk grows, at which part it is most prominent ; or like a round ball upon part of which is a prominence like a woman's nipple, this protrusion being the highest and nearest the sky, situated under the equinoctial line, and at the eastern extremity of this sea. . . . In confirmation of my opinion, I revert to the arguments which I have above detailed respecting the line, which passes from North to South a hundred leagues westward of the Azores ; for in sailing thence westward, the ships went on rising smoothly towards the sky, and then the weather was felt to be milder, on account of which mildness the needle shifted one point of the compass ; and the further we went, the more the needle moved to the Northwest, this elevation producing the variation of the circle which the North-star describes with its satellites ; and the nearer I approached the equinoctial line the more they rose and the greater was the difference in these stars and in their circles. Ptolemy and the other philosophers who have written upon the globe thought that it was spherical, believing that this [western] hemisphere was round as well as that in which they themselves dwelt, the centre of which was in the island of Arin, which is under the equinoctial line between the Arabian Gulf and the Gulf of Persia ; and the circle passes over Cape St. Vincent in Portugal westward, and eastward by Cangara and the Seras ; — in which hemisphere I make no difficulty as to its being a perfect sphere as they describe ; but this western half of the world I maintain is like half of a very round pear, having a raised projection for the stalk, as I have already described, or like a woman's nipple on a round ball. Ptolemy and the others who have written on the globe had no information respecting this part of the world, which was then unexplored ; they only established their own hemisphere, which, as I have already said, is half of a perfect sphere. And now that your Highnesses have commissioned me to make this voyage of discovery, the truths which I have stated are evidently proved, because in this voyage, when I was off the island of Hargin [1] and its vicinity, which is twenty degrees to the North of the equinoctial line, I found the people black and the land very much burnt ; and when after that I went to the Cape Verde Islands I found the people there very much darker still, and the more southward we went, the more they approach the extreme of blackness ; so that when I reached the parallel of Sierra Leone, where, as night came on, the North star rose five degrees, the people there were exces-

---

[1] Arguin, west coast of Africa.

sively black, and as I sailed westward the heat became extreme. But after I had passed the meridian or line which I have already described, I found the climate became gradually more temperate ; so that when I reached the island of Trinidad, where the North star rose five degrees as night came on, there, and in the land of Gracia, I found the temperature exceedingly mild ; the fields and the foliage likewise were remarkably fresh and green, and as beautiful as the gardens of Valencia in April. The people there are very graceful in form, less dark than those whom I had before seen in the Indies, and wear their hair long and smooth ; they are also more shrewd, intelligent, and courageous. The sun was then in the sign of Virgo over our heads and theirs ; therefore all this must proceed from the extreme blandness of the temperature, which arises, as I have said, from this country being the most elevated in the world and the nearest to the sky. On these grounds, therefore, I affirm that the globe is not spherical, but that there is the difference in its form which I have described ; the which is to be found in this hemisphere at the point where the Indies meet the ocean, the extremity of the hemisphere being below the equinoctial line. And a great confirmation of this is, that when our Lord made the sun, the first light appeared in the first point of the East, where the most elevated point of the globe is." — *Hakluyt Society Publications. Select Letters of Columbus.* Tr. by R. H. Major. London, 2d ed., pp. 134-138.

SECTION II.—HOW THE EARTH WAS PEOPLED.

BY M. LE MARQUIS G. DE SAPORTA.

How has the human race been able to spread itself over the whole surface of the globe? Is it the result of different and independent origins in the several continents, or have all men sprung from a common cradle, a "mother-region"? On this point students are divided, Agassiz holding that men were created, and Carl Vogt that they were developed, at different centres, and Quatrefages and the theologians maintaining the unity of their origin. The fact is left that man, the same in all the essential characteristics of the species, has advanced into all the habitable parts of the globe, and that not recently and when provided with all the resources that experience and inventive genius could put at his disposal, but when still young and ignorant. It was then that, weak and almost naked, having only just got fire and a few rude arms with which to defend itself and procure food, the human race conquered the world and spread itself from within the Arctic Circle to Terra del Fuego, from the Samoyed country to Van Diemen's Land, from the North Cape to the Cape of Good Hope. It is this primitive exodus, as certain as it is inconceivable, accepted by science as well as by dogma, that we have to explain, or at least to make probable ; and that in an age when it is only after the most wonderful discoveries, by the aid of the most powerful machinery for navigation, through the boldest and most adventurous enterprises, that civilized man has been able to flatter himself that he has at last gone as far as infant man went in an age that is so far removed from us as to baffle all calculations.

We must insist on this point, for it brings into light an obstacle which those who have tried to trace out the connection between widely separated races and to determine the course that had been followed by tribes now separated by oceans and vast expanses have hitherto found insurmountable ; for, if man is one — to which we are ready to agree — we must assign a single point of departure for his migrations. In these migrations, man has gone wherever he could, and, at every spot he has occupied and settled, has acquired characteristics peculiar to the place, and which differentiated him from the men settling in other places. Hence the varieties of human races. Some of these spots seem to have been peculiarly favorable to his advancement, and became centres of civilization. The number of such centres is, however, very limited, and their distribution is significant.

The continental masses are distributed in three principal groups, one feature in the configuration of which must strike every one who carefully examines a map of the world. It will be noticed that they are so expanded toward the North as to touch in that direction or be separated only by narrow passages, and that they also surround within the Arctic Circle a central polar sea with a bordering island-belt. Going down toward the South we find that the three continents, North America, Europe, and Northern Asia, which had approached each other so closely, give place to three appendages, South America, Africa, and Australia, which in their turn gradually taper off to mere points in an illimitable sea, long before they reach the Antarctic Circle. Within this circle the configuration of the land is precisely the reverse of that in the North ; it is that of a solid cap of land around the pole, in the midst of the great ocean.

If we again observe these masses, we shall find that civilization was born in each of them under similar geographical conditions, viz., in the neighborhood of a smaller interior sea, near or rather North of the tropic of Cancer, between 20° and 35° north latitude. The most eastern of the centres is in China, near the Japan Sea. The most western, and apparently the most recent, was along the inner shores of the Gulf of Mexico. The last civilization was in the course of radiation and transformation when the Europeans came to America, and was wholly independent and autonomous ; but, weak and relatively new, it was not able to resist the sudden onset of a stronger race.

Toward the centre of the space whose extremes we have marked out must be placed two other centres of civilization, more ancient than either of the two already named, and in the same zone of latitude — Egypt, in the valley of the Nile, and near the Arabian Gulf, and Mesopotamia, near the head of the Persian Gulf. Thus, each continental mass had its particular centre of civilization, except Asia, which had two — one in the extreme east, the other near the line which joins it to Europe. This peculiar grouping of the chief centres of civilization in such a relation of neighborhood constitutes the most considerable paleoethnic fact that we are able to record. The Nile and the Syrian sea on the west, upper Armenia and the Caspian on the north, the Hindoo-Koosh and the Indus on the east, and the Arabian Sea on the south, bound the region where Cushites, Semites, and Aryans, the first farmers, workers, and founders of cities, the second pastoral people, and the third mountaineers, afterward emigrants and conquerors, met, elbowed each other, and mingled, conquerors and conquered by turns, inventing arts and the use of metals, learning arms and how to organize themselves hierarchically, reaching their ideal through religion, and having in writing the most powerful instrument at the disposition of human intelligence. With them we have the beginning of history, and a continuous chain of social organizations, down to our own days. The growth of civilization in these centres leaves, however, still unaccounted for the diffusion of mankind all over the earth, which took place at a period far anterior to it.

The spread of man throughout Europe and Asia does not offer very great difficulties, for, in consequence of the long distance for which the two continents are joined, Europe is in reality only a dependency of Asia ; and occupation of Europe from Asia is conformable to religious traditions. The difficulties are, however, formidable when we come to America, which we find occupied from one end to the other by races whose unity has struck the best observers. Not only, moreover, did the American man inaugurate on the soil of the New World an original and relatively advanced civilization, but he has left, chiefly in the North, indisputable traces of his presence in the most remote ages. Paleolithic implements have been found in the valley of the Delaware, at Trenton, New Jersey, and near Guanajuato in Mexico, so clearly characterized that they cannot be mistaken, the situation of which at the base of the Quaternary alluvions and their coexistence with elephants and mastodons indicate the existence of a race contemporaneous with that of the gravels of the Somme, having the same industry and doubtless the same manners and physical traits. Whence could this primitive American race, sister to the one that lived in Europe at the same date, have come, unless we suppose a direct communication between the two continents? The difficulty such men would have in crossing the Atlantic and the certainty which soundings give of the antiquity of the ocean remove all possibility of our believing either that the two continents were formerly joined, or that one of them was discovered by some unknown Columbus navigating the ocean a hundred thousand years before the later one.

We are thus in the presence of the problem, always coming up before us, and always escaping us, of the origin of the American man. Evidently it cannot be resolved by invoking an accidental colonization of Asiatic wanderers, or a shipwrecked company; but it is one in which we have to deal with primitive populations flowing as in Europe by successive waves, and attesting the continuous presence of man, whose gradual development and extension have followed in America the same course as on the old continent. The hypothesis of an immigration from Asia by way of the Aleutian Islands to Alaska might be acceptable, did not the certainty of the presence of an indigenous American population in the Quaternary age reduce it to the proportions of a secondary fact. The same is the case with the relations — contradictory, it is true, and therefore suspicious — which some have attempted to establish between the monuments, statues, and graphic signs of Central America and those of Egypt and Buddhistic Asia. These analogies, aside from their insufficiency, must fall before two paramount considerations: first, the certainty of the contemporaneousness of the American man with the great animals of the Quaternary age ; and, second, the relative uniformity of the copper-colored race, so like itself through the whole extent of the continent, except in that part which is occupied by the Esquimaux. The difficulty arises from the fact that the monogenists, having in view a single birthplace and a single point of departure for the whole human race, and placing neither in the New World, have supposed America to have been colonized by European or Asiatic immigrants following the direction of the parallels of latitude. Emigration in this direction at once meets an obstacle in the oceans, which grow wider the farther South we go. The obstacle disappears if we give up the idea of lateral emigrations, and suppose the movement to have taken place in the direction of the meridians from North to South. No obstacle of any kind offers itself to such migrations ; and the relative uniformity of the Americans, from one end of the continent to the other, would never have excited astonishment, if we had not been preoccupied with the idea of their introduction at a later date.

We may remark, on this topic, that the extreme southern points of the three continents are occupied by races which came originally, without doubt, from somewhere else, and which are ranked, in Terra del Fuego, at the Cape of Good Hope, and in Tasmania, among the lowest of the species. These races, advancing in front of the others, have preserved the visible stamp of the relative inferiority of the stock from which they were prematurely detached. We have to believe, in effect, that these three branches — Fuegians, Bushmen, and Tasmanians — so little elevated in their physical, intellectual, and moral traits, have gone and planted themselves so far away only because the unoccupied space opened out before them. Scouts for the rest of mankind, they have reached, step by step, the extreme limits of the habitable land. They must have occupied for the moment, at least, the parts of the intermediate space, but they could not resist the push of the stronger races, and they could not have survived to our time, except under the condition of re-striction to a small area in the most remote tract of their original domain. There is nothing surprising in the fact that MM. Quatrefages and Hamy, having described the most ancient European race of which we have the skulls, that of Canstadt, should have found its analogies only among these same natives of the extreme South — the Bushmen and the Australians.

It will be seen that we are inclined to remove to the circumpolar regions of the North the probable cradle of primitive humanity. From there only could it have radi-ated as from a centre, to spread into several continents at once, and to give rise to successive emigrations toward the South. This theory agrees best with the presumed march of the human races. It remains to be shown that it is equally in accord with the most authentic and most recent geological data, and that, besides man, it is appli-cable to the plants and animals which accompanied him, and which have continued to be most closely associated with him in the temperate regions which afterward became the seat of his civilizing power.

The general laws of geogony favor this hypothesis in a remarkable manner. To make it seem probable, we have only to establish two essential points that will not be seriously contested by any geologist. One is, that the polar regions, which were covered with large trees, enjoyed a climate more temperate than that of Central Europe, and were habitable and fertile to the eightieth degree, underwent a slow and progressive cooling down till the middle of the Tertiary period. Thence refrigeration made rapid progress till the ice gained exclusive possession of the country south of them. Under such circumstances, man as well as the animals and plants would have to remove or perish — to emigrate step by step, or find himself reduced to a daily more precarious state of existence.

The second point is the relative stability of the existing continental masses, and of their distribution around a sea occupying the Arctic Pole ; while the other Pole was occupied with a cap of land surrounded by an immense ocean. The importance of the Arctic Pole in respect to the production of animals and plants, and to their migrations, and the nullity of the other hemisphere in relation to this feature result from such a grouping. The essential point is, that there is nothing capricious in such an arrangement of lands and seas, and that there have been, if not always, at least from a very ancient period, emerged lands occupying a considerable part of the northern hemisphere, advancing very far toward the Pole, and describing around the Arctic Sea a belt of more or less contiguous countries and islands. This is, in effect, what geology teaches. The changes, immersions, and emersions have never been anything but partial and successive, while the skeletons of the continents go back to the most remote ages. There have always been a Europe, an Asia, an America, and Arctic lands. We know certainly that there have always been around the Arctic Pole extensive territories, if not continents, long the home of the same plants as the rest of the globe, and that, beginning with an epoch that corresponds with the end of the Jurassic, the climate, at first as warm there as elsewhere, has tended gradually to become colder. The depression of temperature was at first manifested very slowly, and was far from having attained its present degree in the Tertiary ; for the trees that then grew in Greenland — the sequoias, magnolias, and plane-trees — now attain their full development in Southern Europe, and are not suited with the climate of Central Europe. We are, then, assured of the ancient existence, near the Arctic Pole, of a zone of lands covered with a rich vegetation. The permanent existence of a polar sea is none the less attested by fossils from all parts of the region. The neighborhood of the Pole was long habitable, and inhabited by man in a time near that in which the vestiges of his industry begin to show themselves alike in Europe and America. In passing thus from the Arctic lands to those bordering on the polar circle, and through the latter into Asia, Europe, and America, man would only have taken the road which a host of plants and animal followed, either before him or at the same time, and under the stress of the same circumstances.

It is, in fact, by the aid of migrations from the neighborhood of the Pole that we can generally explain the phenomenon of scattered or disjoined species, a phenomenon identical with the one which man of the Old World and man of the New World present when they are compared. Combining present notions with the indications furnished by the fossils, we discover numerous examples of disjunction — in which allied forms, often hardly distinguishable, have been distributed at the same time in scattered regions, at extremely remote points in the boreal hemisphere, without any apparent connection along the parallels, to explain the common unit. Europe attests by undeniable fossils that it had formerly a host of vegetable types and forms that are now American, which it could have received only from the extreme North. It had, for example, magnolias, tulip-trees, sassafras, maples, and poplars, comparable in all respects to those which grow in the United States. The two plane-trees, that of the West and that of Asia Minor, to which we may add an extinct fossil European plane-tree, illustrate the same phenomenon of dispersion. Europe in the Tertiary period witnessed the growth of a ginko similar to the one in the north of China. It had sequoias and a bald cypress corresponding with the trees of those names that are now growing in California and Louisiana. The beech seems to have been growing in the Arctic circumpolar zone before it was introduced and extended throughout the northern hemisphere. The same is doubtless the case with the hemlock, of which distinguishable traces have been found in Grinnell-land, above the eighty-second degree of latitude, of a date much earlier than that of its introduction into Europe. The well-established presence in both continents of many animals peculiar to the northern hemisphere must be attributed to emigrations, if not from the Pole, at least from countries contiguous to the polar circle. This is obvious in the case of the reindeer, bison, and stag; but it ought to be equally true in respect to animals of more ancient times, and although we have no other direct proofs of it than the abundance of the remains of mammoths in upper Siberia, the same law doubtless includes the elephants and mastodons. We mean here the species of these two genera which were propagated from the North to the South, and were, in America and Europe, the companions of primitive man. The connection of the continental masses with their belt of hardly discontinuous lands around the polar circle gives the key to all these phenomena. The cause on which they depend would be constantly producing radiations and consequently disjunctions of species and races, whatever kingdom we may consider.

Before leaving the questions that touch on the presumed origin of man, we cannot refrain from speaking of the relations which it has been sought to establish between him and the pithecan apes. Primitive man, according to some authors of the transformist school, was an anthropomorphic ape, perfected physically as to his walk and erect attitude, intellectually by the development of his cranial capacity, till the moment when reasoning, or the faculty of abstraction and the power of using articulate language, took in him the place of instinct. Numerous and undeniable anatomical or physiological analogies of the human body and those of the more highly organized monkeys, which have no tails nor callosities on their paws, and whose faces and ways have something singularly human, favor this system, at least in appearance. The pithecans have, however, other contiguities than purely human ones. Their ways are rather analogous than directly assimilable to those of man ; with other adaptations, they seem to have followed a wholly different course of evolution. They are essentially climbers, while man is exclusively a walker, and has always been predisposed to the erect position. The highest monkeys, the anthropomorphous apes, walk badly and with difficulty. When they leave the trees in which they live, their position is a stooping one, and they bend down their toes so as not to touch the ground with the soles of their feet. We have, then, reason not to admit the simian origin of man without decisive proofs. Moreover, the pithecans seem to have been evolved in an inverse direction from man. Rejoicing in the heat, they perish rapidly when brought into the temperate zones, and this is especially the case with the anthropoid apes. Thus, while man, coming from the North, advances toward the South only when the depression of temperature favors his progress in that direction, the monkeys, to which a strong heat is a vital element, were developed in an age when

Europe had a sub-tropical climate, and disappeared from
that continent as soon as the climate became temperate,
so that their departure concides with the arrival of man.
They fled South to find the heat they needed, precisely
when the diminution of the heat opened to man the
region from which it excluded his predecessors.   The
necessity of placing the cradle of the pithecans in a hot
country enables us to separate the monkeys of the Eastern and Western continents into two distinct groups,
marked by differences in dentition important enough to
oblige us to assume an extreme antiquity for their separation.   Both are descended from the lemurians, now
represented only in Madagascar, but of which early Tertiary fossils are found in Europe.   The most recent
lemurians in Europe are found at the end of the Eocene.
It is later, in the Miocene, and that not the lowest, that
we meet pithecans similar to those of the equatorial zone
of the Eastern continent.   At this epoch, which was
nearly that of Oeningen and the Mollassic Sea, which
divided Europe from East to West, a subtropical climate
still prevailed in the centre of the continent, and the
palm-trees extended up into Bohemia, along the northern
banks of the great interior sea.   By favor of this temperature the monkeys occupied Europe to near the forty-
fifth degree, but without going above it, to disappear forever as soon as it became cool enough for men and
elephants.

The *Mesopithecus Pentelici*, of which M. Gaudry has discovered twenty-five individuals at Pikermi, was small,
walked on its four paws, and lived on twigs and leaves.
The *Dryopithecus* of St. Gaudens had the characteristics
of the highest anthropomorphs, with the bestial face of
the gorilla; but it is to this animal that M. Gaudry is inclined to attribute the flints, intentionally chipped, according to the Abbé Bourgeois, of the Beauce limestone,
at Thénay in the St. Gaudens geognostic horizon.   The

Pliopithecus of Sansan (Gers) resembles a gibbon. To find the present analogues of the *Pliopithecus* and *Dryopithecus* of Miocene Europe, it is necessary to go across the tropic of Cancer to about 12° North latitude, or more than thirty degrees South of the locality of these fossils. If, as is probable, the same interval existed between the perimeter frequented by the European anthropomorphs and the natal region in which man was originally confined, we shall find the latter in the latitude of Greenland, at 70° or 75°. This is indeed an hypothetical calculation, but it is based on a double argument hard to refute.

We can reach almost the same conclusion by a little different reasoning. The abundance of large-flaked instruments in the contiguous valleys of the Somme and the Seine marks the existence at that point of external conditions evidently favorable to the diffusion of man, whose race was then multiplying for the first time. The flora of that epoch, as observed near Fontainebleau, indicates the presence of conditions similar to those now existing in the south of France, near the forty-second degree of latitude. Now, to reach, starting from the forty-second degree, the nearly tropical regions where palm, camphor, and southern laurel trees are associated together, we have to go twelve or fifteen degrees South, to the thirtieth or twenty-eighth degree of latitude, where we see the same climatological conditions existing as prevailed in Miocene Europe when it was hardly warm enough for the anthropomorphic apes. Between these conditions and those which seem to have been first favorable to the growth of the human race there existed a space of twelve or fifteen degrees of latitude. But when palm-trees were growing near Prague, and camphor-trees grew as far North as Dantzic, man, if he existed then, might have lived without inconvenience beyond or around the Arctic Circle, within equal reach of North America and Europe, which he was destined to people. — *Translated for the Popular Science Monthly from the Revue des Deux Mondes.*

29

SECTION III.—THE RECEPTION ACCORDED TO "THE TRUE KEY."

As indicated in the text, the view of Ancient Cosmology presented in chapter first of Part fourth is entirely at variance with that of all our standard authorities. Professor Packard, of Yale College, remarks, "If it is true, all our books and maps are wrong, and we must admit that all scholars have been mistaken in their understanding of the ancient records." In like manner, one of the foreign periodicals editorially observes, "If it is correct, a most striking proof is given of the possibility of many successive generations of archæologists, scientists, and scholars failing to catch the entire drift and spirit of ancient legends and literature in their cosmic teachings and relations." Under these circumstances the ordinary reader seems entitled to some further information before being asked to give it his adherence.

The new view, then, was first published in the columns of "The Independent," New York, August 25, 1881. In March of the following year a second and enlarged edition appeared in "The Boston University Year Book," vol. ix. Soon after a third edition was issued as a pamphlet by Messrs. Ginn and Heath, of Boston. In each case it was entitled "The True Key to Ancient Cosmology and Mythical Geography," and was illustrated by the diagram which stands as frontispiece to this work.

Copies of the paper in each of its successive editions were promptly forwarded — usually with a brief personal note — to the most competent scholars in the universities of Athens, Rome, Berlin, Leipsic, Heidelberg, Bonn, Leyden, London, Oxford, Cambridge, Edinburgh, Belfast, and Dublin. As might be expected an interesting and varied correspondence ensued. Of many of the letters the writer does not feel that he has the right to make any public use ; but in printing the following extracts he believes that he violates no proprieties.

A. H. Sayce, of the University of Oxford, one of the most distinguished of living professors of Comparative Philology, after reading a preliminary sketch, wrote to the author as follows : —

Provisionally, I may say that your view seems to me eminently reasonable and likely to clear up several difficulties. Certainly it throws light on the voyage of Odysseus, more particularly on the visit to Hades.

I look forward to the appearance of your book, which will be of great value to students of the past.

In more recent communications Professor Sayce has used still stronger expressions of personal acquiescence.

The following are all from letters written before the publication of " Homer's Abode of the Dead."

Right Hon. William E. Gladstone, author of " Homeric Studies," " Juventus Mundi," " Homeric Synchronism," etc. : —

I have received with much interest and pleasure the communications you have been good enough to address to me on the Homeric Cosmology. Very long ago I became convinced that Homer proceeded, not on the idea commonly assigned to him, of the earth as a plane, but on the conception of a spherical or convex surface. My views have long been set forth : fundamentally, I am at one with you, and when (if ever) my time of leisure shall arrive, I shall try to learn whether, in the points where you differ from or go beyond me, you have not been the more thorough and accurate of the two.

Robert K. Douglas, of the British Museum, and Professor of Chinese in King's College, London : —

I read your Key with great interest ; and, without having made any special study of the subject, I must say that to my mind it explains most satisfactorily the Homeric Cosmology.

Richard Dacre Archer-Hind, Fellow of Trinity College, Cambridge, England : —

I must say that your explanation of ancient cosmology seems to me very simple and natural. It certainly throws a flood of light upon several points which were before very obscure. I am glad to hear that it is approved by so distinguished an Orientalist as Dr. Rost, Librarian of the India Office, London.

C. P. Tiele, D. D., Professor of the History of Religions in the University of Leyden, Holland : —

After perusing your paper a second time, I cannot but express my opinion that your hypothesis is very plausible and ingenious. The conception of the world as a sphere is not so young as is generally thought. . . . I think you are right in identifying the wide Olympus with the highest heaven. . . . Your description agrees very well with the ancient cosmography of the Babylonians. With you I am satisfied that there is no real difference between mythical Olympus and heaven, and that all earthly Olymps (as there are several of them) are only localizations of the same heavenly abode of the gods.

Howard Crosby, D. D., LL. D., ex-Chancellor of the University of New York : —

Your Key to Ancient Cosmology is to me most satisfactory. I believe you have made a valuable discovery.

W. D. Whitney, LL. D., Professor of Sanskrit and Comparative Philology, Yale College : —

I have looked with some care through your exposition of your view respecting the ancient conceptions of the cosmos, and find it very ingenious and suggestive, and worthy of careful comparison with the expressions of ancient authors on the subject.

Dr. Charles R. Lanman, Professor of Sanskrit, Harvard University : —

The Key I have read once more, and think it is very simple, ingenious and adequate for the explanation of a great variety of heretofore perplexing allusions.

W. S. Tyler, D. D., LL. D., Professor of the Greek Language and Literature, Amherst College : —

Permit me to thank you for the paper. Perhaps no one key will unlock all the chambers of the labyrinth of ancient cosmology and mythical geography. But I believe yours comes the nearest to it of any that has yet been found.

William A. Packard, Professor of the Latin Language and Literature, College of New Jersey, Princeton : —

Dr. Warren's pamphlet gives the result of ingenious and able research, which claims very careful consideration. It does seem to act very widely as a solvent in interpreting ancient cosmogonies. Its elucidation of Homeric expressions is very striking.

Stephen D. Peet, Editor of " American Antiquarian and Oriental Journal : " —

I believe that you have struck a very rich field in your pamphlet on the ancient cosmology. I have long surmised that there was something back of the astrology of the ancients which had exerted a great influence on the religious conceptions, and even on the literary and speculative thoughts of the ancients, but have to thank you for putting together the facts so as to discover the key.

J. Henry Thayer, D. D., late Professor of Greek and N. T. Interpretation, Andover Theological Seminary, now Professor of the same in Harvard University Divinity School : —

Allow me to express my great interest in your Key to Ancient Cosmology. It gives one a sense of relief amounting to satisfaction at its very first perusal. I shall take great interest in teaching it.

James Freeman Clarke, D. D., author of " Ten Great Religions," etc. : —

It seems to me to throw much light on many passages in the classic writers. . . . I cannot help thinking that your view will be a key to unlock many obscure passages.

The seven following extracts fairly illustrate the mass of the communications received since the publication of "Homer's Abode of the Dead," which paper was issued in advance of the present volume simply as a further illustration of the correctness and utility of "The True Key." Each is from the pen of a European scholar of first rank, and the last of them from one of the most widely known of German Egyptologists. Not having as yet permission to use the names of the writers, they are here withheld.

I thank you very much for sending me the "Boston University Year Book," containing your interesting article on the Underworld of Homer.

Homeric interpretation long and (I think) absurdly placed the way to the Underworld in the West; but I am glad at least to acknowledge that from the West—that is, from you and your country — much light has been thrown upon the Underworld of Homer.

In 1868 I went a long way, in a work then published, towards the doctrine that the entrance to the Underworld was beneath the solid earth-mass, as, in 1858, I had endeavored to destroy the prevailing notion about the road by the West.

I regard with amazement the mass of false interpretations of Homer which a quarter of a century ago I found prevailing, and of which I think we are gradually getting rid.

One very great source of aid has been the opening up of Egyptian and Assyrian knowledge, and from this quarter I believe that more aid will yet be drawn.

With you I think that the supposed inconsistencies of Homer about the Underworld are really ascribable wholly, or in the main, to his interpreters.

Many thanks for your letter and for the interesting paper in the "Boston University Year Book" which has followed it. The illustration of your theory which is furnished by the Voyage of the Egyptian Sindbad is very striking, and must be most gratifying to you. I can find no objection to your view except those suggested by the original meaning of the words *Amenti* and *Erebos* (Assyrian *eribu* = *'erebh*); and I am therefore inclined to subscribe to all that Professor Tiele has written you in regard to it. That in Homer the earth is supposed to be a sphere, with Olympos above and Tartaros below, clears up every difficulty.

I read your paper with great interest and pleasure. Now again you have put your favorite thesis so clearly and forcibly that I incline more and more to your opinion. I only wait, before surrendering, for some leisure to go accurately over the principal facts and citations.

I have read your paper with great interest. Your explanation makes things clear, at any rate, though I must read the Odyssey again before venturing to affirm that you see things as Homer saw them.

Accept my best thanks for your "Year Book" for 1883, with its excellent and interesting dissertation upon "Homer's Abode of the Dead." Not being a Homerologist, I am hardly entitled to express an opinion, but your argument seems to me conclusive.

Your paper has an especial interest for me, inasmuch as it shows that there was less difference between the cosmography of Homer and the cosmographies of his successors than we had been brought to suppose. (*The modest writer of the foregoing is one of the most eminent Hellenists of Cambridge, Eng.*)

I have to thank you for your new contribution to our knowledge with reference to the conceptions of the ancients as to the shape of the earth. Your paper on the " Navel of the Earth " is full of interesting and important information. My only doubt is whether the time has come for such wide generalizations as you propose. However, our science wants centrifugal as well as centripetal forces, and a discoverer must not be afraid of places marked " Dangerous."

HOCHGEEHRTER HERR COLLEGA :
Freundlichen Dank für Ihre gütigen Zeilen und den sie begleitenden interessanten Aufsatz. Ihre Hypothese ist höchst überraschend, und würde, sollte sich ihre Richtigkeit auf ganz feste Füsse stellen lassen, in der That mit einem Male Ordnung in eine besonders krauss verwirrte Frage bringen. . . . Sobald es Ihnen nachzuweisen gelingt, dass in der Volksvorstellung der Griechen aus früherer Zeit die Erde kugelförmig

war, werden Sie die Schlacht gewonnen haben, und Niemand wird es fürder wagen dürfen die Stimme gegen Ihre Ansicht zu erheben. Es will mir nicht unmöglich scheinen, Spuren solcher Anschauung zu finden, zumal da die Egypter ganz gewiss schon früh Kenntniss von der Kugelgestalt der Erde besassen. . . . Trotz dieser Bedenken hat mich Ihr Aufsatz lebhaft interessirt. Leider werde ich aus Gesundheitsrücksichten den Orientalisten-Congress zu Leyden nicht besuchen dürfen ; es sollte mich aber freuen, wenn die von Ihnen so geistreich angeregte interessante Frage während desselben zur Discussion käme.

More and more decided are the latest verdicts of American scholars. The following are a half dozen specimens from a considerable collection.

The Rev. A. P. Peabody, D. D., LL. D., Professor Emeritus in Harvard University : —

I have read not only with pleasure, but also with profit, your essay on Homer's "Abode of the Dead." Your theory accords with my impression, and makes that impression — before vague and with less than sufficient reason — definite and well grounded.

C. C. Everett, D. D., Dean of the Theological Faculty of Harvard University, and Professor of Comparative Theology : —

So far as Homer is concerned, your view is certainly fitted to remove grave difficulties.

J. R. Boise, D. D., LL. D., Professor in the Baptist Union Theological Seminary, Chicago : —

The able and learned article on Homer's "Abode of the Dead " has interested me deeply, and I believe your view is the correct one.

Edwin Post, Ph. D., Professor of Latin, Indiana Asbury University, Greencastle, Ind. : —

I have recently re-read your monograph on Ancient Cosmology, and I am more and more convinced that your startling hypothesis will be verified more and more by comparative study.

George Zabriskie Gray, S. T. D., Dean of the Episcopal Theological School, Cambridge, Mass. : —

I have read your treatise with great interest, and desire to thank you for your work. It seems to me that your theory meets the test of all theories, that of accounting for the facts that cannot otherwise be reconciled. Besides thus reconciling the statements of ancient authors regarding the world and the underworld, your theory enables us to see in their writings many new and fruitful suggestions regarding matters hitherto unnoticed and unsuspected. Trusting that this treatise may receive the attention and currency which it so eminently deserves, I remain, etc., etc.

Rev. A. B. Hyde, D. D., Professor of Greek in Allegheny College, Meadville, Pa. : —

I seem to have found in you a guide in a "mighty maze." Homer has been so long waiting, not for an observer, but for some one to teach us how to observe, a seer to show us how to see. The more I reflect upon your scheme of his cosmology, the more I am struck with its beauty and accuracy; that is, its harmony with the Homeric utterances.

The following does not exactly belong in this place, but, coming from an inspired prophet of God, it seems entitled to a somewhat exceptional treatment. The writer's name indicates a Polish nationality, and his peculiar use of the German language somewhat confirms the supposition that he was not to the manner born. His authoritative announcement of the early restoration at the North Pole of the "curseless" primeval Paradise is well calculated to relieve any undue melancholy into which any of our converts, meditating upon the lost Eden, may chance to fall : —

KÖNIGSBERG, IN PREUSSEN, *den 2ten Mai,* 1884.

WERTHGESCHÄTZTER HERR PROFESSOR! — Mit freudigem Staunen lese ich heute in der hiesigen Hartungschen Zeitung folgende Mittheilung: "Die Lage des Paradieses ausfindig zu machen, das ist jetzt das Thema um welches sich das Gespräch in den eleganten Salons der geistigen Aristokratie Boston's, des amerikanischen Athens' dreht, seitdem Professor Dr. Warren der dortigen Universität, in einer langen wissenschaftlichen Abhandlung bewiesen, dass nur allein am Nordpol das Paradies gelegen haben kann. Den Einwand wie ein Mensch am Nordpol bei solcher Kälte Adam heitzen konnte, widerlegt der fromme und gelehrte Mann dadurch, dass es jedenfalls früher dort wärmer gewesen sei. Dr. Warren ist sehr dafür, eine Expedition auszuschicken, um seine auf 'wissenschaftliche Voranssetzungen' gestützte Schlussfolgerungen zu beweisen."

Diese Mittheilung ist mir aus folgendem Grunde eine freudige-interessante weil, wie Sie es glauben, dass am Anfange der Menschheit das fluchlose Paradies am Nordpol stattgefunden, ich es glaube, dass ein solch fluchloses und noch herrlicheres Paradies eben auch daselbst am Nordpol in nicht ferner Zukunft stattfinden wird.

Ich bitte Sie nun ergebenst, Ihre diese Wissenschaft betreffenden Gründe mir ehestens gefälligst mittheilen zu wollen, um zu ersehen, ob diese Ihre Gründe diese wichtigen Vergangenheits-Zustände betreffend, mit den meinigen, die eine noch wichtigere Zukunft betreffen, auf eben demselben Standpunkt der heiligen Schrift und der Geographie beruhen. Ich bin kein Studirter der Weltwissenschaft, also auch nicht der Geographie, und ebenso wenig ein menschlich Studirter der Theologie, jedoch aber ein "göttlich-studirter" Theologe. Kraft dieser meiner göttlichen Ausbildung oder unmittelbar von Gott mir gegebenen Offenbarung—die auch Blicke in die Tiefen der Gottheit mitsichführt, ist auch dieses bis vor einigen Jahren verborgen gewesene Geheimniss der nahen Zukunft mir entsiegelt in Uebereinstimmung der heiligen Schrift und der Geographie.

Auf diese religiöse und natürliche Wahrheit sicher mich stützend und berufend, bin ich mit Ihrer Anschauung ganz übereinstimmend, dass am Nordpol das in Folge des Sündenfalles zerstörte Paradies stattgefunden hat.

Ich hoffe dass wir beiderseits auf dem Grunde dieser unserer Uebereinstimmung in nähere Bekanntschaft mit einander nach Gottes Wohlgefallen kommen werden. In diesem Vertrauen zu Ihnen erwarte ich eine baldige Erfüllung meiner eben an Sie gerichteten Bitte, — mit Hochachtung,

     Ergebenst,   —— ——.

SECTION IV. — THE EARTH AND WORLD OF THE HINDUS.

(Illustrating pp. 129–133 ; 148–154 ; 183, etc.)

THAT the mythological cosmos of the modern Hindus was originally constructed upon the basis of a geocentric system of the planetary heavens I cannot doubt. Its " concentric oceans " are simply the interplanetary spaces mythologically pictured and described. Its "concentric continents" are those invisible solid, concentric, " crystalline spheres " which revolved about the common axis of the Pythagoreo-Ptolemaic universe, and were presided over by the different visible planets. In both systems the Earth is not only the centre of the planetary revolution, but also *the centre of each planetary sphere itself.* How entirely incorrect the flat-world interpretation ordinarily given us is [1] could hardly be more forcibly shown than it is in the following extract : " Priya Vrata, by the wheel of whose car the Earth [or better, the World] was divided into seven continents, had thirteen male children. Six of these embraced an ascetic life ; the rest ruled the seven divisions of the Earth [World.] To Agnidhra was assigned the Jambu-dwípa [the Earth] ; to Medhátithi, Plaksha ; to Vápushmát, Sálmali ; to Jyotishmat, Kúsa ; to Dyutimat, Krauncha ; to Bhavya, Sáka ; and to Savala, Pushkara. With the exception of the sovereign of Jambu each of the six other kings is said to have had seven sons, among whom he divided his kingdom into seven equal parts. These seven divisions in each of the six continents are separated by seven chains of mountains and seven rivers lying breadthwise, *and placed with such inclinations with respect to one another that if a straight line be drawn through any chain of mountains or*

[1] See picture in Dr. Scudder's *Tales for Little Readers about the Heathen.* New York, 1849 : p. 48.

rivers and its corresponding mountains or rivers on the other continents, and produced toward the central island, it would meet the centre of the Earth." [1]

All Puranic descriptions of the Earth are by no means consistent with each other, but the following from the Vishnu Purana can readily be understood if read in the light of the illustrative cuts already given : —

Parásara. — You shall hear from me, Maitreya, a brief account of the earth. A full detail I could not give you in a century.

The seven great insular continents are Jambu, Plaksha, Sálmali, Kusa, Krauncha, Sáka, and Pushkara ; and they are surrounded, severally, by seven great seas, — the sea of salt water (Lavana), of sugar-cane juice (Ikshu), of wine (Surá), of clarified butter (Sarpis), of curds (Dadhi), of milk (Dugdha), and of fresh water (Jala).

Jambu-dwípa is in the centre of all these. And in the centre of this (continent) is the golden mountain Meru. The height of Meru is eighty-four thousand Yojanas ; and its depth below (the surface of the earth) is sixteen (thousand). Its diameter at the summit is thirty-two (thousand Yojanas), and at its base sixteen thousand ; so that this mountain is like the seed-cup of the lotos of the earth.

The boundary mountains (of the earth) are Himavat, Hemakúta, and Nishadha, which lie south (of Meru) ; and Níla, Sweta, and Śringin ; which are situated to the north (of it). The two central ranges (those next to Meru, or Nishadha and Níla) extend for a hundred thousand (Yojanas, running east and west). Each of the others diminishes ten thousand (Yojanas, as it lies more remote from the centre).[2] They are two thousand (Yo-

---

[1] Babu Shome, " Physical Errors of Hinduism." *Selections from the Calcutta Review*, No. xv., April, 1882.

[2] In our diagram of the Hindu *Varshas*, p. 152, the length of the outer partition-ranges diminishes at about the rate here required. In the only other I have ever seen, — one shown me by Professor

janas) in height, and as many in breadth. The Varshas (or countries between these ranges) are: Bhárata (India), south of the Himavat mountains; next, Kimpurusha, between Himavat and Hemakúta; north of the latter, and south of Nishadha, is Harivarsha: north of Meru is Ramyaka, extending from the Nila or blue mountains to the Sweta (or white) mountains; Hiranmaya lies between the Sweta and Sringin ranges; and Uttarakuru is beyond the latter, following the same direction as Bhárata. Each of these is nine thousand (Yojanas) in extent.

Ilávrita is of similar dimensions, but in the centre of it is the golden mountain Meru; and the country extends nine thousand (Yojanas) in each direction from the four sides of the mountain. There are four mountains in this Varsha, formed as buttresses to Meru, each ten thousand Yojanas in elevation. That on the east is called Mandara; that on the south, Gandhamádana; that on the west, Vipula; and that on the north, Supárswa. On each of these stands severally a Kadamba-tree, a Jambu-tree, a Pippala, and a Vata; each spreading over eleven hundred (Yojanas, and towering aloft like) banners on the mountains. From the Jambu-tree the insular continent Jambu-dwípa derives its appellation. The apples

Max Müller in a modern Sanskrit tractate, whose author's name I regret to have lost, — all the ranges were represented as parallel with the Nila and Nishadha. Moreover, as the whole surface of Jambu-dwípa was represented as a circular flat disk, the second of the two successive outer ranges was much more than the required one tenth shorter than its predecessor. Besides this, Jambu-dwípa is repeatedly described in this same Purana as a globe, and should be so treated in all graphic representations.

Postscript. Since the above was written a long search for Capt. Wilford's diagrams in vol. viii. of the *Asiatic Researches* (London, 1808) has been crowned with success. His perpetual vacillation between what he considers the primitive and proper flat earth of "the Pauranics" and the spherical earth of the astronomers is the chief source of his manifold embarrassments. A second and subordinate source of endless trouble is his effort to interpret mythical geography in the terms of geography actual.

of that tree are as large as elephants. When they are rotten they fall upon the crest of the mountain ; and from their expressed juice is formed the Jambu river, the waters of which are drunk by the inhabitants ; and, in consequence of drinking of that stream, they pass their days in content and health, being subject neither to perspiration, to foul odors, to decrepitude, nor organic decay. The soil on the banks of the river, absorbing the Jambu juice, and being dried by gentle breezes, becomes the gold termed Jámbunada (of which) the ornaments of the Siddhas (are fabricated). The country of Bhadráswa lies on the east of Meru, and Ketumála, on the west; and between these two is the region Ilávrita. On the east (of the same) is the forest Chaitraratha ; the Gandhamádana (wood) is on the south ; (the forest of) Vaibhiája is on the west ; and (the grove of India, or) Mandana is on the north. There are also four great lakes, the waters of which are partaken of by the gods, called Aruńoda, Mahábhadra, Ásitoda, and Mánasa.

The principal mountain ridges which project from the base of Meru, like filaments from the root of the lotos, are, on the east, Sítánta, Mukunda, Kurarí, Mályavat, and Vaikanka ; on the south, Trikútá, Sisira, Patanga, Ruchaka, and Nishadha ; on the west Sikhivásas, Vaidúrya, Kapila, Gandhamádana, and Járudhi ; and on the north Sankhakúta, Ŕishabha, Hamsa, Nága, and Kálanjara. These and others extend from between the intervals in the body, or from the heart, of Meru.

On the summit of Meru is the vast city of Brahmá, extending fourteen thousand leagues, and renowned in heaven ; and around it, in the cardinal points and the intermediate quarters, are situated the stately cities of Indra and the other regents of the spheres. The capital of Brahmá is inclosed by the river Ganges, which, issuing from the foot of Vishnu, and washing the lunar orb, falls, here, from the skies, and after encircling the city

divides into four mighty rivers flowing in opposite directions. These rivers are the Sítá, the Alakanandá, the
Chakshu, and the Bhadrá. The first, falling upon the
tops of the inferior mountains, on the east side of Meru,
flows over their crests, and passes through the country of
Bhadráśwa, to the ocean. The Alakanandá flows south,
to (the country of) Bhárata, and, dividing into seven
rivers on the way, falls into the sea. The Chakshu falls
into the sea, after traversing all the western mountains
and passing through the country of Ketumála. And the
Bhadrá washes the country of the Uttarakurus, and empties itself into the northern ocean.

Meru, then, is confined between the mountains Níla
and Nishadha (on the north and south), and between
Mályavat and Gandhamádana (on the west and east). It
lies between them, like the pericarp of a lotos.

The countries of Bhárata, Ketumála, Bhadráśwa, and
Uttarakuru lie, like leaves of the lotos of the world, exterior to the boundary mountains. Játhara and Deva-
kúta are two mountain ranges, running north and south,
and connecting the two chains of Níla and Nishadha.
Gandhamádana and Kailása extend, east and west, eighty
Yojanas in breadth, from sea to sea. Nishadha and Pári-
yátra are the limitative mountains on the west, stretching, like those on the east, between the Níla and Nishadha ranges. And the mountains Triśṛinga and Já-
rudha are the northern limits (of Meru), extending, east
and west, between the two seas. Thus I have repeated
to you the mountains described by great sages as the
boundary mountains, situated in pairs on each of the
four sides of Meru.

Those also which have been mentioned as the fila-
ment mountains (or spurs), Sítanta and the rest, are exceedingly delightful. The valleys embosomed amongst
them are favorite resorts of the Siddhas and Cháranas.
And there are situated upon them agreeable forests and

pleasant cities, embellished with the palaces of Lakshmí, Vishńu, Agni, Súrya, and other deities, and peopled by celestial spirits ; whilst the Yakshas, Rákshasas, Daityas, and Dánavas pursue their pastimes in the vales.

These, in short, are the regions of Paradise, or Swarga, the seats of the righteous, and where the wicked do not arrive even after a hundred births. In (the country of) Bhadráśwa, Vishńu resides as Hayasíras (the horse-headed) ; in Ketumála, as Varáha (the boar) ; in Bhárata, as the tortoise (Kúrma) ; in Keru, as the fish (Matsya) ; in his universal form, everywhere : for Hari pervades all places. He is the supporter of all things ; he is all things. In the eight realms of Kiṁpurusha and the rest (or all exclusive of Bhárata), there is no sorrow, nor weariness, nor anxiety, nor hunger, nor apprehension ; their inhabitants are exempt from all infirmity and pain, and live (in uninterrupted enjoyment) for ten or twelve thousand years. Indra never sends rain upon them ; for the earth abounds with water. In those places there is no distinction of Kŕita, Tretá, or any succession of ages. In each of these Varshas there are, respectively, seven principal ranges of mountains, from which, O best of Brahmans, hundreds of rivers take their rise. (*From H. H. Wilson's Translation of the Vishnu Purana.*) [1]

For further accounts of Puranic geography see Wilford's " Sacred Isles in the West," ch. iii. ; " Geographical Extracts from the Puranas," in " Asiatic Researches," vol. viii.

---

[1] The parentheses and vowel marks in the foregoing are Wilson's.

SECTION V. — GRILL ON THE WORLD-PILLAR OF THE RIG VEDA.

(Illustrating pp. 136 ; 141 ; 144-146 ; 152 ; 155-158, etc. Also the Pillar of Atlas, pp. 350-358.)

" MIT diesem Namen — *Skambha* — der so viel als Pfeiler, Säule, bedeutet, verbindet sich die Vorstellung eines den Himmel oder die Welt tragenden Körpers. Diese Vorstellung hat innerhalb des Veda eine allmählische Ausbildung erfahren. In Rigveda ist der Skambha ursprünglich als eigentliche Säule, als hölzerner Pfeiler gedacht und ist so im Grund nur ein concreter Ausdruck für des Himmels Veste (vgl. IV., 13, 5 ; VIII., 41, 10). Es findet sich aber schon daneben die lebendigere Auffassung, dass derselbe ein Pflanzenstengel ist, wobei der Mythus an die Somapflanze denkt. Hierbei erscheint der Skambha als mit Saft gefüllt (*âpûrna am̐çu*, vgl. IX., 74, 2 ; 86, 46), und es ist damit ein Bild des Himmels gewonnen, das das doppelte Moment des Festen (Aufrechten) und Flüssigen glücklich in sich vereinigt. Diese Anschauung tritt nun viel entwickelter im Atharvaveda wieder auf. Hier ist der Skambha zunächst als der Eine Grundpfeiler und Tragbalken des Weltgebäudes geschildert in den alle einzelnen Theile desselben eingelassen sind, und der das gesammte Queergebälke durchzieht (*aviç, praviç*). Himmel, Luft und Erde mit all ihren Körpern und Elementen, mit dem ganzen Kreislauf ihrer Phänomene und Katastrophen, — alles ruht auf dieser Unterlage, vom Praĝâpati darauf gegründet (X., 7, 7, 2 ff., 35). Auch die Gesammtheit der Götter wird von dieser Weltsäule getragen (X., 7, 13). An diese architektonische Auffassung reiht sich auch im Ath. Veda die Vorstellung eines *Baumes*, von dessen Aesten die Rede ist, dessen Aesten die Götter selbst sind (vgl. X., 7, 21, 22, 38), und der einen Schatz bergen soll. Selbst in animalischer Form

30

wird der Skambha dargestellt, so dass seine einzelnen Körpertheile unterschieden werden (X., 18, 19, 33, 34). Ja schliesslich geht der Mythus so weit, dass er diesen Weltpfeiler oder Weltbaum nicht bloss beseelt denkt, sondern geradezu mit der Weltseele (Purusha) mit dem obersten Brahman, mit dem Praĝâ pati (dem Weltschöpfer) identificirt (X., 7, 15, 17, 8, 2), und die hierin enthaltene Personification tritt noch entschiedener zu Tag, wenn der Skambha sogar mit Indra zusammenfällt (X., 7, 29, 30). Mit Recht ist der elementare Skambha mit dem Atlas der Griechen und den Säulen des Herakles verglichen worden. Wie aber M. Müller angesichts des Skambha und der oben vorgeführten Zeugnisse die Behauptung aufstellen kann : "Es ist kein Beleg dafür vorhanden, dass irgend etwas der Auffassung der Yggdrasil ähnliches je den vedischen Dichtern in den Sinn kam" (Essays, Deutsch, II., 184 [Chips, vol. ii., 204]), ist mir unverständlich. Vergleiche auch die Behandlung des Skambhamythus bei de Gubernatis Mithologia Vedica, pp. 273-299.

Aus der späteren Entwicklung der indischen Mythologie nenne ich noch besonders die Darstellung des Weltbaumes oder himmlischen Baumes in dem paradiesischen, bei der Quirlung des Oceans entstandenen, Pâriĝâta (Korallenbaum, Erythrina Indica), der durch Krishna auf Wunsch seiner Gattin Satjabhâmâ Indra entrissen wurde. Die Beschreibung des Baumes, sowie seiner Entführung erscheint im Purâna (Vishnu, Bhâgavata) noch einfach (vgl. Vish. P. bei H. H. Wilson, pp. 585-588), sehr ausführlich dagegen und mit einzelnen Abweichungen im Harivaṁça. Er hat nach diesem die Eigenschaft, "de satisfaire tous les désirs. Vous n'aurez qu'à penser, et aussitôt par la vertu de celle fleur, qui saura s'entendre et se multiplier, vous aurez des guirlandes, des couronnes, des festons, des parterres entirs. Cette fleur remédie à la faim, à la soif, à la maladie, à la vieillesse, etc. Bien plus, source de bonheur et de gloire elle est encore un gage de vertu ; intelligente et raisonnable, elle perd son éclat avec l'impie, et le conserve avec la personne attachée à son devoir." — Siehe, 'Harivansa,' trad. par Langlois, II., 3, 12. (J. Grill, "*Die Erzväter der Menschheit,*" vol. i, p. 358, 9.)

SECTION VI. — HOMER'S ABODE OF THE DEAD.[1]

(Illustrating Chapters i. and vii. in Part Four ; Chapter ii. in Part Six, and other passages.)

So herrscht gleich über den Ort wo die Unterwelt zu denken sei ein merkwürdiger Zwiespalt. — PRELLER.

Bei Homer ist eine doppelte Ansicht von der Lage des Todtenreiches zu erkennen, einmal unter der Erde, und dann wiederum auf der Oberfläche des Bodens in dem ewigen Dunkel jenseits des westlichen Ocean. Die Ansichten von den beiden Hades fliessen beständig durcheinander. So weit aber die mit jedem verbundenen Vorstellungen zu sondern und einzeln aufzufassen möglich ist, müssen wir sie darzulegen im Folgenden versuchen. — VÖLCKER.

WHERE does Homer locate the realm of Hades? In the whole broad field of Homeric scholarship it would be difficult to find a more fascinating question. Few have been more written upon. The literature of the subject is itself almost a library. No mythologist, no commentator upon the poet, no class-room interpreter even, can evade the question ; and yet, in their answers, the Homeric authorities of all modern times, whatever their nationality, present only a pitiable spectacle of helpless bewilderment. Classifying these various interpreters according to the answers they respectively give to the question propounded, they stand as follows : —

First, a class who content themselves with the general assertion that the earth of Homer was a "flat disk," and that his Hades, like that of the ancients generally, was undoubtedly conceived of as a dark recess or cavern in the bosom of this earth-disk. Anything in the Odyssey

---

[1] Printed in advance in *The Boston University Year Book*, vol. x.

or elsewhere inconsistent with this view is simply a play of poetic fancy.

Second, a class — if class it be — who say with the genial Wilhelm Jordan, " Das Hadesreich der Odyssee ist die von der Sonne abgekehrte Rückseite der Erdscheibe, die ἀντίχθον, Gegenerde, eines weit späteren Zeitalters. Von der ζείδωρος ἄρουρα und vom Götterhimmel aus betrachtet bleibt es allerdings Unterwelt, ὑπὸ κεύθεσι γαίας, aber nicht als Erdinneres, sondern als jenseitige Oberfläche." [1] Here the earth is still a flat disk ; but Hades, instead of being within it, is simply its under or reverse side.

Third, a class who locate the shadowy realm on the same plane with the inhabited earth, but in the far West, just *inside* the Ocean-stream. This includes all commentators who, locating Hades above ground in the West, place Kirkè's isle in the same quarter, and hold that Odysseus did not cross over the Ocean-stream.

Fourth, a class who locate it in the far West, just *outside* the Ocean-stream. This includes all commentators who, locating Hades above ground in the West, place Kirkè's isle in the same quarter, but hold that Odysseus crossed the Ocean-stream. [2]

---

[1] Fleckeisen's *Jahrbücher*, 1872, vol. cv., pp. 1–8.

[2] Rinck, *Die Religion der Hellenen*, Th. ii., p. 459 : " Bei Homer ist das Schattenreich noch keine Unterwelt, sondern jenes liegt ausser dem von der Sonne beschienenen Bereich der Erde, jenseits des Okeanos." Here, and in some other writers, along with a retention of the unity of the authorship of the *Iliad* and *Odyssey*, we find an intimation that the perplexing discrepancy in Greek representations of Hades is due to a gradual translocation of it from the far West to the interior of the earth, in consequence of advancing geographical knowledge. Perhaps a separate class should have been introduced, consisting of the representatives of this view. But had this been done, yet a fourteenth class would have been necessary to include those who, with Charles Francis Keary, exactly reverse the process, and make the oldest Greek Hades interterranean, and the trans-oceanic one at the West a later product. *The Mythology of the Eddas.* London, 1882 : p. 14.

Fifth, a class who locate it in the far East, just inside the Ocean-stream. This class includes all who place Kirkè's isle in the East, and hold that Odysseus did not cross the Ocean-stream in visiting the superterranean Hades.

Sixth, a class who locate it in the far East, just outside the Ocean-stream. This includes all who place Kirkè's isle in the East, and hold that Odysseus crossed the Ocean-stream in visiting the superterranean Hades.

Seventh, a class who try to harmonize the conflicting representations by making the one set of expressions relate to a Hades in the bosom of the flat earth, and the other set of expressions relate to "the entrance" of the passage leading down to it from the world of living men. This class is again subdivided into four sub classes, according as they maintain a *cis-oceanic* or *trans-oceanic* location of this mouth of Hades, and place it to the *East* or to the *West* of the poet.

Eighth, a class who hold that the difficulty is in the poet himself, he having got two incompatible mythologies mixed up together.

Ninth, a class who try to solve all discrepancies by assigning the different representations in the two poems, and in different parts of the same poem, to different ages and to different authors.

Tenth, a class who query whether or no it be not admissible to hold that Homer had two realms of Hades, — the one "subterranean," and the other "beyond the Ocean."

Eleventh, a class who, with Altenburg and Gerland, resolve the whole story of Odysseus' descent to Hades into an astronomical myth;[1] or with Cox see in it simply a mythologico-poetic expression for the prosaic fact that the Sun, the "lord of day," returning after his morn-

[1] "Odysseus in der Unterwelt." *Archiv für Philologie*, 1840, pp. 170–188. G. K. C. Gerland, *Altgriechische Märchen in der Odyssee.* Magdeburg, 1869 : p. 50.

ing and noontide wanderings to his western home, sometimes finds it necessary to make his way behind dark
clouds.[1]

Twelfth, a class who point out the manifest difficulties
of the problem, but frankly profess their utter inability to
present a solution.

Of the more important of the maps of "the world according to Homer," those of Bunbury, Völcker, and For-
biger are constructed according to the view of class
fourth; that of Ukert, according to the view of that division of class seventh who locate the Hades portal in
the far West, just inside the Ocean-stream; that of Gladstone,[2] according to the view of that division of class
seventh who locate the Hades portal in the far East, just
inside the Ocean-stream. Völcker, however, is inclined
to believe in two Homeric Hades-realms, — the one interterranean, the other at the West superterranean and
trans-oceanic.

Such are the multifarious, contradictory, confused, and
despairing answers given to our question by the most
learned and eminent of Homeric scholars. It would be
an easy task to fill a volume with citations illustrating
these various positions, and the ingenious but mutually
destructive arguments by which their respective advocates have sought to establish them. It will be more
profitable to turn from such a Babel of ideas, over which
the darkness of Hades itself seems to have fallen, and
inquire what the poet himself has to say on the subject.

The region of the dead is represented in Homer as
one of perpetual night. Its name is Erebos.[3] From the

---

[1] *Mythology of the Aryan Nations,* vol. ii., 171–180.

[2] Mr. Gladstone has more recently abandoned the flat-earth theory,
and tentatively advocated *an interterranean Hades with its mouth
downwards.* See his *Primer,* London and New York, 1878, pp. 54–
57; and *Homeric Synchronism,* London, 1876, p. 231. Perhaps this
view also should have been included in the foregoing classification.

[3] "Dénomination assyrienne." Félix Robiou, *Questions Homé-*

name of the divinity presiding in it, it is generally called
the house or abode of Aïdes (Hades).[1] That it was conceived of as *underneath the earth* appears from the perpetually recurring expressions, both in the Iliad and in
the Odyssey, relating the descent into and ascent out
of it.[2] In certain passages it is in fact expressly spoken
of as "under the earth;"[3] in others, as "under the recesses of the earth."[4] Hence Aïdes himself is styled
Ζεὺς καταχθόνιος, "the Subterranean Zeus."[5]

In the Battle of the Gods there is a vivid picture of this
underworld and of its trembling king : —

riques. Paris, 1876 : p. 13. The Shemitic origin of this term is significant. It prepares us to find an agreement between the Homeric
and the Assyrio-Babylonian ideas of the realm of the dead. Mr.
Gladstone says, "Long before . . . I had been struck by the predominance of a foreign character and associations in the Homeric
Underworld of the eleventh Odyssey." *Homeric Synchronism.* London, 1876 : p. 213. On the remarkably expressive cuneiform ideo-
graph for *eribu*, see the explanation given by Robert Brown, Jun., in
the *Proceedings of the Society of Biblical Archæology*, May 4, 1880.

[1] This term is also believed to be of Oriental origin, exactly corresponding to the *Bit Edi* of the Akkadians. See the translations of
The Descent of Istar. "Talbot regards, and I think justly, the usual
etymology of Hades — *quasi* Aïdes, '*invisible*' — as an afterthought."
Robert Brown, Jun., *The Myth of Kirkè*, p. 111 n.

[2] *Iliad*, vi. 284 ; vii. 330 ; xiv. 457 ; xxii. 425. *Odyssey*, x. 174,
560 ; xi. 65, 164, 475, 624 ; xxiii. 252 ; xxiv. 10, etc. "Von einem be-
sondern Eingang zu diesem unterirdischen Hades," remarks Völcker
(*Homerische Geographie*, p. 141), "meldet der Dichter nichts ; vielmehr gehen die Seelen, durch nichts gehindert, begraben und unbe-
graben überall unter die Erde." Granting this, there is no ground
for his other assertion, "Dieser Hades ist nicht unter, sondern in der
Erde." The immaterial shade can as easily pass through the whole
globe to an opposite surface as through a thick crust to a central
cavern. But see Mr. Gladstone's *Homeric Synchronism*, p. 222 :
"There is not in all Homer a single passage which imports the idea,
or indicates the possibility, of our passing through the solid earth."

[3] *Iliad*, xxiii. 100 ; xviii. 333.

[4] *Odyssey*, xxiv. 204. Comp. *Iliad*, xxii. 482.

[5] *Iliad*, ix. 457. Comp. iii. 278 ; xix. 259 ; xx. 61. Comp. Herodotus, ii. 122.

Thus the blessed gods inciting, both sides engaged, and among them made severe contention to break out. But dreadfully from above thundered the Father of gods and men, while beneath Poseidon shook the boundless earth and the lofty summits of the mountains. The roots and all the summits of many-rilled Ida were shaken, and the city of the Trojans and the ships of the Greeks. Aïdes himself, king of the nether world, trembled beneath, and leaped up from his throne terrified, and shouted aloud, lest earth-shaking Poseidon should cleave asunder the earth over him, and disclose to mortals and immortals his mansions, terrible, squalid, which even the gods loathe.[1]

But while the abode of Aïdes is thus clearly represented as under the earth, it is nevertheless represented as just across the Ocean-river, and capable of being reached by ship. In the eleventh and twelfth books of the Odyssey, the voyage of Odysseus to this region is described in the same apparently literal nautical terms as is the voyage to the Land of the Lotus-Eaters. And of his interview with the dead, Hayman says, "The whole scene is conceived by the poet as enacted on a geographical extension of the earth beyond the Ocean-stream."[2] There is no hint of any descent into the interior of the earth, no passage through or into subterranean caverns. The journey is as natural in all its aspects as any voyage from one coast of the Atlantic to its opposite.[3] Thus opens the eleventh book : —

[1] *Iliad*, xx. 61 ff. That there may be no question as to the impartiality of the translations given in this paper, the well-known and widely circulated version by Theodore Alois Buckley, of Christ Church, Oxford, is followed. A version giving more accurately the force of the verbs expressing upward and downward motion would in many passages be more favorable to the cosmological view here presented.

[2] Henry Hayman, D. D., *The Odyssey of Homer*. London, 1866: vol. ii., Appendix G 3, p. xvii.

[3] " Von einem Hinabsteigen findet sich keine Spur. Wer beweisen kann, Odysseus sei im Innern der Erde gewesen, der versuche es ! " — Völcker, *Homerische Geographie*, p. 150.

But when we were come down to the ship and the sea, we first of all drew the ship into the divine sea, and we placed a mast and sails in the black ship. And taking the sheep we put them on board, and we ourselves also embarked grieving, shedding the warm tear. And fair-haired Kirkè (Circe) — an awful goddess, possessing human speech — sent behind our dark-blue-prowed ship a moist wind that filled the sails, an excellent companion. And we sat down, making use of each of the instruments in the ship, and the wind and the pilot directed it. And the sails of it passing over the sea were stretched out the whole day; and the sun set, and all the ways were overshadowed. And it reached the extreme boundaries of the deep-flowing Ocean,[1] where are the people and city of the Kimmerians covered with shadow and vapor, nor does the shining sun behold them with his beams, neither when he goes toward the starry heaven, nor when he turns back again from heaven to earth, but pernicious night is spread over hapless mortals. Having come there we drew up our ship, and we took out the sheep, and we ourselves went again to the stream of the Ocean, until we came to the place which Kirkè mentioned.

Here the hero performed the rites and held the consultation which Kirkè had previously prescribed in these terms : —

"O noble son of Laertes, much-contriving Odysseus, do not remain any longer in my house against your will. But first you must perform another voyage, and come to the house of Aïdes and awful Persephonè, to consult the soul of Theban Tiresias, a blind prophet, whose mind is firm. To him, even when dead, Persephonè has given understanding, alone to be prudent, but the rest flit about as shades."

"Who, O Kirkè, will conduct me on this voyage ? No one has yet come to Aïdes in a black ship."

"O noble son of Laertes, much-contriving Odysseus, let not the desire of a guide for thy ship be at all a care to thee ; but having erected the mast, and spread out the white sails, sit down, and let the blast of the North wind carry it. But when thou shalt have passed through the Ocean in thy ship, where

1 That is, the farther shore. See Völcker, p. 145.

is the easy-dug [1] shore and the groves of Persephonè, and tall poplars, and fruit-destroying willows, there draw up thy ship in the deep-eddying Ocean, and do thou thyself go to the spacious house of Aïdes. Here indeed both Pyriphlegethon and Cocytus, which is a stream from the water of Styx, flow into Acheron; and there is a rock, and the meeting of two loud-sounding rivers. There then, O hero, approaching near as I command thee, dig a trench the width of a cubit each way; and pour around it libations to all the dead, first with mixed honey, then with sweet wine, and again the third time with water, and sprinkle white meal over it. And entreat much the powerless heads of the dead, promising that when thou comest to Ithaca thou wilt offer up in thy palace a barren heifer, which-soever is the best, and wilt fill the pyre with excellent things, and that thou wilt sacrifice to Tiresias alone a black sheep, all black, which excels among thy sheep. But when thou shalt have entreated the illustrious nations of the dead with prayers, then sacrifice a male sheep and a black female, turning toward Erebos; and do thou thyself be turned away at a distance, going toward the streams of the river; but there many souls of those gone dead will come. Then immediately exhort thy companions and command them, having skinned the sheep which lie there slain with the unpitying brass, to burn them and to invoke the gods, both mighty Aïdes and dread Persephonè. And do thou, having drawn thy sharp sword from thy thigh, sit down, nor suffer the powerless heads of the dead to go near the blood before thou inquirest of Tiresias. Then the prophet will immediately come to thee, O leader of the people, who will tell to thee the voyage and the measures of the way and thy return, how thou mayest go over the fishy sea." [2]

In the following passage Odysseus narrates how, having arrived "at the place which Kirkè mentioned," he fulfilled her commission : —

---

[1] Buckley well expresses dissatisfaction with this rendering. Völcker translates the term " ein *niedriges* Gestade." It is perhaps the low-down shore as contrasted with the upper or opposite one.

[2] *Odyssey*, x. 488–540.

Then Perimedes and Eurylochos made sacred offerings; but I, drawing my sharp sword from my thigh, dug a trench the width of a cubit each way, and around it we poured libations to all the dead, first with mixed honey, then with sweet wine, again a third time with water, and I sprinkled white meal over it. And I much besought the unsubstantial heads of the dead, promising that when I came to Ithaca I would offer up in my palace a barren heifer, whichsoever is the best, and that I would sacrifice separately to Tiresias alone a sheep all black. which excels among our sheep. But when I had besought them, the nations of the dead, with vows and prayers, then taking the sheep, I cut off their heads into the trench, and the black blood flowed ; and the souls of the perished dead were assembled forth from Erebos, — betrothed girls and youths, and much-enduring old men, and tender virgins having a newly grieved mind, and many Mars-renowned men wounded with brass-tipped spears, possessing gore-besmeared arms, who in great numbers were wandering about the trench on different sides with a divine clamor; and pale fear seized upon me. Then at length exhorting my companions, I commanded them, having skinned the sheep which lay there, slain with the cruel brass, to burn them, and to invoke the gods, both Aïdes and Persephonè. But I, having drawn my sharp sword from my thigh, sat down ; nor did I suffer the powerless heads of the dead to draw nigh the blood, before I inquired of Tiresias.

So far it might appear uncertain whether the hero were really in Hades, or only near it, at some point accessible alike to the living and to the dead. But the lines immediately following show that he was truly in " the house of Aïdes : " —

And first the soul of my companion Elpenor came, for he was not yet buried beneath the wide-wayed earth ; for we left his body in the palace of Kirkè, unwept-for and unburied, since another toil then urged us. Beholding him I wept, and pitied him in my mind; and, addressing him, spoke winged words: " O Elpenor, how didst thou come under the dark west ? Thou hast come sooner on foot than I with a black ship."

Thus I spoke, but he groaning answered me in discourse: " O Zeus-born son of Laertes, much-contriving Odysseus, the evil destiny of the deity and the abundant wine hurt me. Lying down in the palace of Kirkè, I did not think to go down backward, having come to the long ladder; but I fell downward from the roof, and my neck was broken from the vertebræ, and my soul descended to Hades."

In line 69, Elpenor speaks of Odysseus " going *hence from the house of Aïdes ;* " and in line 164, as elsewhere (x. 502; xi. 59, 158; xii. 21; xxiii. 324), the expressions leave no chance to doubt that Odysseus' voyage was a genuine *descensus ad inferos.*[1]

Here, then, are the two grand tests of every proposed solution of the problem of the location of the Homeric Hades : —

I. *Its Hades must be underneath the earth ;* and

II. *It must be on the surface of the earth, beyond the Ocean.*

This strange and perplexing difference, not to say contradiction, in the Homeric representations, did not escape the notice of the older commentators and writers on mythology. Especially has it called out the ingenuity of German scholars. F. A. Wolf recognized it, but did not profess to be able to give an explanation. J. H. Voss invented the method of solving the problem by placing Hades itself within the bosom of the earth-disk, but its " entrance " on the westernmost point of Europe on the inner shore of the ocean. Völcker rejected this solution, but, in the absence of a better, cautiously suggested — as we have seen — the possibility of Homer's having held to two kingdoms of the dead, one within the earth, and one

---

[1] See Preller, *Mythologie,* vol. i., pp. 504, 505, where he says that the region visited was "die ganze und wirkliche Unterwelt, nicht etwa bloss ein Eingang in die Unterwelt." See also Völcker, *Homerische Geographie,* § 76.

in the dark trans-oceanic West.[1] Eggers [2] and Nitzsch [3] inclined to the support of the Vossian compromise; and in 1854 Preller could still speak of it as the one "at present chiefly prevalent." [4] Still, as Preller and others urged, nothing in the descriptions of the western Hades corresponds with the idea of a "portal" or "entrance" to a subterranean world extending so far eastward as to be situated under Greece and Asia Minor: [5] hence the latest interpreters have been as free as were the earlier to take their choice among the wild and contradictory conjectures classified at the beginning of this paper. The latest of these guesses is that of Jordan ; and, though it comes within a hair's-breadth of the truth, it has been the most ridiculed of all.[6]

———————

As pointed out in earlier pages, the one false principle which has vitiated and confused all modern discussions of Homeric cosmology is the groundless notion that the earth of Homer is a flat disk. This mistaken presupposition is responsible for the failure of all hitherto attempted demonstrations of the true location of the poet's Hades. Once conceive of the Homeric Cosmos as rep-

[1] This, if allowed, would afford no relief; for, as Hentze says, "the subterranean character of even the Odyssean Hades can by no means be got rid of." Ameis, *Anhang.*, Book X., 508.

[2] *De Orco Homerico*, Altona, 1836. But Eggers located the Hades entrance inside the Ocean-stream, Nitzsch outside.

[3] G. W. Nitzsch, *Erklärende Anmerkungen zu Homers Odyssee.* Hannover, 1840 : Bd. III., p. xxxv., 187.

[4] *Griechische Mythologie*, I., p. 505.

[5] See Preller : *Mythologie*, vol. i., p. 504. Eisenlohr, *Lage des Homerischen Todtenreichs*, 1872. Bunbury contents himself with the cool remark, "It is certainly not worth while to inquire what geographical idea the poet formed in his own mind of this visit to the regions of Hades." (!) *History of Ancient Geography*, vol. i , p. 58.

[6] See Kammer, *Einheit der Odyssee nach Widerlegung der Ansichten von Lachmann-Steinthal, Köchly, Hennings, und Kirchhoff.* Leipsic, 1873 : pp. 486–490.

resented in the accompanying cut of the "World of
Homer," and the problem of the site of Hades is solved
at a glance. It is the southern or under hemisphere of
the upright spherical earth. In this conception, whatsoever is "trans-oceanic" is also and of necessity "subterranean." Now for the first time can it be understood
how Leda and her noble-minded sons can be "on a geographical extension of the earth" on the farther shore of
the Ocean, and at the same time νέρθεν γῆς (Od., xi.
298). In this Cosmos, Hades cannot be beyond the
Ocean without being also underneath the earth. On the
traditional theory of a flat earth, the passage is and
ever must be the palpable inconsistency which Völcker
represents it. Even the theory of two or of twenty
Homers does not reasonably explain it. Precisely so
with the passages relating to Elpenor. His soul at death
goes κατὰ χθονός, yet it is found with the other ghosts in
the shadowy land just across the Ocean-river. So again
with the passages relating to the shades of the slain Suit-
ors. These reach the Underworld (xxiv. 106, 203);
but it is by a route *along the surface of the ground* to the
Ocean-stream, in full sight of the gates of the sun and of
the stars of the Milky Way (xxiv. 9–12).[1] Illustrious
scholars have accused the poet of *Widersprüche gröber
und ärger* than usual in this account;[2] but the whole
trouble has been, not in the poet, but in the poet's interpreters. With the spherical earth, all is consistent and
precisely as it should be. In this reconstructed Homeric
Cosmos, every crosser of the Ocean-stream, whether it be
Hermes, or Odysseus, or Herakles, reaches the groves of
Persephonè and the house of Aïdes. Wherever Kirkè's
isle is located, the "blast of the North wind" will drive
the voyager thence towards the realms of the dead. In
like manner it can now be understood how the stolen

---

[1] Porphyrius, *De antro Nympharum*, 28, explains that stumbling-
block of commentators, "the people of dreams."

[2] Völcker, *Homerische Geographie*, p. 152.

bride of Subterranean Zeus, while descending behind
swift steeds to the Underworld, can yet for a considerable
time behold the starry heaven, the earth, the sunlight,

OLYMPOS.

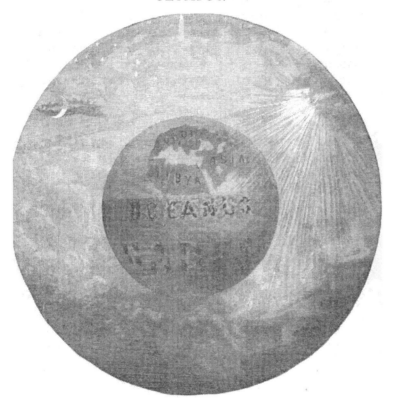

TARTAROS.

The World of Homer.

For a convenient account of this reëstablished world-view of the
ancients, for the use of schools, see *The True Key to Ancient Cosmology and Mythical Geography* (third edition, illustrated, Boston, Messrs.
Ginn, Heath and Co., 1882), from which the cut is taken.

and the fishy sea.[1] Though the god has power to penetrate the solid sphere,[2] it is down no yawning chasm that
his chariot disappears. As far as we can trace him and
his victim, they are still at the surface, simply moving
from the upper to the lower hemisphere.[3] In perfect
accordance with the requirement formulated by Völcker,
Odysseus and his companions descend (xi. 57, 476),
while the ghosts ascend (xi. 38), to reach the meeting-
place on the lower edge of the Ocean-stream. Beautifully
exact and strikingly natural is now the poet's declaration
that Tartaros is "as far below Hades as earth from
heaven," — a declaration as fatal to many of the fifteen or
more traditional explanations of Homer's Hades as it is
to Flach's elaborate and ingenious diagram of the Hades
of Hesiod.[4] With this inverted hemisphere for the kingdom of the dead, Voss need not longer trouble himself
about the mention of "clouds" therein.[5] In fine, with
the correct Homeric conception of the earth and of
Hades, the manifold alleged contradictions of the poet
instantaneously vanish. Better than that, the dual im-

---

[1] *Homeric Hymn to Demeter,* 30–35. Foerster places the origin of
this hymn early in the seventh century before Christ : *Der Raub und
Rückkehr der Persephonè.* Stuttgart, 1874 : pp. 33–39. See Sterrett,
*Qua in Re Hymni Homerici quinque Majores inter se different Anti-
quitate vel Homeritate,* Boston, 1881.

[2] Lines 16–18. Precisely so in the Indian epic, the *Ramayana :* one
and the same point in Hades is reached, whether we accompany
Ansumán digging through the heart of the earth, or follow the goddess Gangâ along the surface of the earth and across the Ocean-
bed. Book I., canto xl. Compare *Odyssey,* xi. 57,58.

[3] The much-debated Nysian field whence the goddess was stolen
was in the land of the gods at the North Pole. Menzel, *Die vorchristliche Unsterblichkeitslehre,* Bd. i., 64–67 ; ii., 25, 87, 93, 100,
122, 148, 345.

[4] *Das System der Hesiodischen Kosmogonie,* Leipsic, 1874.

[5] *Odyssey,* xi. 591. Völcker, while locating *this* Hades above
ground far to the West, is also embarrassed with these clouds, since
his Homeric heaven does not extend over the trans-oceanic region, or
even over the Ocean : p. 151.

ages of Hades, which have so long perplexed and blurred the vision of Homeric interpreters, suddenly resolve themselves into one perfectly focused stereoscopic picture of startling vividness and beauty.

One ground of misgiving and doubt may possibly still occur to cautious minds. "Is it credible," it may be asked, "that the early Homeric Greek, unschooled in the exercise of the scientific imagination, could picture to himself that pendant under-surface of the earth as habitable even by ghosts? Could he so long before 'Newton's day' have gained such knowledge of gravitation as to see how infernal rivers and infernal palaces could cling to an under-hemisphere? That Aristotle and the Greek philosophers of his age were able, we know from their writings;[1] but is it credible that the Greek of the Homeric age was equal to such a task? This proposed conception of Hades requires that we should think of a world where everything is upside down, exactly contrary and antipodal to our own. Can we believe that 'prehistoric men' could achieve such a prodigy of abstract thought?"

A pertinent and perhaps sufficient answer to these questions might be given by pointing to a most curious and instructive funeral-custom among the modern Karens of Burmah. This tribe is certainly not more highly gifted or more highly civilized than were the Greeks of the heroic age, yet they have precisely this Homeric conception of an antipodal Hades. A most competent authority gives us the following account: "When the day of burial arrives, and the body is carried to the grave, four bamboo splints are taken, and one is thrown towards the West, saying, 'That is the East;' another is thrown to the East, saying, 'That is the West;' a third is thrown upwards towards the top of the tree, saying, 'That is the foot of the tree;' and a fourth is thrown downwards, saying,

---

[1] See Dr. H. W. Schäfer, *Entwickelung der Ansichten des Alterthums über die Gestalt und Grösse der Erde*, Leipsic, 1868, quarto.

31

' That is the top of the tree.' The sources of the stream
are pointed to, saying, 'That is the mouth of the stream;'
and the mouth of the stream is pointed to, saying, ' That
is the head of the stream.' *This is done because in Hades
everything is upside down in relation to the things of this
world."* [1]

Striking, however, as would be this answer to the ques-
tioner, a better can be given. The better one points out
to him the foolishness of the assumption that either the
Greeks or the Karens originated for themselves their conceptions of Hades. Both simply inherited from their
fathers the old pre-Hellenic Asiatic idea of an antipodal
Underworld. Ages ago the notion which underlies the
Karen's rites was so prominent in the mind of the East
Aryans that the sudden and inevitable reversal of the
points of the compass, consequent upon entering the Underworld, became a poetic circumlocution to express the
idea of dying: thus, "Before thou art carried away dead
to the Ender by the royal command of Yama, . . . *before
the four quarters of the sky whirl round,* . . . practice the
most perfect contemplation." [2] Ages ago the notion
which underlies the southward voyage of Odysseus led
prehistoric Akkadians, in naming the cardinal points of
the compass, to designate the South as " the *funereal*
point;" and in locating the kingdom of the dead, to place

---

[1] Mason in *Journal of the Asiatic Society*, Bengal, XXXV., Pt. ii.,
p. 28. Spencer, *Descriptive Sociology*, No. 5, p. 23. At least one tribe
of our American Indians at the time of their discovery had a myth
of creation in which the earth was conceived of as a ball. H. H.
Bancroft, *Native Races of the Pacific States*, vol. iii., p. 536. That the
same idea underlay the Hades-conception of the New Zealanders is
plain from various indications. See present work, note on pp. 125,
126.

[2] *Mahâbhârata*, xii. 12,080. Muir, *Metrical Translations from
Sanskrit Writers*, London, 1879, p. 220. " To the gods this sphere
of asterisms revolves toward the right; to the enemies of the gods,
toward the left." *Sûrya Siddhânta*, xii., ch. 55. Comp. Aristotle,
De Cœlo, lib. ii., c. 2.

it *opposite the stars of the south polar sky.*[1] Through all
the lifetime of Babylonia and Assyria, as through all the
lifetime of ancient India,[2] the mount of the gods was at
the summit of the earth at the North Pole; its counterpart — the mount of the rulers of the dead — exactly opposite, beneath the earth, and at the South Pole.[3] Hence
life and light proceeded from the North, darkness and
death from the South.[4] In like manner the Egyptians
had their heaven-touching mountain in the farthest North,

---

[1] Dupuis, *Origine de Tous les Cults*, tom. i., 624. Lenormant,
Chaldæan Magic (English edition), pp. 168, 169. On the significance
of the South in Hindu belief, see Colebrooke, *Essays*, vol. i., pp. 174,
176, 182, 187, vol. ii., pp. 390-392 ; Monier Williams, *Sanskrit Dictionary*, Art. "Yama ;" Muir, *Sanskrit Texts*, vol. v., pp. 284-327 ;
and India literature *passim.*

[2] *Sûrya Siddhânta*, ch. xii. *Journal of the American Oriental Society*, New Haven, 1860, vol. vi., pp. 140-480. Keightley, *Mythology*
(Bohn), p. 240, n. 9.

[3] Of the latter mount, Lenormant correctly says that, in ancient
Chaldæan thought, it is " *située dans les parties basses de la terre*,"
but at times he incorrectly locates it in the West. In like manner
the mountain of the gods — " *le point culminant de la convexité de la
surface de la terre* " — he places not in the North (Is. xiv. 14), but
often in the East or North-east. *Origines de l'Histoire*, Paris, 1882,
tom. ii. 1, p. 134. See also Tiele, *Histoire Comparée des Anciennes
Religions*, Paris, 1882, p. 177, where he speaks of the entrance to
Hades as at the South-west. This is certainly a mistake, for the
Akkadian expression *mer kurra*, " the cardinal point of THE MOUN-
TAIN," must, at least originally, have signified the North. And as to
Lenormant's location of the antipodal mountain of Hades in the
West or South-west, our latest German writer upon the subject, Dr.
Friedrich Delitzsch, an eminent Assyriologist, affirms that in the
cuneiform literature thus far known he has discovered no trace of such
a location. *Wo lag das Paradies?* Leipsic, 1881, p. 121.

[4] "Nach der pythagoräischen, orphischen und neuplatonischen
Lehre brachte der Nordwind Leben der Südwind Tod, wohnten hinter dem Nordwind die Seligen und die Götter als Schöpfer und Er-
halter der Welt, hinter dem Südwind aber die Verdammten und alle
bösen zerstörenden Urmächte." W. Menzel, *Die vorchristliche Unsterblichkeitslehre*, vol. ii., p. 101 ; also pp. 36, 168, 345, and *passim.*
Compare A. Maury, *Histoire des Religions de la Grèce Antique*, Paris,
1869, tom. iii. 354.

and an antipodal counterpart in Amenti, or the abode of the dead.[1] As in ancient India's, so in ancient Egypt's, thought, this world of the dead was exactly the reverse or counterpart of the world of the living.[2] "The tall hill of Hades," like Ku-meru, is therefore a "pendent" one,[3] — the southern or under terminus of the egg of the earth.[4]

[1] For the first, see Brugsch, *Geographische Inschriften altägyptischer Denkmäler,* Leipsic, 1858, Bd. ii., p. 57 ; for the second, *The Book of the Dead, passim.*

[2] See Tiele, *History of the Egyptian Religion* (English edition, 1882), p. 68, "the reversed world : " and the still more forcible expression in his *Histoire Comparée* (Paris, 1882), p. 47, "*le monde opposé au monde actuel.*" Compare *Book of the Dead* (Birch's version), where it is styled "the *inverted* precinct ; " and Thompson's *Egyptian Doctrine of the Future State,* wherein Hades is described as "the *inverted* hemisphere of darkness," and where it is said to be "evident that the leading features of the Greek Hades were borrowed from Egypt." *Bibliotheca Sacra,* 1868, pp. 84, 86. Still more recently Reginald S. Poole has remarked, "Now that we recognize the Vedic source of a part of the Greek pantheon, and its generally Aryan character, we may fairly look elsewhere for that which is not Vedic. If embalming were derived from Egypt, why not the ideas which the Greek saw surrounding the custom, — the pictures of the Underworld, with its judgment, its felicity, and its misery? The stories which Homer makes Odysseus tell, when he would disguise his identity, show the familiarity with Egypt of the Greeks of the poet's time." *The Contemporary Review,* London, 1881, July, p. 61. It would be better to say that Homer's Hades, while agreeing with the Egyptian and Babylonian and Vedic, was not necessarily "borrowed" from either of these peoples, but more likely agreed with the Egyptian, Babylonian, and Vedic, simply because in each case there was a common inheritance, — a survival of still more ancient ideas of prehistoric ancestors.

[3] *Records of the Past,* vol. x., p. 88.

[4] Tiele, *History of the Egyptian Religion,* p. 67 : "The heaven (at night) rests upon the earth, like a goose brooding over her egg." Chabas, Lieblein, and Lefévre have each maintained that the ancient Egyptians were acquainted with the spherical figure of the earth ; while Maspéro, despite his language in *Les Contes Populaires de l'Égypte Ancienne* (Paris, 1882, pp. lxi.–lxiii.), in a private letter of still more recent date admits the possibility that the Egyptians held to such a view as long ago as eighteen centuries before the Christian era. In this connection it may be useful to state that Professor

The assertion sometimes made, that the Egyptian Amenti was just over the hill to the west of Abydos,[1] is only worthy of such cosmologists as Popsey Middleton, or the still more illustrious author of the "Zetetic Astronomy."

About a thousand years before Abraham went down into Egypt, — at least, that is the date assigned by Egyptologists, — a scribe engrossed upon a papyrus a fair copy of a tale of shipwreck. It is now one of the treasures of St. Petersburg. At the Congress of Orientalists, held in Berlin in the year 1881, its existence was first made known to the modern world through the translation then submitted by M. Golénischeff. The tale proves to be a kind of anticipation of the voyage of Odysseus to the realm of Aïdes. As in the Odyssey, it is the ship-commander himself who narrates his adventures. There is no imaginative and poetic vagueness about the details. The ship was one hundred and fifty cubits long, forty broad. The crew consisted of one hundred and fifty men. Upon the Ocean he is wrecked, his crew lost ; he himself, however, is driven upon an island in the neighborhood of the nether world of the dead. Indeed, the place itself was called "The Isle of the Double ; " and it was, as Maspéro believes, peopled by Shades invisible to the voyager only because he was as yet in the body. The king of the island was a huge serpent, thirty cubits long, and possessed of a wonderful beard.[2]

Tiele informs the present writer that he has abandoned his conjecture touching *Cher-nuter,* expressed in his *Vergelijkende Geschiedenis van de Egyptische en Mesopotamische Godesdiensten,* Amsterdam, 1872, p. 94 ; French edition, 1882, p. 51 ; English edition, 1882, p. 72.

[1] As, for example, by Marius Fontane, *Histoire Universelle, Les Égyptes,* Paris, 1882, p. 154. The following is particularly timely : "While at Abydos I explored the mountain cliffs to the westward in the hope of finding early tombs in them. In this, however, I was disappointed, as I came across only a few tombs of the Roman period." Professor A. H. Sayce in letter from Egypt in *The Academy,* London, Feb. 2, 1884, p. 84.

[2] *Les Contes Populaires de l'Égypte Ancienne,* pp. 145–147. On the

In what direction lay this mysterious land ?

Not in the West, where all our Egyptologists persist in locating Amenti, but *in the South.* Directly *up the Nile,* and out into the Ocean at its head-waters, lay the voyager's track. As in the case of Odysseus, so many centuries later, it was the blast of the North wind which bore him thither.[1]

In conclusion, if both the ancient Egyptians [2] and Chaldæans [3] believed that like as the stars of the northern hemisphere are set over the realm of the living, so *the stars of the southern hemisphere are set over the realm of the dead;* if in ancient Hindu thought " the gods in heaven are beheld by the inhabitants of hell *as they move with their heads inverted;*" [4] if in Roman thought —

conflicting views of Egyptologists as to the interpretation of terms designating the points of the compass, see *Zeitschrift für ägyptische Sprache,* 1865, 1877, etc.

[1] The universality of the ancient belief that disembodied souls must cross a body of water to reach their proper abode has attracted the attention of Mannhardt, and led him to remark, " Da auch die keltische, hellenische, iranische und indische Religion diese Vorstellung kennt, so ist es von vorn herein wahrscheinlich, dass dieselbe über die Zeit der Trennung hinausgeht." *Germanische Mythen,* Berlin, 1858, p. 364. This is a far more reasonable explanation than the fanciful attempt of Keary in the work already cited, and in his paper before the Royal Society of Literature entitled *Earthly Paradise of European Myths.*

[2] Creuzer-Guigniaut, *Religions de l' Antiquité,* tom. ii., p. 836. Comp. the language of the recently discovered epitaph of Queen Isis em Kheb, mother-in law of Shishak, King of Assyria (*circa* 1000 B.C.) : " She is seated all beautiful in her place enthroned, among the gods *of the South* she is crowned with flowers." *The Funeral Tent of an Egyptian Queen,* by Villiers Stuart, London, 1882, p. 34. Notwithstanding this, Mr. Stuart, a few pages later, — so powerful is the influence of tradition, — alludes to Amenti as located in the West (p. 49, also p. 27). But the inscription continues : " She is seated in her beauty in the arms of Khonsou her father, fulfilling his desires. He is in Amenti, the place of departed spirits." Comp. p. 33.

[3] Diodorus Siculus, ii. 31, 4. Lenormant, *The Beginnings of History,* New York, 1882, pp. 568, 569.

[4] Garrett, *Classical Dictionary of India,* Art. " Naraka." See also Obry, *Le Berceau de l' Espèce humaine,* p. 184 n.

" Mundus, ut ad Scythiam Rhipæasque arduus arces
Consurgit premitur Libyæ devexus in austros :
Hic vertex semper sublimis, *at illum*
Sub pedibus Styx atra videt, Manesque profundi ; " [1]

if in Greek cosmology the tall Pillar of Atlas is, as Euripides makes it, simply the upright axis of earth and
heaven,[2] — then the earth of the ancients is incontestably
A SPHERE, and Hades its under-surface. The "flat disk"
notion is itself a myth, and a myth without foundation.
In ancient thought, in a sense unrecognized even by the
writer of the words, was it true, —

" The world of Life,
The world of Death, are but opposing sides
Of one great Orb." [3]

SECTION VII. — LATEST POLAR RESEARCH.

THE recent happy issue of the last of the three re-
lief-expeditions sent out by the United States government
for the rescue of Lieutenant Greely and his starving
band of heroes has given unusual popular interest to the
great international undertaking in which he and his men
were so perilously engaged. Still very few, comparatively speaking, understand the scope and promise of this
first really adequate and hopeful scheme for the investigation of Terrestrial Physics near the Pole. Mr. O. B.
Cole, in 1883, described its inception and purpose as follows : —

The representatives of ten nations besides our own are engaged in it ; the fields of observation are in both the Arctic

[1] Vergil, *Georgics*, i. 240, ss.

[2] Peirithous, 597, 3-5, ed. Nauck. Comp. Aristotle, *De Anim.
Motione*, c. 3. Samuel Beal, *Four Lectures on Buddhist Literature in
China*. London, 1882 : p. 147. Lüken on Atlas in *Traditionen des
Menschengeschlechtes*. Münster, second edition, 1869. Also *The True
Key to Ancient Cosmology*, pp. 13-21.

[3] Morris, *The Epic of Hades* (fourteenth edition). London, 1882 :
p. 230.

and Antarctic, as well as the intermediate regions of the globe; there have been established eighteen Polar stations, and upwards of forty auxiliary stations ; the observations have been made during the year which will end with the present month — that is, between September 1, 1882, and September 1, 1883; they have been made and recorded daily, and bear upon the same identical points of inquiry. This scheme of observation originated with Lieutenant Charles Weyprecht, an Austrian·explorer of fame, who, however, did not live to see it carried into execution. He first broached it at a meeting of German naturalists and physicists held at Gratz on September 18, 1875. The plan was formally approved at a meeting of the International Meteorological Congress held in Rome in the spring of 1879, and its details were perfected at other meetings of the same body held in Hamburg, October 1, 1879, and at Berne, August 7, 1880. Finally, on August 1, 1881, ten delegates, of whom General Hazen, chief of the United States Signal Service, was one, met at St. Petersburg and organized an official Polar Commission. All the members of this commission had authority to act for their respective governments.

The Polar stations were assigned among the nations as follows : The United States, at Lady Franklin Bay, Grinnell Land, and Point Barrow, Alaska; Great Britain and Canada, at Fort McRae and Fort Resolution, on the Great Slave Lake, in British America ; Denmark, at Godthaab and Upernavik, on the west coast of Greenland ; Germany, at Hogarth Inlet, Cumberland Sound ; Austria, at Young Foreland, Jan Mayen Island, north of Iceland ; Finland, at Soudan Kyla, in Lapland ; Holland, at Dickerson Haven, mouth of the Yenisee River, in Russia; Norway, at Bossekop, northwestern coast of Norway; Sweden, at Mosel Bay, Spitzbergen ; and Russia, at Moller Bay, Nova Zembla, and Lighthouse Point, at the mouth of the Lena River. The Antarctic stations are those of Germany, on the South Georgia Islands : France, at Cape Horn ; Italy, at Punta Arenas, in Patagonia ; and the Argentine Republic, at Cordoba. The Polar stations are all within thirty degrees of the North or the South Pole, and the auxiliary stations are spread over the rest of the habitable globe. In his original presentation of the scheme Lieutenant Weyprecht remarked that the unsatisfactory scientific results of the various Arctic and Antarctic expeditions are owing mainly to two causes : first, that the primary object of these expeditions has been geographical discovery, while scientific investigation was secondary; and, secondly, that these individual voyages have been of an isolated character, and hence the observations made are necessarily deficient as compared with what would be gained by a properly scientific investigation, which should obtain, for combination and comparison, memoranda of magnetic and meteorological observations simultaneously made in all parts of the world under a uniform system. Such an investigation, he said, would be feasible only by the united action of the great nations of the world.

By the plan adopted, the following schedule of work was agreed upon for each of the several stations : Meteorological observations : temperature of the air, temperature of the sea, barometric pressure, humidity, direction and force of wind, kind, amount, and motion of the clouds, rainfall, and weather and optical phenomena. Magnetic observations : absolute declination, absolute inclination, absolute horizontal intensity, variations of declination and inclination, and variations of horizontal intensity. All these observations were considered obligatory, and were to be made at each station hourly each day, excepting on the 1st and 15th of each month, when the readings were to be made every five minutes. The following observations were considered desirable, and doubtless have generally been made : Variations of temperature, with height, solar radiation, evaporation, galvanic earth currents, parallax of the aurora, spectroscopic observations on the aurora, ocean currents, tidal observations, structure of ice, density of sea-water, atmospheric electricity, and the force of gravity. The several expeditions were started in season to arrive at their respective stations by the date assigned for beginning, September 1, 1882. . . .

The station of the party of Lieutenant Greely at Lady Franklin Bay is the most northerly one of the whole, and is but about eight degrees south of the Pole. It is very difficult of access on account of the masses of ice that collect in Baffin's Bay. It was arrived at in a vessel by Lieutenant Greely, though the start was made a year in advance of most of the other expeditions, under an apprehension that the vessel might be stopped by ice, and a long journey have to be made overland. The consequence is that the observations of this party began in the fall of 1881. It was the intention, however, to remain two years, and various stores were laid in and arrangements were made accordingly. Early in the summer of 1882 a steamer was sent by the government with supplies for the party, but was unable to reach them because of the ice. The supplies were left at points designated beforehand by Lieutenant Greely, whence he could convey them to headquarters by sledges. Another party was started this summer, and if they cannot reach him by navigation will employ sledges and push north till they meet him. He has instructions to retreat this season by sledge in the contingency of the non-arrival of a vessel, and to come down the coast of Grinnell Land. Either by vessel or on these coast-line sledge journeys the two parties will undoubtedly meet, and probably something definite will be heard from them by the end of September.[1] . . .

Point Barrow is on the northern or Arctic Ocean shore of Alaska, in latitude 72° north. The party stationed here is in charge of Lieutenant P. H. Ray. A relief vessel visited the place in the summer of 1882, and found all well. The observers reported that the preceding winter had been long and severe, but not exceeding in these respects what had been expected. Hourly meteorological observations had been kept up uninterruptedly from October 17, 1881, and magnetic observations from December 1. From that date to August 1, 1882, over 90,000 readings of the magnetic instruments were taken, and a corresponding amount of meteorological work had been done.[2]

Last summer, just before the world had learned of the rescue of Lieutenant Greely, the commanders of all the different stations, Greely alone excepted, held a conference in Vienna, and congratulated each other and the scientific world upon the success achieved. The recovery of the extremely valuable observations of the then missing officer has now crowned and completed the

[1] Soon after the above was written came the disastrous news of the destruction and failure of the second relief expedition.

[2] Summary of a paper read before the Boston Scientific Society (from the *Boston Daily Advertiser*). See also A. Bellot, "Observatoires Scientifiques Circumpolaires," in *Bulletin de la Société de Geographie*, Paris, 1 Trimestre, 1883, and the current scientific periodicals. The last-cited article has a valuable map of the international system of stations. For an imaginary discovery of the North Pole, see Thos. W. Knox, *Voyage of the Vivian.* New York, 1884.

grandest and most beneficent enterprise in which the Christian nations have for centuries, if indeed ever, engaged. Most remarkable, perhaps, of all is the fact that in these several expeditions more than five hundred men, of various nationalities, were kept more than a full year within the Arctic Circle, transported thither and returned, and yet, but for a single mistake in provisioning one of the parties, not one life would have been sacrificed. What could be fuller of promise with respect to the future of polar exploration?

It is to be feared that stratigraphic and paleontologic questions have had too little consideration on the part of the scientific commissions which have planned the latest (as well as the earlier) Arctic expeditions. Whoever has read the fascinating pages of Heer's "Flora Fossilis Arctica," and Count Saporta's "Monde des Plantes avant l'Apparition de l'Homme" (see his chart opposite p. 128), and Baron Nordenskjöld's exceedingly interesting researches and studies in Spitzbergen, cannot well avoid the conviction that the pick and shovel and hammer, intelligently applied anywhere within the Arctic Circle, are almost certain to give us facts of inestimable value both to natural science and to archæology.

> *The world hath lately made such comet-like*
> *Advance on Science, we may almost hope,*
> *Before we die of sheer decay, to learn*
> *Something about our infancy. . . .*
> . . . . *All* HERE
> *Thou seest hath holden fellowship with gods ;*
> . . . *These rocks retain*
> *Their caverned footsteps printed in pure fire.*
> *Those were the times, the ancient youth of Earth,*
> *The elemental years, when Earth and Heaven*
> *Were one in holy bridals, — royal gods*
> *Their bright immortal issue ; when men's minds*
> *Were vast as continents, and not as now*
> *Minute and indistinguishable plots*
> *With here and there acres of untilled brains ; when lived*
> *The great original, broad-eyed, Sunken Race*
> *Whose wisdom, like these sea-sustaining rocks,*
> *Hath formed the base of the world's fluctuous lore.*
>   PHILIP JAMES BAILEY.

SECTION VIII. — THE TRUSTWORTHINESS OF EARLY TRADITION.

" Is memory capable of preserving through successive
generations the facts of history, or whatever else peoples
are continuously interested in knowing ?   At first one is
apt to say ' No,' remembering how seldom two people can
agree in their recollection of even the briefest saying or
commonest occurrence.   But look into the matter.   Note
how the power of memory differs in different people, and
how it may be cultivated, and especially how it strength-
ens when systematically depended on, while, when little
is left to it, it weakens.   It is a small fact, but not without significance, that among the first things which children are set to fix in their memories, apart from any idea
of sacredness, are long series of historical names, dates,
and events, — English kings, American colonists and
presidents, — far exceeding in difficulty those Israelitish
histories which Kuenen thinks cannot be trusted because
only preserved by memory.   This shows that it is less a
question of the power of memory than of how far memory
is looked on as sacred, and guarded so as to hand on its
contents unimpaired.   As for evidence of the power of
memory, what better can we desire than the well-known
fact of the transmission of the Iliad, with its 15,677 lines,
for generations, perhaps for centuries, before it was even
written ?   Yet even that is a mere trifle compared with
the transmission of the Vedas.   The Rig Veda, with its
1017 hymns, is about four times the length of the Iliad.
That is only a part of the ancient Vedic literature, and
the whole was composed, and fixed, and handed down by
memory, — only, as Max Müller says, by ' memory kept
under the strictest discipline.'   There is still a class of
priests in India who have to know by heart the whole of
the Rig Veda.   And there is this curious corroboration
of the fidelity with which this memorizing has been car-

ried on and handed down : that they have kept on transmitting in the ancient literal form laws prohibiting practices that have nevertheless become established. Suttee
is now found to be condemned by the Vedas themselves.
This was first pointed out by their European students,
but has since been admitted by the native Sanskrit scholars. Nothing could show more clearly the faithfulness
of the traditional memory and transmission. It has, too,
this further bearing on the date of the so-called Mosaic
legislation : it shows that the fact of customs existing in
a country for ages unchallenged does not prove that laws
condemning such customs must necessarily be of later
origin. But there is more that is instructive in the transmission of this Vedic literature. There has been writing
in India for twenty-five hundred years now, yet the cus-
todians of the Vedic traditions have never trusted to it.
They trust, for the perfect perpetuation and transmission
of the sacred books, to disciplined memory. They have
manuscripts, they have even a printed text, but, says Max
Müller, 'they do not learn their sacred lore from them.
They learn it, as their ancestors learnt it thousands of
years ago, from the lips of a teacher, so that the Vedic
succession should never be broken.' For eight years in
their youth they are entirely occupied in learning this.
'They learn a few lines every day, repeat them for hours,
so that the whole house resounds with the noise ; and
they thus strengthen their memory to that degree that,
when their apprenticeship is finished, you can open them
like a book, and find any passage you like, any word, any
accent.' And Max Müller shows, from rules given in
the Vedas themselves, that this oral teaching of them was
carried on, exactly as now, at least as early as 500 B. C.[1]

"Very much the same was it with those Rabbinical
schools amid which the Talmud gradually grew up. All
of that vast literature, exceeding many times in bulk

[1] [See F. Max Müller, *Origin and Growth of Religion.* New York
edition, pp. 146–161.]

Homer and the Vedas and the Bible all together, was, at any rate until its later periods, the growth of oral tradition. It was prose tradition, too, which is the hardest to remember, and yet it was carried down century after century in the memory; and long after it had been all committed to writing, the old memorizing continued in the schools. Indeed, it has not entirely ceased even now, for my friend Dr. Gottheil, of New York, tells me that he has had in his study a man who thus knows the entire Talmud by heart, and can take it up at any word that is given him, and go on repeating it syllable by syllable, with absolute correctness.

"In the presence of such facts, surely we must be prepared to revise our ideas of what memory is capable of, — ideas derived from the very limited uses for which we usually depend on it now. Such facts show that memory, consolidated into tradition, is perfectly competent at least to act as an accurate instrument for transmitting along many generations whatever men are very anxious to have remembered. It is simply a question of being anxious and of taking special care."

After other interesting and impressive illustrations, drawn from the history of peoples in the most diverse states of culture, the writer closes as follows: " If there is anything in these facts which I have collected they mean at least this: that we may take up again the discarded traditions of the old heroic ages, and of the world's morning time, with far more confidence than has been usual of late years. Homer will be read with a new interest, and Herodotus, and — best of all — the world-old histories of the Bible. I know they will not give us detailed narratives by which this or that point can be proved, or names or dates to be learned off as school-boy tasks. But they will give us glimpses of the ancient days; pictures here and there of such men and women as loved and fought in those old buried cities of Hissarlik, or meditated by the Ganges, or wandered from Chaldea with Abraham, or followed Moses out of· the mighty empire of Egypt into those wild solitudes of Sinai, — pictures of life; landmarks of great deeds and thoughts and worships and laws ; a dawn to the history, not of abstract theories, nor of dazzling sun-myths, but of real peoples and real men." (*Brooke Herford in The Atlantic Monthly for August,* 1883.)

INDEX

OF AUTHORS REFERRED TO OR QUOTED.

INDEX OF SUBJECTS.

CPSIA information can be obtained
at www.ICGtesting.com
Printed in the USA
BVHW041537230720
584416BV00006B/289